COGNITIVE-BEHAVIORAL THERAPY
WITH COUPLES AND FAMILIES

COGNITIVE-BEHAVIORAL THERAPY WITH COUPLES AND FAMILIES

A Comprehensive Guide for Clinicians

FRANK M. DATTILIO

Foreword by Aaron T. Beck

THE GUILFORD PRESS
New York   London

© 2010 The Guilford Press
A Division of Guilford Publications, Inc.
72 Spring Street, New York, NY 10012
www.guilford.com

Printed in the United States of America

This book is printed on acid-free paper.

Last digit is print number: 9   8   7   6   5   4   3   2   1

Library of Congress Cataloging-in-Publication Data

Dattilio, Frank M.
  Cognitive-behavioral therapy with couples and families : a comprehensive guide
for clinicians / Frank M. Dattilio.
    p. cm.
  Includes bibliographical references and index.
  ISBN 978-1-60623-453-2 (hardcover : alk. paper)
  1. Family psychotherapy.   2. Marital psychotherapy.   3. Cognitive therapy.
I. Title.
  RC488.5.D34 2010
  616.89′156—dc22
                                                                                2009030662

To my wife, children, and grandchildren.
You are truly the light of my life.

About the Author

Frank M. Dattilio, PhD, ABPP, is one of the leading figures in cognitive-behavioral therapy (CBT) in the world. He holds faculty positions with the Department of Psychiatry at Harvard Medical School and the University of Pennsylvania School of Medicine. He is also in the private practice of clinical and forensic psychology and marital and family therapy in Allentown, Pennsylvania. Dr. Dattilio is listed in the National Register of Health Service Providers in Psychology; is board certified in both clinical psychology and behavioral psychology with the American Board of Professional Psychology; and is a clinical member of the American Association for Marriage and Family Therapy. He has also served as a visiting faculty member at several major universities throughout the world.

Dr. Dattilio trained in behavior therapy through the Department of Psychiatry at Temple University School of Medicine under the supervision of the late Joseph Wolpe, MD, and was awarded a postdoctoral fellowship through the Center for Cognitive Therapy at the University of Pennsylvania School of Medicine, where he worked closely under the supervision of Aaron T. Beck, MD.

Dr. Dattilio has more than 250 professional publications in the areas of couple and family problems, anxiety and behavioral disorders, and forensic and clinical psychology. He has presented extensively on CBT throughout the United States, Canada, Africa, Asia, Europe, South America, Australia, New Zealand, Mexico, the West Indies, and Cuba. His works have been translated into more than 27 languages and are used in more than 80 countries. Among his many publications, Dr. Dattilio is coauthor of the books *Cognitive Therapy with Couples*, *The Family Psychotherapy Treatment*

Planner, and *The Family Therapy Homework Planner*; coeditor of the *Comprehensive Casebook of Cognitive Therapy*, *Cognitive-Behavioral Strategies in Crisis Intervention*, *Cognitive Therapy with Children and Adolescents: A Casebook for Clinical Practice*, and *Comparative Treatments for Couple Dysfunction*; and editor of *Case Studies in Couple and Family Therapy: Systemic and Cognitive Perspectives*. He has filmed several professional videotapes and audiotapes, including the popular series "Five Approaches to Linda," and serves on the editorial boards of a number of professional journals, nationally as well as internationally, including the *Journal of Marital and Family Therapy* and *Contemporary Family Therapy*. Dr. Dattilio is the recipient of several professional awards for outstanding achievement in the fields of psychology and psychotherapy. He resides in Allentown, Pennsylvania, with his wife, Maryann, and regularly visits his three adult children and eight grandchildren.

Foreword

I am delighted that Frank Dattilio has embarked on the challenge of producing a truly comprehensive text on cognitive-behavioral therapy with couples and families. As we rapidly approach the fifth decade of cognitive therapy's introduction into the psychotherapeutic arena, it is evident that the modality has grown exponentially throughout the world as one of the most popular and effective approaches in contemporary mental health treatment. Since the development of cognitive therapy's application with couples, which took root in the 1980s, there has been a proliferation of research on relationship discord and the role of cognitive processes as they affect emotion and behavior. In the late 1980s and throughout the 1990s, the application of cognitive therapy was expanded to encompass family dynamics, as well as the role that schema plays in the process of change.

In *Love Is Never Enough* (Beck, 1988), I made the practical application of the cognitive therapy approach available to the general public, which helped to increase the general awareness of the power of cognitive therapy in the course of treating relationship distress. Frank Dattilio, who is a former student of mine and a major proponent of the application of cognitive therapy with couples and families, has been instrumental, along with a number of other colleagues, in promoting cognitive therapy's acceptance in the field of family therapy. His well-received book *Case Studies in Couple and Family Therapy: Systemic and Cognitive Perspectives* (Dattilio, 1998a) has helped to integrate cognitive therapy into the mainstream of contemporary family therapy and to bolster its acceptance among couple and family therapists around the world.

The widespread adoption of the cognitive therapy approach may be attributed to many factors, foremost of which is that cognitive therapy has been subjected to more controlled outcome studies than any other therapeutic modality. The research evidence supporting its efficacy is encouraging to all those working in the field of couple and family therapy, particularly given the increasing demand for evidence-based treatments. Cognitive therapy also tends to appeal to clients who value a pragmatic and proactive approach to solving problems and building the skills that are vital to reducing relationship dysfunction. Further, the approach emphasizes a collaborative relationship between therapist and client(s), which is a posture that has become more and more appealing to contemporary couple and family therapists.

The current volume provides an updated review of the development of cognitive therapy as applied to couples and families. There is important new emphasis on how one's family of origin influences belief systems in relationships, as well as on schema in relationships and the restructuring of dysfunctional belief systems. Ample case material and the inclusion of special populations make this book highly readable and broadly relevant. Specific sections on methods of clinical assessment and interventions provide readers with a hands-on approach for dealing effectively with various types of dysfunction in relationships. In sum, this book is an excellent resource for mental health professionals of all therapeutic modalities.

AARON T. BECK, MD
University Professor of Psychiatry
University of Pennsylvania School of Medicine
and
The Beck Institute, Philadelphia

Preface

Recent data suggest that 43% of couples will divorce within the first 15 years of marriage, with second marriages having an even higher likelihood of failure (Bramlett & Mosher, 2002). Couple and family problems account for approximately half of all visits to psychotherapists' offices. Recent surveys tell us that most therapists who specialize in family therapy work primarily with couples (Harvard Health Publications, 2007). Unfortunately, the track record for success in professional couple therapy has not been impressive (Gottman, 1999). More than 30% of couples completing conjoint therapy fail to show long-term improvement (Baucom, Shoham, Mueser, Daiuto, & Stickle, 1998). Nowhere has this finding been underscored more than in the ambitious Consumer Reports Survey undertaken in the mid-1990s, which indicated that, among consumers of psychotherapy, those who participated in family therapy were the least satisfied (Seligman, 1995). In contrast, other research comparing couple therapy with no treatment at all concluded that couple therapy unequivocally increased satisfaction more than no treatment (Christensen & Heavey, 1999).

So, with all of the fine contemporary modalities of couple and family therapy available to us, along with the current thrust of evidence-based therapies, why is there still so much discontent among consumers?

There are a number of likely explanations for this discouraging outcome. One may be that spouses or family members hold rigid beliefs about their partners or relatives and the potential for change in the relationship. Much of couple and family therapy involves the members coming in each week and describing their fights and disagreements. The therapist calms them down and helps them to spell out their feelings and listen to each other. They feel better and go home, and then function well until they have their next fight. Couples and families are not easy to change. The individual personalities of the family members are often quite complex and can involve behavioral patterns that interlock poorly. Many come to therapy wanting not to change, but to be vindicated and perhaps have their partners or other family members change. They often avoid taking a hard look at themselves and committing to what they need to change in themselves, such as in the case of those maintaining unrealistic expectations about their relationships. Unless family members can be helped to see their own roles in the problems that plague them, they will have no motivation to change. In addition, many couples and families drag their feet when it comes to entering into treatment. In studies undertaken with couples seeking divorce, less than one-fourth reported that they sought help from a marriage counselor before initiating divorce proceedings (Albrecht, Bahr, & Goodman, 1983; Wolcott, 1986). When those who failed to seek treatment were questioned about the reason, they frequently cited the unwillingness of the spouse (33%), their disbelief that anything was wrong, or their conviction that it was simply too late for any type of intervention (17%) (Wolcott, 1986).

This book presents a comprehensive model of cognitive-behavioral therapy (CBT) with couples and families. It addresses areas of neurobiology, attachment, and emotional regulation, placing specific emphasis on schema restructuring against the backdrop of a systems approach. In addition, this book gets into the nitty-gritty aspects of working with difficult families who are stuck in rigid thought and behavioral patterns that clinicians often find arduous to treat.

Over the years, cognitive-behavioral couple and family therapy has evolved into a precisely focused and integrative approach. It is nicely adaptable by practitioners of differing modalities. In fact, in recent surveys, more than half of all practitioners said that they most often use CBT in combination with other methods (Psychotherapy Networker, 2007). The concept of schema has been expanded greatly beyond traditional CBT with couples and families and, in many ways, has been one of the cornerstones in facilitating change. CBT places a heavy emphasis on the importance of belief systems and those elements that so profoundly influence emotion and behavior.

When I began using cognitive-behavioral strategies with couples and families more than 30 years ago, I encountered considerable opposition from family therapists who espoused the more traditional models in the field. They often criticized the CBT approach as being "too linear" or "superficial" and failing to address the concept of "circularity, or some of the underlying dynamics," found with relationship dysfunction (Nichols & Schwartz, 2001; Dattilio, 1998a). Many of my colleagues also felt that CBT ignored the emotional component of family members and was concerned only with thoughts and behavior. Eventually, I realized that there was some merit to my colleagues' criticism. Their feedback encouraged me to rethink how the CBT approach could be refined to embrace these important components during the course of treatment. The manner in which CBT with couples and families had initially been portrayed, unfortunately, left many with the impression of a wooden and inflexible approach, despite the fact that the majority of the interventions were very effective and integratable with other modalities. Some of the earlier work with couples and families, for example, failed to consider the systemic dimension of treatment or to highlight how a person's belief system was influenced by his or her family of origin (Dattilio, 1989; Dattilio & Padesky, 1990). However, since that time I have been strongly influenced by my colleagues Norman Epstein and Donald Baucom, who enhanced the CBT approach in working with couples so as to include a greater focus on emotion. They have both contributed a great deal to the empirical literature. Their work has also influenced my development and the expansion of my approach in applying CBT to families. Some of the more recent scholarly work in this area has also embraced an expanded model against the backdrop of a systems perspective and the highlighting of the emotional component of treatment. This revised model offers the flexibility to integrate other modalities of treatment (Dattilio, 1998a, 2005a, 2006a), which serves to broaden the scope of the approach.

The impetus for writing this book was twofold—to provide a more contemporary version of CBT with couples and families and to enhance its effectiveness through a specific emphasis on schema. Since the early 1990s there has been a substantial amount of empirical as well as clinical/case literature published on CBT with couples and families that has changed the landscape of what was once considered traditional CBT. This text offers some of the basic components of CBT, yet applies them with a greater emphasis on schema identification and restructuring. Some of the content of this book is based on the fine work of Jeffrey Young and colleagues (Young, Klosko, & Weishaar, 2003), but is greatly expanded in order to reflect an appreciation for relationship dynamics and systemic interaction that are found in clinical work with individuals.

This book was a challenge to write for several reasons. First, there has been a burgeoning of professional literature in the past 20 years on various aspects of couple and family therapy, much of which, although important, exceeds what can fit into a single text. Hence, synthesizing what is essential and what is not became a major endeavor. This book is therefore designed to offer the reader a comprehensive guide to the practice of CBT with families without listing study after study, but using a greater focus on clinical practice.

Second, the field of psychotherapy in general has gravitated toward evidence-based practice (Sue & Sue, 2008). Hence, documentation is required to be much more empirical than previously—when practitioners could simply write about what they themselves found to be effective in treatment without having to provide rigorous scientific evidence. Anecdotal writing no longer carries the same weight in the field that it once did. However, a major problem with reporting on empirical evidence is that the text often becomes so bogged down with references that the emphasis on clinical practice is lost.

It became a juggling act for me to attempt to remain scientific while crafting a text that is interesting and shows the details of clinical practice. I hope this book offers you an expanded and contemporary version of CBT with couples and families that is useful to clinicians, yet fills a much needed void in the cognitive-behavioral literature, as well as in the field of couple and family therapy in general.

Author's Note

Throughout this book, the term *couple* is used for any partnership (married or unmarried) and *family* for any partnership with children.

Acknowledgments

With the passage of time, I have come to realize how fortunate I have been to study under some of the greatest minds in the history of our field. As a neophyte, I had the distinct honor of coming under the tutelage of the late Joseph Wolpe, who, in addition to imparting his own clinical wisdom, exposed me to many eminent guest lecturers at his Philadelphia training center in the late 1970s. Among these esteemed guests were the late Viktor Frankl and Anna Freud. It was during my training with Wolpe that Aaron T. Beck expressed an interest in my work and offered me a postdoctoral fellowship through the Center for Cognitive Therapy and the University of Pennsylvania School of Medicine in the early 1980s. My years of training in traditional behavior therapy and, later, in cognitive therapy prepared me well for what would eventually become a fruitful career in the field of couple and family therapy. I subsequently had the wonderful opportunity to share many collegial teaching and writing experiences with such prominent figures as Arthur Freeman, Donald Meichenbaum, Norman Epstein, Harry Aponte, James Framo, Cloé Madanes, Arnold Lazarus, William Glasser, and Peggy Papp, to name a few. My experiences with these colleagues helped to shape my clinical acumen as a cognitive-behavioral therapist, as well as a couple and family therapist, and for that I thank them immensely. I also thank the thousands of couples and families with whom I have worked throughout the world who have helped me to shape my clinical skills to what they are today. Without them, my clinical expertise and theoretical beliefs would be insular.

Compiling a major text such as this is not possible without the aid of many talented assistants. I owe a tremendous debt of gratitude to my colleague Michael P. Nichols, whose tireless effort and superb editorial guidance has helped to shape this text into its present form. Jim Nageotte and Jane Keislar at The Guilford Press also deserve acknowledgment for their guidance on the project from beginning to end. Suzi Tucker has also been immensely helpful in providing feedback and guidance on my writing style. I must also thank Seymour Weingarten, Guilford's Editor-in-Chief, who has always been extremely supportive and patient with my ideas over the past two decades. It is because of Seymour's open-mindedness and flexibility that this and many other projects in the past have become a reality.

A hearty thanks is also extended to my research assistants, Kate Adams and Katy Tresco, and more recently, Amanda Carr, who spent many hours conducting endless literature searches and collecting reprints. I also thank my personal secretaries, Carol Jaskolka and Roseanne Miller, for their long hours of typing and their excellent computer skills. Their expertise in coordinating all of the details with this book is appreciated more than they will ever know.

Finally, I owe the greatest acknowledgment to my loving wife, Maryann, and my children and grandchildren, who endured my many absences during the preparation of this book. They have all taught me the true meaning and beauty of being a husband, father, and grandfather.

Contents

1

Introduction

OVERVIEW OF CONTEMPORARY
COGNITIVE-BEHAVIORAL THERAPY
WITH COUPLES AND FAMILIES

Cognitive-behavioral therapy (CBT) with couples and families has now entered the mainstream of contemporary family therapy and prominently appears in the majority of major textbooks in the field (Sexton, Weeks, & Robbins, 2003; Nichols & Schwartz, 2008; Goldenberg & Goldenberg, 2008; Becvar & Becvar, 2009; Bitter, 2009).

In a national survey conducted within the past decade by the American Association for Marriage and Family Therapy (AAMFT), marriage and family therapists were asked to report "their primary treatment modality" (Northey, 2002, p. 448). Of the 27 different modalities that were mentioned, the most frequently identified modality was cognitive-behavioral family therapy (Northey, 2002). More recently, an additional survey, partnered with Columbia University, reported that of the 2,281 responders, 1,566 (68.7%) stated that they most often use CBT in combination with other methods (Psychotherapy Networker, 2007). This data is telling and reflects the utility and effectiveness of CBT with couples and families.

Applications of CBT to problems with intimate relationships were introduced almost 50 years ago with Albert Ellis's early writings on the important role that cognition plays in marital problems (Ellis & Harper, 1961). Ellis and his colleagues proposed that relationship dysfunction occurs when individuals (1) hold irrational or unrealistic beliefs about their partners and the relationship and (2) make negative evaluations when the partner and

1

relationship do not live up to unrealistic expectations. When these negative cognitive processes occur, the individual is likely to experience strong negative emotions (anger, disappointment, and bitterness) and to behave in negative ways toward the partner. The principles of Ellis's rational–emotive therapy (RET) were applied to work with distressed couples, challenging the irrationality of their thinking (Ellis, 1977; Ellis, Sichel, Yeager, DiMattia, & DiGiuseppe, 1989). However, despite the popularity of RET as a form of individual and group treatment for many individual problems, RET with intimate relationships received only a lukewarm reception from couple and family therapists during the 1960s and 1970s. These decades marked the early development of the field of couple and family therapy, which was spearheaded by theorists and clinicians who eschewed models that focused on psychological processes and linear causality in favor of family interaction patterns and the circular causal concepts of systems theory (Nichols & Schwartz, 2008). Ellis's emphasis on individual cognition and the generally linear nature of his "ABC" model, in which irrational beliefs mediated individuals' emotional and behavioral responses to life events, was seen as incompatible with a family systems approach.

LEARNING THEORY PRINCIPLES

Another major development in psychotherapy during the 1960s and early 1970s involved behavior therapists' utilization of learning theory principles to address various problematic behaviors of children and adults. Later, behavior principles and techniques that were used successfully in the treatment of individuals were applied to distressed couples and families. For example, Stuart (1969), Liberman (1970), and Weiss, Hops, and Patterson (1973) described the use of social exchange theory and operant learning strategies to facilitate more satisfying interactions in distressed couples. Similarly, Patterson, McNeal, Hawkins, and Phelps (1967) and others (e.g., LeBow, 1976: Wahler, Winkel, Peterson, & Morrison, 1971) applied operant conditioning and contingency-contracting procedures to help parents control the behavior of aggressive children. This operant approach offered solid empirical support and became popular among behaviorally oriented therapists, but still received little recognition from couple and family therapists.

The behavioral approaches shared with family systems approaches a focus on observable behavior and the factors in interpersonal relationships that influence it. However, there were fundamental differences that made behavior therapies unappealing to many couple and family therapists. First, the behavioral model, with its emphasis on stimulus and response, tended to be too linear for systemically oriented therapists. Second, the systems theorists believed that an individual's symptomatic behavior served a function in the family, which seemed compatible with behaviorists' notion of "functional analysis" of antecedents and consequences of problematic behaviors. Family therapists commonly focused more on the individual's symptoms as having symbolic meaning for a larger family problem. Thus, even though early forms of behavioral family therapy did attend to the reciprocal influences that parents' and children's behavior have on each other, couple and family therapists tended to consider them relatively linear and simplistic when it came to accounting for complex family interactions. The early behavioral approach to family therapy was highlighted by specifying family problems in concrete, observable terms, and with the design of specific empirically based therapeutic strategies. These strategies were subjected to empirical analysis of their effects in achieving specific behavioral goals (Falloon & Lillie, 1988).

Robert Liberman (1970) contends that neither the family therapist nor the family he or she was treating needed to particularly understand the family dynamics in order to make a change in the family system. Liberman believed that a careful behavioral analysis was all that was required.

The late Ian Falloon (1998), however, encouraged behavioral couple and family therapists to adopt an open-systems approach that examined the multiplicity of forces that might operate within a family. He stressed a focus on the physiological status of the individual, as well as his or her cognitive, behavioral, and emotional responses, along with the interpersonal transactions that occur within the family, social, work, and cultural-political networks. "No single system is the focus to the exclusion of others" (p. 14). Hence, Falloon advocated for a more contextual approach, whereby each potentially causative factor should be considered in relation to other factors. This contextual approach was elaborated by Arnold Lazarus (1976) in his multimodal assessment approach. Ironically, family system approaches have focused almost exclusively on intrafamilial dynamics, viewing extrafamilial stress factors as almost irrelevant. The goal of a behavioral analysis is to explore all systems operating on each spouse or family member that contribute to the presenting problems. It is for this reason that pioneering behavioral family therapist Gerald Patterson (1974) stressed the need for assessment to occur in different settings, such as in adjunctive agencies or in school or work environments.

As behaviorally oriented therapists added the components of communication and problem-solving skills training to their interventions with couples and families (e.g., Falloon, 1988; Falloon, Boyd, & McGill, 1984; Jacobson & Margolin, 1979; Stuart, 1980), those interventions were often adopted by traditional family therapists. One reason for this integration seems to be that systemic therapists have commonly considered communication processes to be central in family interaction and have valued structured techniques for reducing the number of unclear messages family members send to one another.

However, there were still differences between the assumptions of systemic therapists and those of behavioral therapists about the role of communication in family functioning. Drawing from the legacy of concepts such as the *double-bind* hypothesis (Bateson, Daveson, Haley, & Weakland, 1956), which posited that contradictory and constraining messages from parents contribute to the development of psychotic thinking, systemically oriented therapists viewed communication training as a means of reducing the homeostatic function of an identified patient's disturbed behavior within the family. The double-bind theory has since been refuted (Firth & Johnstone, 2003; Kidman, 2007).

Research on family communication and mental disorders has not supported the view that disordered communication causes mental disorders, but rather that it acts as a stressor on an individual's biological vulnerability to a disorder (Mueser & Glynn, 1999). Behavioral family therapists such as Falloon and associates (1984) focused on altering unclear and negative family communication that acts as one of the major life stressors and increases the likelihood that symptoms of psychopathology will be exhibited. Research on *expressed emotion*, or the degree to which family members exhibit criticism, hostility, and emotional overinvolvement with a member diagnosed with a major mental disorder, demonstrated that such conditions within the family decreased the probability that the identified patient would improve with treatment and increased the likelihood that he or she would experience relapses (Miklowitz, 1995). Furthermore, behavioral family therapists viewed the clear, constructive expression of thoughts and emotions, empathic listening, and efficient problem-solving skills as crucial for the resolution of conflicts among family members, including couple conflicts and parent–child conflicts. Findings by researchers in several countries indicated that behaviorally oriented therapy that included communication and problem-solving skills training produced significant improvement in family functioning (Mueser & Glynn, 1999). Furthermore, studies on couple communication by researchers such as Christensen (1988) and Gottman (1994) indicated the importance of reducing avoidant behaviors, in addition to aggressive acts, between distressed partners. It appears that a lack of awareness of these developments has perpetrated the idea that behavior therapy is simplistic.

As behaviorally oriented therapists developed more comprehensive approaches to modifying family interactions that contribute to distressed relationships, their methods became more appealing to couple and family therapists whose work was guided by systems theory (Falloon, 1988). Nevertheless, schools of family therapy that have emphasized the modification of behavior patterns (e.g., the structural-strategic and solution-focused approaches) typically continued to use interventions that were different from those used by behavioral couple and family therapists (e.g., directives, paradoxical prescriptions, and unbalancing interventions, such as temporarily siding with one family member).

COGNITIVE THERAPY PRINCIPLES

It was not until the late 1970s that cognitions were introduced as a component of treatment within a behavior paradigm (Margolin & Weiss, 1978). Behavior therapists initially viewed cognitive techniques with disdain, perceiving them to be difficult to measure with any degree of reliability. This thinking, however, gradually changed with the release of new research results. Behavioral researchers such as Jacobson (1992) and Hahlweg, Baucom, and Markman (1988) provided examples of the systematic use of cognitive strategies in couple therapy: teaching spouses to recognize precipitants of disagreements and to subsequently restructure their behaviors. This was later followed up by a number of researchers, most specifically Baucom and Epstein (1990).

During the 1980s, cognitive factors became an area of increasing focus in the couple research and therapy literature. Cognitions were addressed in a more direct and systematic way by behaviorally oriented therapists (e.g., Baucom, 1987; Dattilio, 1989; Eidelson & Epstein, 1982; Epstein, 1982; Epstein & Eidelson, 1981; Fincham, Beach, & Nelson, 1987; Weiss, 1984) than by adherents of other theoretical approaches to couple and family therapy. Clearly, family members' thought processes have been considered important in a variety of family therapy theoretical orientations (e.g., reframing in the strategic approach, "problem-talk" in solution-focused therapy, and life stories in narrative therapy). However, none of the original mainstream family therapy approaches has used the concepts and systematic methods of CBT to assess and intervene with cognition in intimate relationships. Traditional family therapists looked at cognition, but only in very simple ways, such as addressing the specific thoughts that family members expressed and their obvious conscious attitudes. However, cognitive therapists were busy developing more thorough and complex ways to deal with family members' underlying belief systems that drove interaction with one another.

Established cognitive assessment and intervention methods derived from individual therapy were adapted by cognitive-behavioral therapists for use in couple therapy to identify and modify distorted cognitions that partners experience about each other (Baucom & Epstein, 1990; Dattilio & Padesky, 1990). As in individual psychotherapy, cognitive-behavioral interventions for couples were designed to enhance partners' skills for evaluating and modifying their own problematic cognitions, as well as skills for communicating and solving problems constructively (Baucom & Epstein, 1990; Epstein & Baucom, 2002).

Similarly, behavioral approaches to family therapy were broadened to include family members' cognitions about one another. Ellis (1982) was one of the first to introduce a cognitive approach to family therapy, using his RET approach. At the same time, Bedrosian (1983) applied Beck's model of cognitive therapy to understanding and treating dysfunctional family dynamics, as did Barton and Alexander (1981), which evolved into what later became known as functional family therapy (Alexander & Parsons, 1982). During the 1980s and 1990s the cognitive-behavioral family therapy (CBFT) model saw a rapid expansion (Alexander, 1988; Dattilio, 1993; Epstein & Schlesinger, 1996; Epstein, Schlesinger, & Dryden, 1988; Falloon et al., 1984; Schwebel & Fine, 1994; Teichman, 1981, 1992), and CBFT is now featured as a major treatment approach in family therapy textbooks (e.g., Becvar, 2008; Goldenberg & Goldenberg, 2000; Nichols & Schwartz, 2008; Bitter, 2009).

THE INTEGRATIVE POTENTIAL
OF COGNITIVE-BEHAVIORAL THERAPY

Unfortunately, there are very few empirical outcome studies on CBT with families. Faulkner, Klock, and Gale (2002) conducted a content analysis on articles published in the marital/couple and family therapy literature from 1980 to 1999. The *American Journal of Family Therapy, Contemporary Family Therapy, Family Process*, and the *Journal of Marital and Family Therapy* were among the top journals from which 131 articles that used quantitative research methodology were examined. Of these 131 articles, fewer than half involved outcome studies. None of these studies that were reviewed considered CBT. A more recent scan of the professional literature indicates that this statistic has remained consistent (Dattilio, 2004a).

However, cognitive-behavioral couple therapy (CBCT) has been subjected to more controlled outcome studies than has any other therapeutic modality. There is substantial empirical evidence from treatment outcome studies with couples to indicate the effectiveness of CBT with relationships, although most studies have primarily focused on the behavior interventions of communication training, problem-solving training, and behavior contracts, with only a handful examining the impact of cognitive restructuring procedures (see Baucom et al., 1998, for a review that employed stringent criteria for efficacy). Baucom et al.'s (1998) review of outcome studies indicated that CBT is efficacious in reducing relationship distress. A smaller but growing number of studies on other marital and family therapy approaches, such as emotionally focused (Johnson & Talitman, 1997) and insight-oriented couple therapies (Snyder, Wills, & Grady-Fletcher, 1991), suggest that they have comparable, or in some cases, even better outcome results than the cognitive-behavioral approaches. Additional studies are necessary to enable us to draw conclusions about the relative efficacies of these empirically supported treatments, but there is encouraging support for cognitive-behavioral, emotionally focused, and insight-oriented therapies as treatments that can be helpful to many distressed couples (Davis & Piercy, 2007).

There has been less research on generic applications with individual disorders, such as schizophrenia and child conduct disorders. Outcome studies have demonstrated the effectiveness of behaviorally oriented family interventions (psychoeducation and training in communication and problem-solving skills) with such disorders (Baucom et al., 1998), although cognitive interventions, per se, have not been evaluated. As increasing emphasis has been placed on empirically validated treatments in the mental health field, the cognitive-behavioral approach has gained popularity and respect among clinicians, including couple and family therapists (Dattilio, 1998a; Dattilio & Epstein, 2003; Epstein & Baucom, 2002; Davis & Piercy, 2007). Sprenkle (2003) has noted the application of more rigorous outcome criteria in research on couple and family therapy, and the movement of the field in general toward a more evidenced-based discipline. In addition, there appears to be more attention given to case-based reports within the family therapy literature. Traditionally, case-based research has not been considered as scientific by many in the field, owing to the lack of controlled conditions and objectivity. However, case study materials can serve as the basis for drawing causal inferences in properly designed clinical cases (Dattilio, 2006a) and, in many ways, seem to be preferred among students and trainees.

In a text edited by Dattilio (1998a), an overwhelming majority of experts on various theories of marital and family therapy acknowledge the helpful addition of cognitive-behavioral techniques to their particular approaches to treatment. Many of these experts actually indicated that they incorporate many of the same techniques in their approaches, but identify them by other terms.

The growing adoption of cognitive-behavioral methods by couple and family therapists appears to be due to several factors in addition to the research evidence supporting their efficacy. First, CBT techniques tend to appeal to clients, who value the pragmatic, more proactive approach to solving problems and building skills that the family can use to cope with future difficulties (Friedberg, 2006). Further, CBT emphasizes a collaborative relationship between therapist and client, a stance that is increasingly popular in postmodern approaches to couple and family therapy. Recent enhancements of CBT for intimate relationships (see Epstein & Baucom, 2002, for a detailed presentation) have broadened the contextual factors that are taken into account in the couple's or family's physical and interpersonal environment (e.g., extended family, the workplace, neighborhood environment, national socioeconomic conditions). For example, recent exploration has involved integrating CBT with other interventions such as dialectical behavior therapy (DBT) in treating emotional dysregulation in intimate relationships (Kirby & Baucom, 2007).

CBT has become a mainstream theoretical approach and continues to evolve through the creative efforts of various practitioners. The cognitive-behavioral model has always been amenable to change, given its emphasis on empiricism and maximizing clinical efficacy through research identifying what works and what does not. Because of its adaptability and the degree to which it shares with many other models of treatment an assumption that change in couple and family relationships involves shifts in the cognitive, affective, and behavioral realms, CBT has great potential for integration with other approaches (Dattilio, 1998a; Dattilio & Epstein, 2005).

Some works have underscored the integrative power of cognitive-behavioral approaches in the treatment of individuals (Alford & Beck, 1997), as well as of couples and families (Dattilio, 1998). Cognitive-behavioral therapists also have increasingly integrated concepts and methods derived from other theoretical orientations; for example, the concepts of system boundaries, hierarchy (control), and a family's ability to adapt to developmental changes, emphasized in structural family therapy (Minuchin, 1974), are prominent in Epstein and Baucom's (2002) work with couples.

Because couples and families embody a complex set of dynamics that are directly or indirectly related in a causal network, it is essential to consider conducting CBT against the backdrop of a systems approach. That is, factoring in the circularity and multidirectional flow of influence among family members is important to the effectiveness of the intervention. The systemic nature of family functioning requires that the family be considered as an entity composed of interacting parts. Consequently, to understand any behavior in a family relationship, one must look at the interactions between the members, as well as the characteristics of the family as a unit. Similarly, a cognitive-behavioral perspective focuses on the interaction among family members with a particular emphasis on the interrelated nature of family members' expectancies, beliefs, and attributions. In this sense, then, both CBT and systemic traditional family therapy share an emphasis on multidirectional, reciprocal influence and the necessity of looking at behaviors in that particular context.

Although cognitive-behavioral concepts can usually be integrated with certain models, there may be some models that are fundamentally incompatible with CBT. For example, solution-focused therapists largely ignore current and historical aspects of families' presenting problems, instead emphasizing efforts to implement desired changes (see Nichols & Schwartz,

2001, for a review). Although cognitive-behavioral therapists also want to identify and build on clients' existing strengths and enhance their problem-solving abilities, they assess and intervene with cognitive, affective, and behavioral aspects of problematic patterns that often are ingrained and difficult to change. Thus, practitioners of alternative approaches need to determine the extent to which cognitive-behavioral concepts and methods enhance, or are counter to, key aspects of their models. As researchers continue to test the effects of adding interventions derived from other models to cognitive-behavioral procedures, the potential for integration in clinical practice should increase.

2

The Mechanics of Change
with Couples and Families

COGNITIVE PROCESSES

Perceptions

What you selectively notice and what you attend to is what makes up
your experience.
                          —WILLIAM JAMES, 19th-century philosopher

We all have perceptions about people and about life in general. Perceptions involve those aspects of a person or a situation that fit into categories that have particular meaning to us. In couple and family relationships,
perceptions pertain to how we interact and how we perceive a spouse or
family member throughout the course of our interactions. For example, a
husband may see his wife, or even one of his siblings, as being "touchy"
or "over sensitive." Consequently, because perceptions determine how we
attend to people, they often supersede other cognitions, such as attributions, expectancies, and assumptions, which are outlined in the following
section. At the same time, these other cognitions go on to later affect and
influence our perceptions and, in turn, may change our perceptions. As a
result, perceptions are susceptible to change, depending on new information we may encounter. Yet, depending on the impact of our experiences,
perceptions may be difficult to alter. For example, if a man initially perceives his wife as being a generally "unselfish" person, then he will likely
incorporate this perception into his general view of her. Consequently, as
he goes on to experience further events with her, the new information will

always be judged in light of that initial perception, and he will ignore or forgive numerous "selfish" acts.

Sometimes, perceptual bias may occur, depending on the course of a person's experiences with his or her partner or family members. Some of these biases are outlined in the discussion that follows.

Expectations and Standards

Cognitive processes are the backbone of the cognitive-behavioral approach to relationship dysfunction. Baucom, Epstein, Sayers, and Sher (1989) developed a typology of cognitions that frequently surface during the course of relationship distress. Although each type is a normal form of human cognition, each is susceptible to distortions (Baucom & Epstein, 1990; Epstein & Baucom, 2002). These processes include:

1. *Selective attention.* The individual's tendency to notice only certain aspects of the events occurring in relationships and to overlook others (e.g., focusing on the partner's words and ignoring his or her actions).
2. *Attributions.* Inferences about the factors that have influenced a partner's actions (e.g., concluding that a partner failed to respond to a question because he or she wants to control the relationship).
3. *Expectancies.* Predictions about the likelihood that particular events will occur in the relationship (e.g., that expressing feelings to one's partner will result in the partner's getting angry).
4. *Assumptions.* Beliefs about the general characteristics of people and relationships (e.g., a wife's assumption that men don't need emotional attachment).
5. *Standards.* Beliefs about the characteristics that people and relationships "should" have (e.g., that partners should have no boundaries between them, sharing all of their thoughts and emotions with each other).

Because there is typically so much information available in any interpersonal situation, some degree of selective attention is inevitable, but the potential for couples and family members to form biased perceptions of each other is an important area of focus. Inferences involved in attributions and expectancies are also normal aspects of human information processing involved in understanding other people's behavior and making predictions about their future behavior. However, errors in these inferences can have harmful effects on couple and family relationships, especially when one person attributes another's actions to negative characteristics (e.g., malicious intent) or misjudges how others will react to his or her own actions.

Assumptions are adaptive when they are realistic representations of people and relationships, and many standards that individuals hold, such as moral standards about the wrongness of abusing others, contribute to the quality of family relationships. Nevertheless, inaccurate or extreme assumptions and standards can lead individuals to interact inappropriately with others, as when a parent holds a standard that children's opinions and feelings are not to be taken into account as long as they live in the parent's house.

Beck and his associates (e.g., Beck, Rush, Shaw, & Emery, 1979; J. S. Beck, 1995) refer to moment-to-moment stream of consciousness ideas, beliefs, and images as automatic thoughts—for example, "My husband left his clothes on the floor again. He doesn't care about my feelings" or "My parents are saying 'no' again because they aren't willing to help me out." Cognitive-behavioral therapists have noted how individuals commonly accept automatic thoughts at face value. Although all five of the types of cognition identified by Baucom et al. (1989) can be reflected in an individual's automatic thoughts, cognitive-behavioral therapists have emphasized the moment-to-moment selective perceptions and the inferences involved in attributions and expectancies as most likely to be within a person's awareness. Assumptions and standards are thought to be broader underlying aspects of an individual's worldview, considered to be schemas in Beck's cognitive model (Beck et al., 1979; J. S. Beck, 1995; Leahy, 1996).

The cognitive model proposes that the content of an individual's perceptions and inferences is shaped by relatively stable underlying schemas, or cognitive structures, such as the personal constructs first described by Kelly (1955). Schemas are like road maps that people follow to lead them through life and through their relationships. They are assumed to be relatively stable and may, at times, become inflexible. Many schemas about relationships and the nature of family interactions are learned early in life from primary sources such as family of origin, cultural traditions and mores, the mass media, early dating and other relationship experiences. The *models* of self in relation to others that have been described by attachment theorists appear to be forms of schemas that affect individuals' automatic thoughts and emotional responses to significant others (Johnson & Denton, 2002). In addition to the schemas that partners or family members bring to a relationship, each member develops a schema specific to the current relationship.

As a result of years of interaction among family members, individuals often develop jointly held beliefs that constitute a family schema (Dattilio, 1994). To the extent that the family schema involves cognitive distortions, it may result in dysfunctional interactions. An example of this may be family members who collectively view one sibling as being unreliable. They may habitually step in to do things for their sibling, thereby enabling unreliable behavior, which leads to its continuation.

Schemas about relationships are often not clearly articulated in an individual's mind, but exist as vague notions of what is or should be (Beck, 1988; Epstein & Baucom, 2002). Once developed, they influence how an individual subsequently processes information in new situations. For example, they influence what the person selectively perceives, the inferences he or she makes about the causes of another's behavior, and whether he or she is pleased or displeased with the family relationships. Existing schemas may be difficult to modify, but repeated new experiences with significant others have the potential to change them (Epstein & Baucom, 2002; Johnson & Denton, 2002). In many ways, they are like phobias that are rarely challenged. People just avoid the things to which they are phobic. If a father firmly believes that his daughter should marry within their own culture, then he may remain steadfast to this belief unless some new information changes his belief system, such as his seeing firsthand how happy his daughter is with the mate she chose. Schemas usually change when the new information is powerful enough to modify people's beliefs.

Common Cognitive Distortions with Couples and Families

In addition to automatic thoughts and schemas, Beck et al. (1979) identified cognitive distortions, or information-processing errors, that contribute to cognitions becoming sources of distress and conflict in people's lives. In terms of Baucom et al.'s (1989) typology, they result in distorted or inappropriate perceptions, attributions, expectancies, assumptions, and standards. The following list includes descriptions of these cognitive distortions, with examples of how they may occur in the course of couple and family interactions.

1. *Arbitrary inference.* Conclusions are made in the absence of substantiating evidence, for example, parents whose teenager arrives home a half hour beyond her curfew conclude, "She's up to no good again."
2. *Selective abstractions.* Information is taken out of context, and certain details are highlighted while other important information is ignored. For example, a man whose wife responds to his questions with one-word answers concludes, "She's mad at me."
3. *Overgeneralization.* An isolated incident or two is allowed to serve as a representation of all similar situations, related or unrelated. For example, when a parent declines a child's request to go out with his friends, the child concludes, "You never let me do anything."
4. *Magnification and minimization.* A situation is perceived as more or less significant than is appropriate. For example, an angry hus-

band blows his top upon discovering that the checkbook isn't balanced and says to his wife, "We're in big trouble."

5. *Personalization.* External events are attributed to oneself when insufficient evidence exists to render a conclusion. For example, a woman who finds her husband adding more salt to her meal assumes, "He hates my cooking."

6. *Dichotomous thinking.* Experiences are codified as either black or white, a complete success or a total failure. This is otherwise known as *polarized thinking.* For example, when a husband is reorganizing a closet and his wife questions the positioning of one of the items, the husband thinks to himself, "She's never happy with anything I do."

7. *Labeling and mislabeling.* One's identity is portrayed on the basis of imperfections and mistakes made in the past, and these are allowed to define oneself. For example, subsequent to continual mistakes in meal preparation, a wife thinks, "1 am worthless," as opposed to recognizing her error as being minor.

8. *Tunnel vision.* Sometimes mates see only what they want to see or what fits their current state of mind. A man who believes that his wife "does whatever she wants anyway" may accuse her of making a choice based purely on selfish reasons.

9. *Biased explanations.* This is a type of thinking that partners develop during times of distress, automatically assuming that a spouse has a negative alternative motive behind his or her intent. For example, a woman tells herself, "He's acting real 'lovey-dovey' because he wants a favor from me. He's setting me up."

10. *Mind reading.* This is the magical gift of being able to know what another person is thinking without the aid of verbal communication. Some spouses end up ascribing unworthy intentions to each other. For example, a man thinks to himself, "I know what is going through her mind; she thinks that I am naive about what she's doing."

Selective Attention

In his early work in cognitive therapy for depression, Aaron Beck and associates (Beck et al., 1979) suggested that individuals who experience depression often focus on selective aspects of a situation or event, failing to recognize other aspects that are equally important. This was the basis for Beck's theory that individuals engaged in "biased interpretation." Family members often engage in the same biases, particularly when they are in conflict with each other or when there is tension in a relationship. We often see this perceptual bias in therapy when family members or couples cannot agree on how an event occurred, or what was said during an argument. This bias can involve positive or negative attributes to which individuals give selective attention. A classic example is an adolescent who contends that her parents tell her only what she has done wrong and don't praise her for the good things she does. Partners or family members often complain about selective attention being one of the major areas of dissension in their relationships.

When family members selectively attend to negative aspects of one another, this can have a damaging effect on their relationship. It is no surprise that individuals who engage in such selective attention, or bias, also have low rates of agreement about past conversations, events, or interactions (Epstein & Baucom, 2002). Selective attention can certainly contribute to cognitive distortions and further alienation.

Developing a more balanced perspective on one's partner or family member is often the focus of CBT. When negative interactions occur over a period of time, such biased perceptions can become ingrained and further serve to alienate individuals from each other. A perfect example of this is a young girl who views her sister as the "golden child" in their parents' eyes— the one who can do no wrong. Therefore, she may view her sister as getting away with everything and build up a resentment toward her that evokes her parents' scoldings about treating her sister with more kindness. This may exacerbate her resentment and cause the siblings to become more alienated from each other, sparking future envy and negative sentiments. It is then the goal of the therapist to attempt to restore the balance in order to help the individuals reduce the dysfunction in their relationship.

Three of the more common cognitive processes introduced earlier in this chapter are explained in more detail in the following paragraphs.

Attributions

Most people attribute interactions to a cause-and-effect dynamic, and each of the parties to these interactions has his or her own explanation of the direction of the cause and effect. Specifically, once a family member focuses on certain behaviors of an interaction, he or she develops inferences to explain those behaviors. These inferences are termed *attributions* and serve as explanations for relational events. Attributions are a key component of a person's subjective experience of his or her relationship.

THE CASE OF DAVE AND BRENDA

Dave and Brenda drove to the hospital for the birth of their first child. En route, Dave stopped at the drugstore to buy some aspirin in anticipation that he might develop a headache. Brenda interpreted Dave's decision to stop at the drugstore as being more concerned about fulfilling his own needs than getting her to the hospital on time. Dave's major concern was that he might develop a headache and wouldn't be able to concentrate. He wanted to avoid leaving his wife's side while she was giving birth. Despite his explanations, Brenda clung to her interpretation that his need to stop at the drugstore was a selfish one, which was a biased interpretation and one that went on to trail them for years into the marriage. In fact, every time Brenda accused Dave of being selfish, she would refer to the birth of their first child and Dave's desire to "take care of his own needs" as a point of reference. This banter went on to become a sore subject and tainted the memory of their first child's birth. The event triggered strong and disdainful emotions for both Dave and Brenda, which ended up being a point of contention.

Numerous empirical studies indicate that distressed partners tend to blame each other for problems and attribute each other's negative actions to broad and unchangeable traits more than do nondistressed partners (Bradbury & Fincham, 1990; Epstein & Baucom, 2003). In fact, *attributional bias* is perceived as being responsible for maintaining ongoing distress in disenchanted couples (Holtzworth-Munroe & Jacobson, 1985). Distressed family members have a propensity to perceive other members' negative behavior as due to enduring traits, which reinforces the notion that these behaviors are difficult to change and are likely permanent fixtures. This is often what some family members use to explain or justify their own behavior in response to other members' negative behavior patterns. Consequently, they may be caught in a situation in which they accentuate the undesirable and downplay the desirable, and sometimes even attribute desirable behavior to chance or external factors in the relationship. Consider the relationship between Dave and Brenda: Any time an important event came up, Brenda anticipated that Dave would be focused on his own needs over those of everyone else and, therefore, would look to find fault with his actions, choosing to interpret them as self-serving. Hence, she would engage in cognitive distortions that affected her emotions and behaviors, repeating the cycle of dissension. This concept, obviously, tends to affect problem-solving behaviors, as well as communication, and to fuel further negative behavioral exchange (Bradbury & Fincham, 1990; Miller & Bradbury, 1995).

Expectancies

Attributions that individuals make about one another's behaviors often lead them to make predictions about future behavior. Such attributions create *expectancies*. Expectancies take the form of predictions about the course a relationship is likely to take and tend to become ingrained. Expectancies have a profound effect on people and how they behave. It is not uncommon for families to come to therapy filled with such expectancies, complaining that they have basically "had it" and see no light at the end of the tunnel. Often, one partner may announce that coming to therapy is a "last ditch effort" for the family's sake and have little optimism about the survival of the relationship.

When family members attempt to predict each other's behavioral patterns, they often become less amenable to making any movement toward improvement in the relationship. Negative predictions and expectancies create a sense of hopelessness in couples and families.

THE CASE OF TED AND DORIS

Ted maintained an unshakable belief that his wife, Doris, was a "spoiled brat" during her childhood and was permitted by her parents to do whatever she wanted. It was Ted's contention that Doris's parents overindulged her and reinforced her "unreasonable demands." As a result, once conflict developed in their marital relationship, Ted came to believe that Doris would do whatever she wanted, because her parents continued to support her regardless of her actions. Consequently, Ted saw no chance for change in the relationship. Doris, on the other hand, felt that Ted used his complaint as a convenient excuse that he could pull out any time he wanted to elicit sympathy from others.

Expectancies rarely occur in isolation. They are usually based on some threads of truth, which make them very hard to deny or to challenge. Expectancies and attributions are usually tightly integrated. Some interesting research conducted by Pretzer, Epstein, and Fleming (1991) revealed that in cases in which spouses attributed relationship problems to their own behavior and less to their partner's behavior or extraneous factors, spouses were more likely to predict improvement in their relationship problems for the future. In essence, the more partners insist on blaming each other, the more pessimistic their assumptions become. Epstein and Baucom (2002) have written that selective attention, attributions, and expectancies are integrally related to each other and to emotions. Therefore, if one person in a family selectively focuses on undesirable behaviors in another, then he or she is more likely to view these behaviors as characteristic of that person. Consequently, he or she may perceive the behavior as being unlikely to change, which can lead to pessimistic expectancies for the relationship's future. Moreover, such pessimistic cognitions are likely to spawn unsettling emotions, ranging from depression to anxiety about the future.

Assumptions

Assumptions involve beliefs that family members hold about relationships. Assumptions govern or entail what people think about the world and how others act, which is part of the template they use to navigate their way through life. Everyone in an intimate relationship, be it a family or a couple, maintains a basic template of how his or her spouse or family members function in life. This template delineates moods, actions, behavior, likes, dislikes, and so forth. If a mother views her daughter as a basically good person, who is kind and gentle, then she may make allowances for her daughter if the child snaps impolitely at somebody, contending that she is either "under stress" or "just not feeling well." She does this to explain the inconsistency of her daughter's actions and to allow her to firmly retain the image of a good daughter. This mother's perceptions are not easily disconfirmed, unless a series of major events occur that radically change her perception of her daughter. Unfortunately, the same is true when family members assume the worst about each other.

Family members make assumptions about each other on a regular basis that often involve basic value systems. These value systems are used to govern people's lifestyles. Gordon and Baucom (1999) found that negative events are experienced as traumatic when they disrupt basic assumptions that individuals hold about their partners or family members. For a man to behave in ways that are antithetical to his wife's adoring view of him may devastate or shock her. Epstein and Baucom (2002) indicate that when assumptions are disrupted in relationships, a spouse no longer knows how to interpret his or her partner's behavior, or how to behave him- or herself, because such a disruption is so overwhelming. At no time is this more upsetting than when a spouse has an extramarital affair. Often, an affair causes the betrayed spouse to say things like "I don't know who I'm married to." "This isn't the person I fell in love with." "I would have never dreamed that this could happen!"

THE CASE OF TOM AND JENNIFER

When Tom had a one-night stand with a woman he met at a bar while on a business trip, Jennifer said, "My world was turned upside down." Jennifer went on to say that she struggled to understand why her husband would do such a thing and was surprised to learn from him that he was feeling angry and isolated from her because he was not getting the attention and emotional support he felt he deserved. Tom's statements caused Jennifer to become completely confused about their relationship in general. Subsequently, she remarked, "I feel like I'm living a lie. I was under the impression that our marriage was a whole lot more than it is. Now I don't know what's real." The affair had a similarly destructive effect on Tom and Jennifer's children, especially the teenage daughters who viewed their father as being their "rock" and believed he could "do no wrong." The oldest teenage daughter, Analice, said during a family session, "This has really affected how I trust men in general. I want no part of relationships if this is what can happen."

Assumptions are powerful cognitions that govern our relationships. They aren't usually explicit, and they need to be uncovered and brought into the open.

Standards

As discussed earlier, attributions are explanations of why people do what they do, and expectancies are predictions about how they will act in the future. Assumptions serve as beliefs that individuals hold about the characteristics of their partners and intimate relationships. Unlike attributions, standards are based on principles, on individual beliefs about what should be. Family schemas, also mentioned earlier, emerge from the concept held by family members that there is a certain way families are supposed to act (Dattilio, 1993). Both couples and families typically use standards to evaluate whether each member's behavior is appropriate and acceptable in the relationship. Such standards serve as a rough guideline to follow, based on a historical pattern of expected behavior. Standards may direct how affection should be expressed or how family members should relate to one another. They may also prescribe how external contacts with others outside the relationship should be handled. In essence, standards guide us in how we should be governing our lives with respect to our relationships to one another and to the world. The long-standing belief held by many men has been that a woman belongs at home and should be present with the family and that a man's job is to serve as the breadwinner. This standard is one that has caused a great deal of dissension in relationships, particularly in contemporary society. Consequently, an individual who holds standards about boundaries or roles in marriages and families may be expected to evaluate events in terms of these standards. Therefore, when problems arise in a family situation, they will likely be attributed to boundary issues and the violation of those boundaries (Baucom, Epstein, Daiuto, Carels, Rankin, & Burnett, 1996).

THE CASE OF LORENA AND BART

An example of conflicting standards involves Lorena and Bart. In Bart's family, this was the standard: Whenever you receive a gift from a family member, you keep it or make good use of it. What you don't ever do is give it away to anyone else. This would be a sign of great disrespect to the giver. The standard in Lorena's family, which was of Mexican descent, was this: If someone greatly admires something of yours, you offer it to him or her. So when Lorena received a scarf from her mother-in-law that had been in her husband's family for generations, she had no idea that it would cause so much dissension when she gave the scarf to her own mother, who had admired it. Lorena saw her action as a way to honor both her mother-in-law and her mother. But Lorena's husband and mother-in-law were insulted and saw it as a sign of disrespect.

Standards emanate from a variety of places. They may also develop as a result of exposure to the media, one's religious or cultural experience, one's previous relationships, or social interactions. Standards are probably most germane to family-of-origin experiences. The standards family members hold, and the boundaries describing the appropriate behaviors that they assume, become intricate. Schwebel (1992) suggested that family members establish a sort of "family constitution."

A number of standards address interrelationships among family members, such as the manner in which behaviors and emotions are expressed, and the maintenance of power and control in the family. Schwebel (1992) also suggested standards for the division of labor, how chores are assigned and who does what, dealing with conflict, what is tolerated, how resolution is sought and balance restored, boundaries and privacy, how and what lines are drawn, and who is permitted to do what and when. He also suggested standards for family members' dealings with individuals outside the family unit, such as procedures to be used with extended family members, as well as friends and acquaintances.

There has been some focus in the literature on transgenerational schemas, which often include specific standards that trickle down into marital relationships and subsequently to family interactions (Dattilio, 2005b, 2006a). Much of the early work of the pioneering family therapist Murray Bowen focused on the concept that what we think has been passed down through the generations, which has a significant impact on family tradition and loyalty. Some standards also have a personal quality, as individuals place additional value on the standards they inherited based on their personal experiences and thus strengthen them. These standards typically pertain to things like sexual behavior, honesty, and integrity. This may explain why some research findings support the notion that individuals who share a spiritual or religious orientation tend to have a more fulfilling marriage or family life (Clayton & Baucom, 1998). Baucom, Epstein, Daiuto, and Carels (1996) further found that couples who maintained relationship-oriented standards tended to find their relationships more rewarding. Baucom and Epstein (2002) argue that, in many instances, individuals' standards about intimate relationships are well ingrained and have significant importance. The authors further contend (p. 73) that the importance of relationship standards in individuals' lives seems to vary in at least three ways:

1. The degree to which individuals develop a variety of standards about interpersonal relationships and articulate these standards.
2. The degree to which these internal standards influence their behavior.
3. How emotionally upset they become when their standards are not met.

Baucom, Epstein, Rankin, and Burnett (1996) find that regardless of the particular standards that an individual maintains, he or she tends to be happier if those standards are met in his or her relationship. Hence, within reasonable limits, having one's standards met typically contributes to relationship satisfaction, regardless of the particular standards.

Therefore, it is essential for family therapists to attempt to understand what family members' standards are in regard to their relationships and how they should function. This understanding may be very helpful when they attempt to help their clients explain whether the standards are being met. This concept hit home with me early on in my career while working with a young bicultural couple who expressed severe conflict in the marriage over what the husband considered improper on the part of the wife.

THE CASE OF SAL AND MAUREEN

Sal and Maureen met while Sal was visiting his brother in America. Sal hailed from a small mountain town in central Sicily. Maureen was American born and of Irish descent. Sal and Maureen were married only 1 year when significant cultural differences began to emerge. Maureen was a vibrant redhead who was known to make conversation with almost anyone. Her friends and family often said that "her congeniality was infectious." Sal admitted that Maureen's outgoingness was one of the attributes he fell in love with. But this attribute turned sour for him one day when he arrived home to find Maureen on the patio having a drink with an unmarried male neighbor. This behavior was a major violation of standards in Sicilian families—for a young married woman to entertain another man at home alone with alcohol. Sal was furious that Maureen would do such a disrespectful thing and started calling her a *puttana* (whore). Maureen thought that Sal was being "ridiculous," particularly because her upbringing was quite the opposite, and saw nothing wrong with such social behavior. In fact, it was Maureen's belief that this conflict rested on the issue of trust and that both spouses should have enough trust in each other to believe that he or she would not violate the marital relationship.

There has been much more research on attributions and standards than on the other forms of cognition (see Baucom et al.'s [1989] typology and Epstein & Baucom, 2002, for a review of findings). A sizable amount of research on couples' attributions indicates that distressed couples are more likely than nondistressed couples to attribute their partners' negative behavior to global, stable traits; negative intent; selfish motivation; and a lack of love (see Bradbury & Fincham, 1990, and Epstein & Baucom, 2002, for reviews). In addition, couples in distressed relationships are less likely to attribute a partner's desirable behaviors to global, stable causes. These biased inferences can contribute to family members' pessimism about improvement in their relationships and to negative communication and lack of problem solving.

Clearly, the concepts of assumptions, expectancies, and attributions, as well as standards, overlap just as do many of the cognitive distortions. A therapist treating a family usually has to identify and tease out multiple forces at work, as in the following case.

THE CASE OF NICK AND ALICE

Nick and Alice were a couple in their early 40s who had been married for 15 years. They came to therapy complaining of extreme tension in their relationship due to differences of opinion in regard to their finances. Nick claimed that because of Alice's excessive spending, they were likely facing bankruptcy. Nick and Alice admitted that this was a pattern that had existed for their entire marriage, which Nick believed had finally caught up with them.

The pattern in this relationship was that Alice would spend more than they could afford. Each time she did, Nick would work overtime in order to cover the expenses. Each time he worked more hours and covered the expenses, Alice felt that they were now flush and could safely spend additional monies. Despite their frequent arguments about finances, Nick contended that Alice forced them to live beyond their means. Alice had developed this attitude toward money and consumption early in the relationship. She had been raised as an only child, and her parents provided her with whatever she wanted, regardless of whether or not they could afford it. Nick contended that Alice's parents had started a vicious cycle of her "getting whatever she wanted." Nick felt that he had fallen prey to this cycle when he married Alice. "I just wanted to make her happy, but now I'm on this rapid treadmill of having to work constant overtime because Alice can't say no to herself." When asked why he put up with this, Nick admitted that he feared that Alice would leave him if he didn't indulge her in whatever she wanted. "But now we are probably facing bankruptcy, and I don't know what to do." Alice, on the other hand, felt that Nick was exaggerating. "We always pull out of it," she said. "What's the big deal? He worries too much—and we're not facing bankruptcy." Alice admitted to overspending, but declared, "Hey, we only go around once—what's money for anyway?"

Nick came from a different family environment. His parents were poor and never made much money. "My mother made do on whatever my father brought home and that was it! No bickering about overspending. We always had enough." Hence, the *attribution* in this situation was "We're in debt because Alice can't control her spending, and I enable it because I want to make her happy." Both admitted that this was the cognitive process that operated in the relationship and that they equally contributed to the vicious cycle. Nick further admitted that he was aware of the fact that his willingness to repeatedly "bail them out" by working overtime was an enabling behavior on his part.

As for the *expectancies*, both believed that this cycle of behavior was likely to continue inasmuch as neither of them was willing to change his or her ways. For years, they had both contributed to what had become an ingrained pattern of behavior, which, in many ways, now seemed to be spinning out of control.

The basic *assumption* held by Nick was, "It is what it is." Alice could never say no to herself because she believed that she always had to have what she wanted. Nick was not likely to impose any limitations on Alice's behavior because he was inhibited by his fear of saying no to her, risking her unhappiness and the possibility that she would leave him. Thus, he continued to enable this behavior as a means of avoiding the worst—Alice's leaving him.

Hence, the *standard* in the relationship had been to do little about the situation, although both knew that things should change or be modified. This was particularly so because they had now gotten themselves into so much debt that they risked losing everything. Whereas Alice maintained one standard, that she should be able to spend what she wishes, Nick's standard was that they should be more frugal and engage more in self-denial. This conflict also involved an issue of control for both in the relationship. Interestingly, both parties seemed to ignore a possible middle ground (moderation in spending) and took little responsibility for their behaviors and the overall situation.

Deficits in Communication and Problem-Solving Skills

There is considerable empirical evidence to suggest that members of distressed families exhibit a variety of dysfunctional patterns involving their expression of thoughts and emotions. Poor listening and problem-solving skills have also been identified as factors causing distress (Dattilio & Van Hout, 2006; Epstein & Baucom, 2002; Walsh, 1998). The expression of thoughts and emotions involves self-awareness, an appropriate vocabulary to describe one's experiences, freedom from inhibiting factors such as fear of rejection by the listener, and a degree of self-control (e.g., not succumbing to an urge to retaliate against a person who upsets you). Effective problem solving involves the ability to define the characteristics of a problem clearly, generate alternative potential solutions, collaborate with other family members in evaluating the advantages and disadvantages of each solution, reach consensus about the best solution, and devise a specific plan to implement the solution. Thus, effective family problem solving requires both good skills and goodwill.

Deficits in communication and problem solving may develop as a result of various processes, such as maladaptive patterns of learning during socialization in the family of origin, deficits in cognitive functioning, forms of psychopathology such as depression, and past traumatic experiences in relationships that have left an individual vulnerable to disruptive cognitive, emotional, and behavioral responses (e.g., rage or panic) during interactions with significant others. Research has indicated that individuals who communicate poorly in their couple relationships may exhibit constructive communication skills in relatively neutral outside relationships, suggesting that chronic issues in the intimate relationship are interfering with productive communication (Baucom & Epstein, 1990). These topics are discussed further in Chapter 5.

Excesses of Negative Behavior and Deficits in Positive Behavior between Partners or among Family Members

Destructive and ineffective communication and problem-solving skills are not the only forms of problematic behavioral interaction in distressed couples and families. Members of close relationships commonly direct a variety of types of *noncommunication behavior* toward each other (Baucom & Epstein, 1990; Epstein & Baucom, 2002). These are positive and negative acts (perform a task to achieve a goal, such as completing household chores or failing to do so) that are intended to affect the other person's feelings (e.g., giving him or her a gift or forgetting to give a gift). Although these typically are implicit messages conveyed by a behavior, they do not involve explicit expression of thoughts and emotions. Research has demonstrated that members of distressed relationships direct more negative acts and fewer positive ones toward each other than do those in nondistressed relationships (Epstein & Baucom, 2002). Furthermore, distressed couples are more likely to reciprocate in an unproductive fashion, which can result in an escalation of conflict and distress. Consequently, a basic premise of CBT is that the frequency of undesirable behavior must be reduced and the frequency of more productive behavior must be increased. Because undesirable behavior tends to have a greater impact on relationship satisfaction than does productive behavior (Gottman, 1994; Weiss & Heyman, 1997), it has received more attention from therapists. Although this is a basic concept, it is nonetheless a very important one because each partner in a couple is usually seeking productive interaction in order to fulfill his or her own needs. Therapists can assist couples by using some of the *quid pro quo* strategies described in Chapter 6, which discusses behavioral techniques. These techniques have been demonstrated to be highly effective with couples that are gridlocked in distressed relationships.

Although family theorists and researchers have focused on minor aspects of desirable and undesirable behavior, Epstein and Baucom (2002) propose that, in many instances, relationship satisfaction is based on larger behavioral patterns that have significant meaning for each partner. Some of the larger issues involve boundaries between and around a couple or family, the distribution of power and control, and the amount of time and energy that each person puts into the relationship. As noted earlier, individuals' relationship standards concerning these dimensions are associated with relationship satisfaction and communication, and the family therapy literature suggests that these behavior patterns are core aspects of family interaction (Epstein & Baucom, 2002; Walsh, 1998).

Epstein and Baucom (2002) have also described destructive interaction patterns between members of couples that commonly interfere with the partners' fulfillment of their needs within the relationship. These patterns include mutual (reciprocal) attack, demand–withdrawal (one person pursues and the other withdraws), and mutual avoidance and withdrawal. Therapists often must help clients reduce these patterns individually before they will be able to work together collaboratively as a couple to resolve issues such as different preferences for togetherness versus autonomy. The same may hold true for members of a family as well.

ATTACHMENT AND AFFECT

Models of Attachment and the Secure Emotional Connection

In the 1940s and early 1950s, British psychoanalyst John Bowlby developed what he called *attachment theory*. Bowlby developed this theory from a number of insights, combining object relations theory, post-Darwinian ethnology, modern cognitive developmental psychology, cybernetics (control systems theories), and community psychiatry (Mikulincer & Shaver, 2007).

Since attachment theory's inception, there has been a wealth of research literature addressing the issue of how early childhood attachments affect our lives (Ainsworth, Blehar, Waters, & Wall, 1978; Cassidy & Shaver, 1999; Mikulincer & Shaver, 2007; Mikulincer, Florian, Cowan, & Cowan, 2002; Wallin, 2007). This concept focuses on how couples and family members deal with each other and how that is reflected in their attachment history. Attachment theory can be traced to the pioneering studies of John Bowlby and Mary Ainsworth. Bowlby (1979) believed that human attachment patterns noted in infant–caregiver interactions went on to play a vital role in human development "from the cradle to the grave" (p. 129). Bowlby (1979) was also the first to discuss individual differences in attachment system functioning in the context of romantic and marital relationships. It was Shaver, Hazan, and Bradshaw (1988) who went on to propose the concept that romantic attachment bonds in adulthood were vital, suggesting that they are similar to the bonds that infants form with their primary caregivers. Their work went on to spawn a great deal of research on the attachment styles of couples and the success or failure of their romantic and marital relationships (Johnson & Whiffen, 2003).

Such issues as attachment-related processes affecting the formation, consolidation, and maintenance of long-term romantic relationships and the effect of these relationships on relationship quality, satisfaction, and stability are included in this topic. Bowlby proposed the concept that attachment bonds are characterized by four basic behaviors: (1) proximity seeking, (2) safe haven behavior, (3) separation distress, and (4) secure-base behavior (Bowlby, 1969, 1973). Bowlby believed that these basic behaviors became most evident when one observes the comfort and security that spouses derive from each other, particularly during periods of stress.

Attachment Styles

According to Mary Ainsworth (1967), infants use their attachment figure (usually the mother) as a secure base for exploration. When an infant feels threatened, he or she will turn to the caregiver for protection and comfort. Variations in this pattern are evident in two insecure strategies of attachment. In the *avoidant* strategy the infant tends to inhibit attachment seeking, and in the *resistant* strategy the infant clings to the mother and avoids exploration (Nichols & Schwartz, 2008, p. 108).

Attachment style pertains to the interconnected cognition, emotions, behaviors, and physiology that develop as part of an individual's repertoire in relationships. Attachment styles begin early in life, based on our relationship with our parents or caretakers, and are later transferred, but reformulated, once we become involved in romantic relationships. Hazan and Shaver (1987) proposed the concept that adults form attachments to their partners or spouses and subsequently develop an internal working model of a mature romantic relationship. Further development of the basic theory was expanded by Bartholomew and Horowitz (1991), who suggested that these mature attachment styles are characterized by thought processes, which fit into the basics of a belief or schema; one's view of being worthy or unworthy of love and intimacy and one's view of others as being trustworthy or unreliable. Bartholomew and Horowitz (1991) further expanded this concept into four styles of attachment:

1. *Secure*—the view of oneself as worthy and others as trustworthy, allowing one to be comfortable with intimacy and autonomy.
2. *Preoccupied*—maintaining a negative view of oneself, yet a positive view of others, causing one to become overinvolved in close relationships and depending on others for a sense of self-worth.
3. *Fearful–avoidant*—a negative view of both oneself and others, causing one to be fearful of intimacy and avoiding relationships with other people.
4. *Dismissing*—maintaining a positive view of oneself, but a negative view of others, causing one to avoid relationships with others, preferring to remain independent and shying away from intimate relationships.

Research has supported a positive correlation between adult attachment and relationship satisfaction (Mikulincer et al., 2002). When both partners in a relationship are securely attached, they report the highest satisfaction with their romantic relationship (Senchak & Leonard, 1992).

Further, it has been found that attachment orientation is likely to affect the progression of intimacy in relationships, as well as commitment and tolerance. In their comprehensive textbook on attachment in adulthood, Mikulincer and Shaver (2007) cite studies that indicate that people who suffer from insecurity due to poor attachment are likely to react to a partner's unfavorable behavior with more hostility, dysfunctional anger, and less forgiveness than people who have experienced secure attachments. They also have difficulty in managing interpersonal conflict.

Attachment issues are vitally important in family relationships. Research has demonstrated that ruptured attachment and a negative family environment inhibit children from developing the internal and interpersonal coping skills needed to buffer against certain vulnerabilities and social stressors (Diamond, Diamond, & Hogue, 2007). Therefore, when people are insecure because of attachment difficulties early in life, it affects the extent to which they express respect, admiration, and gratitude to a spouse. This has a profound impact on the maintenance of long-term relationships (Gottman, 1994). Markman, Stanley, and Blumberg (1994) posit that expressing positive regard for one's partner is one of the four crucial relationship values, along with commitment, intimacy, and forgiveness. Clearly, if attachment insecurities reduce the quality of couple relationships, the damage and difficulties can generalize to other family subsystems and affect the functioning of the family as a unit (Paley et al., 2005; Leon & Jacobvitz, 2003). The trickle-down effect proceeding from parents to offspring, can be profound.

Cognitive Processes in Attachment

Just as emotions play an important role in attachment, so do cognitive processes. This is particularly so in regard to addressing attachment issues and making changes in relationships. Young and associates discuss the notion of attachment through early maladaptive schemas. One in particular is the disconnection and rejection domain, otherwise known as the *abandonment schema* (Young et al., 2003). Individuals who maintain this type of schema constantly expect to lose the people closest to them. They fear abandonment, such as through illness, death, or being left for someone else. Somehow they anticipate that they will be left, particularly in a time of need. The signs of this schema are pervasive vigilance and a chronic anxiety about their loved ones. This may also be manifested in the form of sadness or depression. When there is actual loss, it may produce grief or, if the grief is too painful to bear, it may produce rage. People with this schema may also tend to be very "clingy" in relationships or to show possessive or controlling behaviors—jealousy is often used to prevent abandonment. Some individuals may avoid intimate relationships altogether in an attempt to avoid the anticipated pain of being left by another.

Young et al. (2003) also believe that the abandonment schema is frequently linked with other schemas, such as the *subjugation schema*. In this case, an individual believes that if he or she does not do what the spouse wants, the spouse will leave him or her. We saw this earlier in the case example involving Nick and Alice. Hence, there is a sense of relinquishing oneself to the other, sometimes to the point of losing one's own integrity. Abandonment is also frequently linked to the *dependence/independence schema*, in which the individuals are convinced that if the spouse leaves them, they will be unable to function on their own. The following case involves a classic example of this type of schema.

THE CASE OF WILMA AND CHARLES

A middle-aged woman named Wilma was so dependent on her husband that she never argued with him. She was completely passive and never challenged Charles, for fear that he would become disenchanted and leave her. In fact, on one occasion, Wilma learned that Charles was involved in an extramarital affair with his secretary. When Charles admitted his indis-cretion, Wilma begged him not to leave her and even promised that she would not complain about the extramarital relationship, provided that he would always remain in the marriage with her. At times, Wilma would even cover for Charles with the children so that no one would know he was being unfaithful to her. She promised that it would always remain their "little secret." This type of pathological attachment is often rooted in a *rigid abandonment schema* that leads to a person's relinquishing his or her identity and values in order to avoid being alone. When questioned about the rationale for her behavior, Wilma explained, "It's better to tol-erate Charles's having an affair than facing life alone. I couldn't make it alone, and turning a 'blind eye' to his unfaithfulness is a small price to pay for the security of having him in my life." To Wilma, such security was essential to her survival.

Charles, on the other hand, felt that he benefited to some degree from Wilma's fear of rejection because it allowed him to do what he wanted. However, he later also found her dependent behaviors to be a bore and unstimulating.

Schema Restructuring

Addressing issues of attachment often goes hand in hand with addressing issues of emotional regulation. Working on these in therapy requires the cli-ent to examine his or her own schema regarding intimate attachments and the accompanying emotions that often stem from experiences in the client's family of origin. Much of the standard format for schema restructuring is also applied to a person's schemas about the vulnerability of getting close in relationships. Fear of losing one's sense of identity and autonomy may often be the basis of such resistance. This might explain a spouse's reticence to becoming too close and may pertain to early attachment issues in his or her life. The cognitive therapy literature (Beck, 2002; Young, Klosko, & Weishaar, 2003) has emphasized that maladaptive schemas regarding attachment and bonding that develop early within the nuclear family tend to be the strongest, most resistant schemas to change. These schemas are typi-cally strengthened by later life experiences. This is why any examination of early childhood experiences is important in understanding the problems of emotional dysregulation and attachment. The early formation of ingrained beliefs about being abandoned or unlovable is at the hub of resistance and a failure to bond or emote in relationships. The following case of Jenna is a prime example of how such a schema develops. This vignette further shows how cognitive-behavioral techniques were implemented so that the issues in Jenna's relationship with her fiancé, as well as with her father, could be addressed.

EMOTIONALLY CAUTERIZED: THE CASE OF JENNA

Jenna, a 41-year-old woman, presented for therapy with her 48-year-old fiancé, Ken, because she was having difficulty engaging with him emotionally. Jenna explained that she had dated many men over the years, but had never had any long-term relationships. These relationships would last only a few months and end because she was not able to reciprocate emotionally. The majority of the men who dated Jenna became frustrated with her and subsequently ended the relationship, complaining that she was cold and often too rigid for them. Only in the past year and a half did Jenna meet Ken, who seemed to be more tolerant of her behavior and fell in love with her, despite her rigidity. Jenna was very much in love with Ken, but they were experiencing difficulties in the relationship because she had problems with getting emotionally close and was unable to display emotional affection. Jenna went on to explain to me that she was able to be physically intimate with Ken but she struggled with intimacy and wasn't able to respond emotionally to his overtures, such as by telling him that she loved him. For example, both shared with me that when Ken felt affectionate toward Jenna, he would give her a hug. Jenna had difficulty hugging Ken for any prolonged period of time. After a few seconds of embrace, she would push him away. Ken, however, wanted more from Jenna and would become frustrated with her. Jenna also stated that, during their lovemaking, they were able to have sexual relations and be intimate to a point, but it was short lived because Jenna felt guarded about getting too deeply "into it" with Ken.

Despite all of the difficulties that she described to me, Jenna said that she loved Ken very much and felt that he was the first person she had ever wanted to marry. However, although they were engaged, they both worried about Jenna's ever being able to loosen up enough emotionally to fully engage in a lasting intimate relationship.

Jenna's Family of Origin

I decided to spend some time dealing with Jenna's background and investigating her family of origin in an attempt to better understand her family dynamics and how she was raised. Jenna grew up in a Serbian American family in which her father was extremely controlling and dominant. Her mother, however, was passive and meek. Jenna (who tended to be assertive even as a teenager) locked horns with her father and developed a very tense relationship with him. She described herself as "loathing" her father because of his domineering, arrogant style and the manner in which he treated her mother. She never felt that she bonded with her father and, in fact, even referred to him by his first name. Jenna went on to say that she suffered from an eating disorder during her adolescence, as well as some depression. She was eventually so disgusted by her father's arrogance that she left the home at age 18. She went on to do very well as a stockbroker, like her father, but continued to have little to do with him. She regarded him as a "father figure," but resented the manner in which her mother submitted to her father, almost as though she were his servant. (Interestingly, Jenna had a younger brother who was more like her mother and married a woman who was domineering, like their father.)

Consequently, Jenna often said that she was vigilant about being "consumed by men" and never wanted to reveal too much of her vulnerability in relationships. She said that she was "emotionally traumatized" by her father, which caused her to develop an insulation that would not allow men to get close to her. Ken was the first man whom Jenna ever allowed to get as far as he did, and she admitted that this was very difficult for her. Jenna further explained, "I feel like, if I allow him to get too close, I'll lose a part of myself and lose control."

Early Attachment Issues

Much of my work with Jenna revolved around her early attachment issues with her father. She recalled wanting to be "Daddy's little girl" when she was very young, but was never able to live up to his expectations. In many ways, Jenna felt that her father pushed her away by criticizing her and always being extremely demanding of her. She recalled an incident when she was 10 years old. She bought home a report card on which she had earned mostly all As and one B. Her father proceeded to berate her for being so "weak and insolent" as to obtain a B and ruining a potentially perfect record. Jenna recalls that her father was a tyrant and had unreasonable expectations, which she resented. Nonetheless, she still tried to live up to his expectations in order to win his love. In this respect, Jenna learned to never trust men very much and transferred the poor attachment she had with her father to her romantic relationships with men in general. She attempted to compensate by becoming very close to her mother and insulated herself in her relationships with men.

Jenna went on to elaborate that each time she reached out to her father, he "burned" her by criticizing her or denigrating her, thus eroding her self-esteem. When Jenna first began dating, she found that many of her boyfriends did the same thing and basically only wanted to use her for a sexual relationship. These experiences caused Jenna to harden over the years and to insulate herself from getting too close to any male. She developed the schema that she was not worth much to men other than to satisfy their physical needs. This belief system caused her to further harden and insulate herself from any emotion.

I pointed out to Jenna that it was interesting that she chose to see a male therapist who was close to her father's age. This was ironic in the sense that it seemed like an opportunity for Jenna to rekindle a bond with a father figure vicariously through me, yet reject me and consequently her therapy, if I were to get too close. Jenna was very open and honest with me about her feelings, which I interpreted to be her need to reattach to her father. She seemed to trust me, particularly because I was careful never to criticize her.

Focus of Treatment

Among the foci of our work together was to help Jenna learn how to let go and open herself up to Ken. Most of this therapy centered on her request to learn how to feel. Jenna often said, "I want to open myself up emotionally to Ken, but how do you do that when you are 'emotionally cauterized'?" I found this term that Jenna used, "emotionally cauterized" to be very interesting. It surely was a term that described her well. Teaching Jenna to be less defensive became a major challenge in therapy. We worked a great deal on her lack of attachment with Ken and her fear of trusting him. One of the areas I used as a tool was Jenna's sexual relations with Ken. As I gathered information in regard to their sexual intimacy, Jenna informed me that she was able to reach orgasm during vaginal intercourse with Ken. She informed me that this was not a problem and that she enjoyed it. I asked her specifically about how it was that she could allow herself to let go and reach orgasm without feeling guarded and vulnerable. She was unable to explain to me how she could do this, other than to "focus on the moment." I used this as a framework in an attempt to help Jenna let go and experience emotion with Ken. For example, I engaged her in a number of behavioral and cognitive exercises in which I had her deliberately approach Ken and ask him for a hug, at which point I instructed her to deliberately prolong the hug. I also had Jenna examine what it felt like for her to do this and identify specific thoughts she had of vulnerability or loss of control.

During the first exercise, Jenna said that she was able to complete the assignment, but she couldn't put her finger on her thoughts. She simply went blank and felt as though she were becoming emotionally numb. This is not unusual and is referred to as *cognitive avoidance*. I asked Jenna to repeat the exercise on several occasions, but to concentrate on the feel of Ken's body and the warmth of the two of them together, as well as focusing on their respective breathing during the embrace. Over a period of time, I encouraged Jenna to get in touch with a feeling of enjoying being enveloped in Ken's arms, inasmuch as he was so much larger than she, yet, at the same time, recall her sense of "fear and vulnerability." I had her repeat the exposure exercise several times, encouraging her to feel whatever she wanted to feel and refrain from making any judgments about the appropriateness of her feelings.

Over time, I had Jenna reexpose herself for longer periods of time and encouraged her to say out loud what she felt, as well as what her thoughts were about what she was feelings. I also had her engage in a number of other activities, such as deliberately being late for certain activities and going beyond many of the rigid boundaries she had often imposed on herself, such as leaving dishes unwashed in the sink, in order to break her repeated patterns of compulsive behavior.

Family-of-Origin Session

In addition, I proposed inviting Jenna's father into a session so that we could address their relationship. I asked her permission to contact her father and invited him into a conjoint session. Initially, Jenna bristled at this notion and expressed her reservations about how it might go. We went on to discuss some of the potential benefits of such a conjoint meeting, and Jenna eventually agreed to it. Surprisingly, Jenna's father was very open to coming in and told me that he had been distressed for years over his poor relationship with his daughter and would like an attempt to improve it. Jenna was very resistant to this idea, but after some encouragement and support from Ken, she agreed. We initially met with Jenna and her mother and father in order to discuss the family dynamics. Jenna's mother reinforced the idea that, for years, she had been uncomfortable with Jenna's relationship with her father and thought that it was a good idea that they had agreed to meet in therapy.

I conducted several sessions with Jenna and her father, George, in which we talked about their attachment and bond. Jenna's father admitted that there was very little bond because he never knew how to bond with his own mother. His mother was a strict Serbian immigrant, whom he described as being "devoid of emotions." His father had died of heart failure at a very young age. Therefore, it was very difficult for him to express emotions until he met Jenna's mother. Although his wife was very affectionate and supportive, George admitted that he often rejected her overtures because he had difficulty dealing with intense emotion. We discussed how much of this impacted George's relationship with Jenna and talked about the bond that the two had failed to develop. This process took approximately 8 months, but it proved to help Jenna significantly in learning to open up and let herself feel. Jenna was also shocked when her father revealed that he had also entered into individual therapy. This seemed to encourage her to work more diligently on her own issues. Jenna often said, "We just needed to snip off the cauterized edges so that I could feel again." We also discussed the idea that what felt like "numbness" to Jenna was actually her own self-imposed insulation as a mode of protection. She often believed that she was unable to feel because she had never experienced her feelings in the past. I recommended to her that her recollections were a means of protecting herself as a tortoise does by retreating into its shell.

This example underscores the notion of how important early attachment is to a couple's relationship and how injuries during the early attachment period go on to affect later relationships.

The Role of Affect Regulation

Despite common misconceptions, emotion has always played an important part in the therapeutic process of cognitive-behavioral therapy. Because emotions are what therapists typically encounter from the start of the therapy process, it would be difficult, as well as unwise, to ignore them. Families usually enter into treatment after some intense emotional upheaval or crisis has occurred. In a survey of 147 married couples seeking marital therapy, the most common reason given for seeking treatment was problematic communication and lack of affection (Doss, Simpson, & Christensen, 2004). Hence, emotional distance was found to be just as common a reason for seeking couples therapy as communication problems. Much of the research literature tells us that emotions are primarily nonconscious mental processes that create a state of readiness for action, disposing us to behave in a particular way in our environment (Siegel, 1999). The state of readiness is activated by these unconscious mental processes that are later made conscious. Emotions influence the flow of states of mind that dominate a vast number of our mental processes.

Most theories of emotion share some common themes. One is that emotion involves complex layers of processes that are in constant interaction with the environment. At a minimum, these interactions involve the cognitive processes (such as the appraisal or evaluation of meaning), perception, and physical changes (such as endocrine, autoarousal, and cardiovascular changes).

As discussed in Chapter 4, the structure of the brain facilitates an innate capacity to modulate emotion and to organize its state of activation (Gleick, 1987). The mind's ability to regulate emotional processes stems from the brain's capacity to modulate the flow of arousal and activation throughout its circuitry. Primary emotional processes, along with affective expression and mood, can be altered by the brain. A popular concept of emotional regulation refers to the ability of the mind to alter the various components of emotional processing. Siegel (1999) states, "The self-organization of the mind in many ways is determined by the self-regulation of the emotional states. How we experience the world, relate to others, and find meaning in life is dependent on how we come to regulate our emotions" (p. 245). But how much of the cognitive processes are responsible for the regulation as well? There is no doubt that what parents do with children early in their lives greatly affects the outcome of the children's development. Longitudinal research underscores this quite clearly (Milner, Squire, & Kandel, 1998). Both temperament and attachment history contribute to the marked differences that we witness between adults in their ability to regulate their emotions (Siegel, 1999). For example, Dawson (1994) found in studies of infants of clinically depressed mothers that the infants' capacity to experience joy and excitement is markedly reduced, especially if the maternal depression lasts beyond the first year. Such experiences can profoundly shape the general intensity and balance of emotional activation throughout childhood and into adulthood.

The term *emotional regulation* refers to the general ability of the mind to alter the various components of emotional processing. No doubt, the self-organization of the mind, in many ways, is determined by the self-regulation of emotional states. Therefore, how we come to experience the world, relate to others, and find meaning in life are dependent on how we have come to regulate our emotions. Emotion reflects the fundamental way in which the mind assigns value to external and internal events and then directs the allocation of attentional resources to further the processing of these representations.

Emotional Intensity and Emotional Focus

It is often at moments when emotions become most intense that people seem to experience the greatest need to be understood by others—and experience the most intense feelings of vulnerability as well. This may be why many couples and family members act out physically or withdraw when they feel that they are not being heard.

A recently developed approach known as *emotionally focused therapy* (EFT) has been introduced as an intervention for couples (Johnson, 1996, 1998). It is one of the few couple therapies that has demonstrated positive outcomes that persist over time (Johnson, Hunsley, Greenberg, & Schindler, 1999). EFT centers on change and negative interaction patterns that contribute to secure and emotional bonds. The EFT perspective on relationship distress focuses on emotional responses and rigid, self-reinforcing patterns of interaction. The essence of EFT is that troubled couples are seen as interacting with their defenses. In therapy, they learn to let their guard down and reveal their more vulnerable feelings. EFT is a constructionist approach that focuses on the process of how individual partners actively organize and create their ongoing experience and schemas about the identity of self and others in the context of their "interactional dance" (Johnson, 1998). The partners in a couple are viewed as being "stuck" in certain ways of regulating, processing, and organizing their emotional responses to each other, which then constricts the interaction between them and prevents the development of a secure bond. It is the philosophy of EFT that constricted interactional patterns subsequently evoke and maintain states of negative affect, which, obviously, create difficulty in the relationship.

The interesting aspect of EFT is that it gives priority to emotion as a determinant of attachment behavior, which is a positive force for change in couple therapy. Rather than viewing emotion as an aspect to be overcome and replaced by cognitive restructuring, EFT rests on attachment theory and the observation that in an attachment relationship (such as a marriage or other intimate partnership) emotion tends to override other cues; hence the title "emotionally focused." In fact, a problem in integrating CBT techniques with EFT is that EFT views relationships in attachment terms, rather than from an exchange perspective that focuses on rational negotiation and behavioral contracts.

There are many good aspects of the EFT approach, which involve discovering unacknowledged feelings and underlying interactional positions. There is also an emphasis on reframing problems in terms of the cycle of unmet attachment needs and the promotion of owning one's needs, as well as the expanded aspects of self-experience. Many of these aspects can be woven into the cognitive-behavioral approach, particularly through developing a conceptualization regarding the notion of schema and the "emotional schemas" that couple and family members maintain. As stated earlier, the concept of schema has recently been expanded to include multilevel aspects containing details of emotion, physiology, and behavior. An important aspect emphasizes memory structures that involve emotion and other sensory stimuli such as physiological and neural, as well as cognitive and behavioral components (James, Reichelt, Freeston, & Barton, 2007).

The cognitive-behavioral approach integrates aspects of emotion in a manner different from that of EFT. The case of Jenna, discussed earlier in this chapter, illustrates how emotion is addressed from a cognitive-behavioral perspective.

Although the terms *cognitive* and *behavioral* may not appear to imply anything to do with emotions, affective responses are, in fact, a core component of the cognitive-behavioral approach. Cognitive-behavioral techniques have been criticized for placing insufficient emphasis on affect and emotion, causing them to be dismissed by some as superficial (Webster, 2005; Dattilio, 2005e). However, this is a common misperception and misportrayal of CBT. The theory behind CBT supports the idea that cognitions heavily influence emotion, physiological reactions, and behaviors and that a reciprocal process exists among these domains (Dattilio & Padesky, 1990). CBT is concerned with the complex and interdisciplinary relationships among thoughts, feelings, behaviors, and biophysiology. It has chosen a specific method with which to address these components in the pursuit of helping couples and family members change. The processing of emotion is viewed as crucial for survival and is as highly influential as cognitive schemas in the processing of information. In his early work, Beck (1967) proposed that individuals respond to stimuli through a combination of cognitive, affective, motivational, and behavioral responses and that each of these systems interacts with the others. Most therapists recognize the limitations of psychotherapeutic interventions, particularly with couples and families. The manner in which CBT processes affect and addresses emotion during the course of therapy is what makes it unique within the psychotherapeutic arena. Epstein and Baucom (2002) provide a detailed description of problems that involve either deficits or excesses in individuals' experiencing of emotions within the context of their intimate relationships, as well as in their expression of those feelings to their significant others. The following is a brief summary of those emotional factors in couple and family problems.

Some individuals pay little attention to their emotional states. This can result in the individuals' feeling overlooked in their close relationships. Alternatively, an individual who fails to monitor his or her emotions may suddenly express them in a destructive way, such as by abusive behavior toward his or her spouse or family members. The reasons for an individual's being unaware of emotions vary, but may include learning from experience in his or her family of origin that expressing feelings is "inappropriate" or "dangerous." Consequently, individuals may develop a fear that expressing even mild emotions will lead to losing control of their equilibrium (perhaps associated with posttraumatic stress disorder or another type of anxiety disorder), or have an expectation that their family members simply do not care how they feel (Epstein & Baucom, 2002).

In contrast, some individuals have difficulty regulating their emotions, and they experience strong levels of emotion in response to even relatively minor life events. Unregulated experiencing of emotions such as anxiety, anger, and sadness can decrease an individual's satisfaction with couple and family relationships and can contribute to the person's interacting with family members in ways that facilitate and increase conflict. Factors contributing to unregulated emotional experiences may include past personal trauma (e.g., abuse, abandonment), growing up in a family in which others failed to regulate emotional expression, and forms of psychopathology such as borderline personality disorder (Linehan, 1993).

THE CASE OF MATT AND ELIZABETH

Difficulty with regulating emotional expression was the case with Matt and Elizabeth, who sought couple counseling after Matt had an extramarital affair. This crisis brought to the surface some of the underlying issues in the couple's relationship, issues the two of them had been enduring for quite some time. Matt eventually decided to disclose his indiscretion to his wife because his guilt was so overwhelming. When Matt revealed his infidelity, he and Elizabeth experienced a brief period of what Elizabeth called a "hysterical bonding" to each other and became physically and emotionally intimate for approximately 1 week. I have found that this is not an unusual reaction for some couples who deal with a crisis by attempting to establish closeness or clinging to each other. I have seen this with many couples in similar situations during my years of practice. Despite their obvious crisis, Matt and Elizabeth informed me that they both felt that they had always had a strong intellectual bond with each other and shared the same sense of adventure. This was important and had been a strong point in the relationship in the past. This is why Matt's affair came as such a shock to Elizabeth, because she didn't understand what was missing from their relationship.

Problems in the Relationship

During the initial phases of therapy, we attempted to look at the differences contributing to some of the emotional problems in the relationship. Matt was raised in a family that was much less emotionally expressive than Elizabeth's family. Family members had to sort of account for their behaviors by explaining themselves. There was very little closeness between family members. Emotions were something that Matt simply had difficulty expressing and felt more comfortable burying. Elizabeth, however, came from a family in which she was used to expressing her emotions and having them validated. She also came from a completely different environment in which she experienced a positive attachment to her parents.

Elizabeth's crying regarding Matt's extramarital affair opened the door for Matt to express his support for her. He tried to show his support to Elizabeth the best way he could. Both had fallen into a pattern that made it difficult for them to express emotions to each other. Usually, Elizabeth became hurt and upset about something that had occurred in the relationship, perhaps something Matt had done or said in the past. She started by looking for some expression of emotion from him, but he would not show his feelings. Consequently, Elizabeth became guarded, got angry, shut down, and became resentful. When Elizabeth did this, Matt struggled with her resentment. He felt that Elizabeth "walled herself off" and became defensive, thus contributing to their alienation. Given the way he was raised, Matt interpreted this as a personal attack on him, which, in many respects, it certainly was. Elizabeth's defensiveness caused him to become defensive as well, to withdraw and go off on his own. He recalls that his family was very unemotional. "Any time there was any type of conflict at all, you would have to try to figure out what the other person was thinking and doing." He said, "People in my family just didn't communicate their emotions. It was like we were emotionally stunted."

All of this contributed to constant alienation between Matt and Elizabeth. Elizabeth said that when such alienation occurred, "we would just both go to our own safe place and wait until some time passed rather than talking to each other." I talked to Matt and Elizabeth about how this situation was analogous to the building up of plaque in the lining of a person's arteries that hardens over time and restricts blood flow, which is how most heart attacks occur. I explained to them that as this emotional gridlock in their relationship evolved over time, they alienated each other more and more until they became hardened in expressing any emotions at all. This was hypothesized as one of the reasons that Matt may have stepped outside the relationship—because he felt that he needed to connect with another person and was also angry about what was going on in his relationship with Elizabeth.

Elizabeth stated that her greatest frustration in her relationship with Matt was that she always had to point things out to him. "Nothing happens on its own," complained Elizabeth. Matt's explanation was that he couldn't deal with Elizabeth's anger, so he simply avoided it, something he was used to doing all of his life.

Much of our work together in couple therapy was to allow for the gradual exchange of emotions over several months. Interestingly, this was facilitated through the use of both cognitive and behavioral strategies. This is particularly important because Matt was more of a cognitively oriented individual, although both Matt and Elizabeth described themselves as "intellectual types." Despite the fact that Elizabeth was more emotional, a common ground was reached by focusing on behavioral interaction initially and then moving on to increased emotional exchange. Consequently, having them make some modifications in the way in which they avoided each other on simply a behavioral level allowed some leeway for us to eventually address the issues of their thoughts about change and attaching a specific emotion to it. For example, instead of the couple separating physically when things became tense, I suggested that Matt hold Elizabeth's hand in silence prior to expressing any verbal statements. This, at least, served to keep them engaged in a less threatening way.

During one of the therapy sessions, we discussed Matt's unpleasant physiological response to expressing any sensitivity at all. He feared having to put his "intellectual abilities" on hold and described himself as similar to a "deer caught in the headlights of an oncoming car." "Expressing emotion means opening up my vulnerability and puts me 'out of my element.' Without intellectual skills, I feel lost." This was clearly an issue of emotional regulation for Matt, because he tended to bottle his emotions inside and feared that if he "allowed himself to feel," his emotions would all tumble out in an "emotional cascade." He described it as an "all or nothing" situation, an aspect that I would later point out to him as being a cognitive distortion. This was particularly so in the case of expressing anger, which I hypothesized to be behind his infidelity.

Interestingly, Elizabeth responded to Matt's description by seeing it as a manipulation. "When Matt does show any emotion, it's overwhelming and he will express it in response to me expressing my emotions. If I get upset and try to express it to him, he then becomes very withdrawn and cuts me off and then it's 'all about Matt'." Matt would also attack Elizabeth by getting angry with her whenever she expressed emotion, which would cause "me to withdraw," as Elizabeth stated it. "He would then try to hurt me by ignoring me. This is what his brother would do to him when they were growing up."

Course of Treatment

Much of my work with this couple involved discussing methods for regulating their emotions on both a cognitive and an affective level and adjusting their behaviors accordingly. During one session, Elizabeth raised the issue of Matt's being unable to comfort her when she needed it. She stated, "He has no idea what to do." Matt would place his head on her shoulder, thinking that he was comforting her when, in fact, Elizabeth needed to place her head on his shoulder. Matt replied, "How can I do that when she is sitting in a single chair? She facilitates no overtures for me to do that."

Much of helping them learn to comfort each other was to almost choreograph their movements with behavioral exercises, showing them exactly what the other needed physically, as well as emotionally. It was at that point that Elizabeth raised another issue: "When this is scripted, it seems phony. Why doesn't he know what to do?" This is where cognitive restructuring entered our work, as I helped her realize that this was a distortion and that she could not expect Matt to know what to do all the time. The distortion was the belief that something must always be spontaneous in order for it to be genuine. Part of facilitating a healthy, flowing relationship is the partners' being able to let each other know what they need—even if that means structuring it as a choreographed dance. I emphasized to them that spontaneity is likely to come later, but initially it may have to be scripted until they both learn what the other needs. Part of their behavioral homework assignment was to have Matt and Elizabeth write down exactly what they needed from each other when they are being comforted. This included consistent emotional and behavioral displays, such as physically stroking each other or a smile here and there. Sometimes, nothing needed to be said verbally, but just one putting his or her arms around the other, or stroking his or her hair, was sufficient for nonverbal communication.

In addition to the way in which an individual experiences emotions, the degree and manner in which he or she expresses those emotions to others can significantly affect the quality of couple and family relationships. Whereas some individuals inhibit their expression, others express feelings in an uncensored manner. Possible factors in unregulated emotional expression include past experiences in which strong emotional displays were the only means of effectively gaining the attention of significant others or temporary relief from intense emotional tension, and limited skills for self-soothing. In our discussion, Elizabeth explained to me that Matt would sometimes get depressed and stay in bed for days. He would want Elizabeth to "nurse-maid him" and sit with him. Surprisingly, Elizabeth had never received this kind of treatment from her own parents. "My parents never nursed us, even when we were physically ill." It was a pride issue, and it was understood that you "toughed it out—so we just took care of ourselves." Matt recalled that the only time his parents took care of him was when he was sick. So he admitted to seeking comfort from Elizabeth most when he was ill. This disgusted Elizabeth because her parents were intolerant of this behavior, and she viewed it as a sign of weakness. She would become frustrated with what she saw as Matt's self-pity. Having them change this type of interaction was an objective of treatment. During the course of our sessions, we discussed alternative behaviors for Matt that were not offensive to Elizabeth. Part of a homework assignment was for Matt to try this new behavior and for Elizabeth to give him verbal feedback.

Sometimes, the inhibited individual's family members find it convenient not to have to deal with the person's feelings; in other cases, family members are frustrated by the lack of communication and they may pursue the person, which can result in a circular demand–withdraw pattern such as we saw with Matt and Elizabeth. In contrast, some family members who receive unregulated emotional expression commonly find it distressing and either respond aggressively or withdraw from the individual. If an individual's unbridled emotional expression is intended to engage others to meet his or her needs, the pattern can often backfire (Epstein & Baucom, 2002; Johnson & Denton, 2002).

Quite often, families come to treatment with a focus on their emotional concerns. Emotions are the outward expressions of inner turmoil and interpersonal conflict. Emotions may also have interesting interconnections with cognitive processes and behavior, which sometimes makes it difficult to discern what is going on with a particular individual or couple. Most people explain their bonds with their spouses or family members by virtue of how they feel toward them. In many respects, individuals often say that their emotions are what lead to a variety of thoughts and behaviors and guide their interactions through the relationship and through life in general.

Palmer and Baucom (1998) conducted a study in which they viewed the manner in which marriages lasted and the spouses' reflections on those components that contributed to couples remaining together. The authors indicated that distressed couples sought treatment because they were deeply unhappy about the absence of both positive and negative emotional responses from their partners. In essence, spouses need to see a balance of emotion from their partners.

Gottman (1999) stressed the importance of differentiating between feelings of anger and a sense of contemptuousness. Anger in an emotional exchange between spouses or family members may not be derisive, but, when added to the expression of criticism and contempt, changes into something negative. The focus here is working with these feelings that involve destructiveness because of the strong interpersonal exchange. This makes a case for the role of cognition, in that emotions that involve a negative sentiment or attitude toward one's spouse or family members may be perceived as an emotional–cognitive dynamic. It is no doubt typically the negative emotions that individuals come bearing to treatment and are usually what they cite as being the cornerstone of discontent.

Secondary to the need to identify negative emotions in relationships is the importance of determining the roots and pervasiveness of these emotions. Momentary emotions that dissipate and do not pervasively erode the course of a relationship may be differentiated from those that remain more consistent and are debilitating. For example, the anger that one family member feels for another, which is followed by ongoing contentiousness and a derisive display of behaviors, may be said to be more pronounced then the simple situational anger that one person may feel for another. In addition, the expression of certain emotions can be destructive, even if they occur infrequently, if they are associated with profound events that may be long remembered by the other person. For example, a wife who became angry with her husband for making a remark about her excessive spending of money retaliated by telling several friends at a dinner party about an incident when he was unable to perform sexually. Despite the fact that both of their angers subsided at the dinner party, the husband went on to feel humiliated in front of his friends and often brought up the issue to his wife to indicate how cruel she could be.

Positive versus Negative Moods

There has been quite a bit of research in the professional literature on the notion of "positive and negative moods," or affectivity in relationships. Some of the early studies by Watson and Tellegen (1985) address the issue of positive and negative affects as fundamental emotions that are specific to situations, as well as general tendencies over time. Schuerger, Zarrella, and Hotz (1989) further studied the stability of emotions over varying time periods, indicating that positive affectivity yields higher relationship stability than does negative affectivity. Beach and Fincham (1994) also elaborated on positive and negative affects in relationships, indicating that individuals who experienced high levels of positive affect also displayed a better sense of well-being and social dominance, as compared with those with high levels of negative affectivity. Consequently, Beach and Fincham (1994) inferred that individuals with positive affect are more responsive to situations that produce positive moods, social interaction, and sexual intimacy, than those who are higher in negative affectivity. The latter are more likely to experience anxiety, sensitivity to rejection, and sadness. To no one's surprise, affectivity clearly has a profound effect on day-to-day mood and the individual's environment. Further research has borne out this hypothesis, particularly that of researchers such as Cook et al. (1995), who found that, in a longitudinal study of marital stability, those spouses who remained together had a tendency to be more positive, less influenced by external sources, and more stable and steady, as compared with those who eventually divorced. The couples that remained together also influenced each other positively, whereas those who faced divorce influenced each other in a negative direction.

Experiencing and Expressing Emotions

During an initial couple therapy session, Gloria complained that she never knew what her husband, Gus, felt. "Sometimes it's almost like living with a stranger." When Gus was asked about his response to his wife's complaint, he said, "How can I express what I can't feel? It's as though I am emotionally void."

Before you can express an emotion, you have to experience it. This is a problem area that therapists often encounter with one or more family members during the course of treatment. Obviously, personality structures greatly affect the manner in which individuals experience and express their emotions. Some personality-disordered individuals may experience an emotion, but in a fragmented manner. Therefore, they are not specifically sure what they feel. Their experience of an emotion may take time to unfold, and when they express the emotion, they may do so over a period of time.

Anger is an emotion that is expressed in varying ways. Individuals may express anger or frustration in passive–aggressive ways, such as by spending beyond the limits they have agreed on with their partners, or even simply writing checks without recording them (causing a check to bounce because of insufficient funds) and, in this way, aggravating their partners. Others may express their anger more overtly by doing physical damage to items or screaming and displaying rage. Still others express their anger verbally, yet without physically damaging anything or injuring anyone.

The complexity that develops in couple and family relationships is often due to the responses of others to these expressions, which often serve to form a pattern of negative exchange. Many family members often adapt to a partner's or family member's patterns of emotional expression in a way that either quells or provokes conflict. It is when negative feelings, such as contempt, are expressed in a relationship interaction that a negative outcome is likely to follow. This was the profound result found in John Gottman's studies (1999), in which he determined that the single best predictor of divorce was the amount of contempt expressed as partners interacted with each other. He determined that contempt was a global sentiment that evolved over the course of a relationship and was expressed at particular moments of distress or conflict. Gottman further discovered that when individuals expressed an emotion, such as anger, immediately, they were more likely to resolve their issues than those who sustained a lingering sense of contempt for the other person. This is often why it is important, during the course of relationship therapy, to facilitate the expression of emotion by helping individuals to get in touch with their feelings and express them appropriately, rather than bottling them up only to be released later in a destructive fashion. In the case discussed earlier, involving Matt and Elizabeth, the use of cognitive and behavioral techniques to better regulate Matt's emotional expression was essential in improving their relationship. Once he learned to better regulate his anger by using cognitive self-talk and expressing it before it built up, the emotional exchange in the relationship greatly improved and reduced the couple's day-to-day tensions.

Therapeutic approaches based on attachment theory and social learning theory agree that individuals often avoid experiencing threatening or unacceptable emotions or replace them with less threatening or more acceptable ones (Kelly, 1979). Psychodynamic perspectives refer to this as a defense mechanism, which individuals use to avoid unacceptable feelings. They may even convert them to a reaction formation, which involves expressing the opposite of what they really feel. Johnson and Greenberg (1988) suggest that expressing emotions can be a major way to regulate attachment and a related sense of security, such as closeness and intimacy. Hence, a partner may express tender emotions of caring and warmth to his or her spouse or family member as a way of eliciting greater intimacy and security from the other person. Obviously, if this is met with rejection, secondary or reactionary emotions, such as anger, rejection, and dissatisfaction, may emerge. This may be used to guilt-trip the other into responding positively or serve as a means of chastisement and expressing injury. Often, difficulties arise when one individual in a relationship is comfortable with less emotional expression than the other, which obviously can create some distance in the relationship.

Thoughts and Beliefs about Emotional Expression

One of the hallmarks of the cognitive-behavioral approach to working with relationships involves cognitions about the expression of emotion. CBT posits that individuals maintain different thoughts and beliefs about experiencing and expressing their emotions, which govern the manner in which their emotional display unfolds.

There is considerable debate in the professional literature as to whether emotions affect cognition more than cognitions affect emotion. As discussed earlier, the emotionally focused theorists, such as Johnson and Greenberg (1988), have proposed that emotions are at the root of what individuals experience and that they may tend to develop cognitions secondary to these emotions. Cognitive-behavioral therapists, however, place more credence in the notion that individuals develop beliefs that lead to the experience of certain emotions and, particularly, how they express them. It is not uncommon for women to feel more comfortable than men about expressing their emotions and the importance they place on them (Brizendine, 2006). Hence, the beliefs about how one should express emotions are very important in relationships. Secondary to this is the issue of whether certain individuals lack the adequate skill to express those emotions, particularly if they haven't expressed them in the past. Being unable to be in touch with their emotions, with what they are experiencing at the moment, and incorporate these internal sensations into an external display may be a serious handicap for some men.

Difficulty in expressing emotions in a modulated fashion with appropriate levels of intensity and display may also be an area in which many people have difficulty. This is often observed in individuals who display an unwillingness to regulate their emotional expression, particularly when they feel angry and justified in being angry. Many feel that if they don't vent their emotions in a forceful or direct manner, they may become ill by holding them in.

Epstein and Baucom (2002) discussed how individuals in distressed relationships may have poor emotional regulation without any personality disorder, particularly because they appear to experience anger in dichotomous terms. That is, they may feel the need to display their emotions, such as anger, in an "all-or-nothing" fashion. Hence, addressing emotional regulation may be critical. The professional literature is quite lean in regard to research on emotional regulation in distressed relationships, but there has been some material written on strategies for addressing emotional regulation (Heyman & Neidig, 1997).

As mentioned previously, emotions are viewed by most theorists as being integrally related to cognitions and behaviors. To assume that cognition and behavior do not accompany emotion would be naive. Logical thinking implies that they influence each other mutually. So the real question is, what is the best way to intervene? In practice, interventions can probably start with either feelings or cognitions, but therapists who concentrate on feelings should also remember to address cognitions, and vice versa. Albert Ellis (1982) first suggested that people generally act after cognitive processing occurs. It is on the basis of such cognitions that an individual responds emotionally. Yet other theorists have purported that various mood states are related to different styles of information processing (Bless & Bohner, 1991; Bless, Hamilton, & Mackie, 1992; Johnson & Greenberg, 1988). Hence, it is perceived that when individuals are in a negative mood they are likely to engage in more cognitive introspection. Research has indicated that negative emotions, such as brooding, may clearly initiate cognitive processing and that negative moods, pessimism, and the like, lead to a state of mind that may be consuming, such as in a spouse who is always looking on the dark side and maintaining a "doom and gloom" attitude (Gottman, 1994).

Gottman (1994) found that a negative mood initiates negative cognitive processing, which then leads to selective re-attending to negative events. From this selective re-attending, negative attributions develop and lead to negative expectancies for the future. Beck described this as a *negative frame*, which renders individuals vulnerable to viewing a situation in a biased light. Research suggests that negative mood seems to result in more focused and detailed cognitive processing (Epstein & Baucom, 2002). These researchers found that mood has a tendency to influence memory by biasing interpretations and recall of stored memories of negative situations or negative events. The cycle of gridlock that many couples and families enter when emotionally distressed may make them prone to recall negative memories about interactions as opposed to positive ones with each other.

A good example of this occurs when I ask couples to use one-word adjectives to describe their discontent with their partners. Later, when asked to use one-word adjectives to describe what attracted them to each other, the words may often be the inverse of the words used to describe what was troubling them about their partners.

THE CASE OF JEFF AND MARGE

When Jeff was asked to describe in one-word adjectives what irritated him about his wife, Marge, he listed the following: *frivolous, superficial, irresponsible, impulsive, emotional,* and *flighty.* Later, he listed the following one-word adjectives as describing what attracted him to Marge: *wonder-*

ful, charming, carefree, spontaneous, lively, and *playful.* When these were aligned, the following lists appeared:

IRRITATING QUALITIES	ATTRACTIVE QUALITIES
Frivolous	Wonderful
Superficial	Charming
Irresponsible	Carefree
Impulsive	Spontaneous
Emotional	Lively
Flighty	Playful

When Jeff saw how these descriptive adjectives lined up, he admitted that some of them in the first list may have been the same qualities in the second list, but were being viewed in a different light because of his mood and perception at the time. Jeff, like many members of couples, was stuck in a negative frame. His view of Marge had become affected by his negative frame of mind. Thus, what he once perceived to be appealing qualities of his partner were now distasteful.

Emotional states have a profound effect on relationships. There is no doubt that emotions are a critical part of family relationships and often set the tone for daily interactions. It is important, however, that family members maintain a balance between positive and negative emotional exchanges at various levels so that there is little bias in one direction or the other. A major focus of the cognitive-behavioral approach is monitoring the way in which family members behave in response to negative emotional exchanges. In the text *Enhanced Cognitive-Behavior Therapy for Couples,* Epstein and Baucom (2002) provide a detailed summary that delineates various cognitive and emotional factors that help to color an individual's experience of his or her intimate relationships. In their summary, the authors clearly outline the important interplay between cognitions and emotions (pp. 103–104).

Difficulty in Adapting to Life Demands Involving Individuals, Relationship Issues, or the Environment

The enhanced cognitive-behavioral approach to families integrates aspects of family stress and coping theory (e.g., McCubbin & McCubbin, 1989) with traditional cognitive-behavioral principles. Families are faced with a variety of demands to which they must adapt, and the quality of their coping efforts is likely to affect the satisfaction and stability of their relationships.

Demands on a couple or family may derive from three major sources: (1) characteristics of the individual members (e.g., a family has to cope with a member's depression), (2) relationship dynamics (e.g., the members of a couple have to resolve or adapt to differences in the two partners' needs, as when one is achievement- and career-oriented and the other focuses on togetherness and intimacy), and (3) characteristics of the interpersonal environment (e.g., needy relatives, a demanding boss) and physical environment (e.g., neighborhood violence or rural isolation). Cognitive-behavioral therapists assess the number, severity, and cumulative impact of various demands that a couple or a family is experiencing, as well as its available resources and skills for coping with those demands. Consistent with a stress and coping model, the risk of couple or family dysfunction increases with the degree of demands and deficits in resources. The family members' perceptions of demands and their ability to cope also play a prominent role in the stress and coping model. Therapists' skills in assessing and modifying distorted or inappropriate cognition can be very helpful in improving families' coping skills.

THE ROLE OF BEHAVIORAL CHANGE

Social Exchange Theory

Social exchange theory has always been an important component of cognitive-behavioral treatment of families. Most empirically based couple therapies have their foundations in behavioral couple therapy, which focuses on directly changing behavior by maximizing positive exchanges and minimizing negative exchanges (Jacobson & Margolin, 1979; Weiss et al., 1973). This concept is particularly important inasmuch as most unhappy couples report higher daily frequencies of negative events than of positive events (Johnson & O'Leary, 1996).

Social exchange theory centers on the costs and benefits associated with relationships. It emphasizes that there is technically a downside to particular social conditions, such as being married or single, and there are moments when the downside may predominate in the mind of an individual, causing him or her to view the social condition with regret. Social exchange theory was first conceived by Homens (1961) and later elaborated on by Thibaut and Kelley (1959). Thibaut and Kelley applied the concept of social exchange to the dynamics of intimate relationships, in which they identified patterns of interdependency. Social exchange theory is based on economic theories and views couple interaction through the lens of an exchange of costs and rewards. Simply stated, costs are reasons why a relationship would be considered undesirable, whereas rewards pertain to reasons that partners would remain in a relationship. If you think about your own spousal relationship, you may discover many costs and rewards.

Some costs may be your spouse's bad habits, such as excessive spending of money or his or her temperament. However, these costs may be strongly outweighed by the rewards, which may consist of the spouse's kindness, sensitivity, and his or her constant loyalty and support. It is the balance of costs and rewards that often helps couples to determine whether or not they are satisfied in a relationship.

The same holds true for family members. Siblings are likely to be courteous to one another if they perceive that the same level of courtesy will be extended to them. Give and take is often what quells family conflict and can restore balance in familial interactions.

The general notion of a cost–benefit ratio serves a number of significant purposes. The level of satisfaction within a marital or couple relationship and the commitment to remain together or to separate may be viewed in the context of perceived rewards relative to the costs.[1]

A main concept of social exchange theory is the tendency of individuals to compare the rewards they are receiving with the perceived alternatives. Such a comparison is a complex process involving interrelated cognitive phenomena, which include perception, labeling, and expectation. Consequently, a woman whose husband was disloyal to her may think, "He's only done this one time and it won't likely happen again." Consequently, she weighs the "cost" of living with the injury (memory of the betrayal) against the cost of living without her husband and concludes that the former outweighs the latter. The reward of such thinking may be the means of avoiding the possible outcome of a separation.

A spouse's expectation of appropriate, desirable, and acceptable behavior forms the standard against which his or her partner's behavior is measured. Such expectations derive from the individual's sense of self, personal value system, and past social experiences. Someone with low self-regard may evaluate his or her spouse's behavior as appropriate, desirable, and acceptable, whereas an individual with higher self-regard may view the same behavior as the opposite. Failure to share major financial decisions may be of little consequence for the individual who does not value that behavior. Spouses' expectations of one another has also been an important variable in the determination of comparison levels when analyzing marital satisfaction (Baucom & Epstein, 1990).

A key component of interdependence is the degree to which a spouse seeks rewards within the relationship rather than independently or outside the union. The coordination of a couple's efforts to contribute to each other's objectives depends on the extent to which they seek to satisfy each

---

[1] In the case of family members, it may be slightly different, because they don't always have a choice as to whether they want to remain together. Because family members are born into their families of origin and don't choose their relatives, their situations present few options.

other's needs and objectives within the relationship. Even though a couple may function with a significant level of interdependence, one or both partners may desire to have some outcomes met independently, or outside the marriage.

Kelly (1979) indicated that there will likely be ongoing shifts in couples' interdependence over time, in terms of how and to what extent they seek satisfaction of their goals and needs in the relationship. There can be a potential conflict in regard to several aspects, which the author outlined as follows:

1. *Mutuality of dependence*—are the spouses mutually interdependent in an outcome area, or is one spouse unilaterally dependent?
2. *Degree of dependence*—the higher the dependence, the greater the intensity.
3. *Correspondence of outcome*—does the outcome an individual desires depend on his or her own options, the spouse's options, or a combination of the two?

Kelly (1979) also stressed what he called the *comparison level for alternatives*. Distressed spouses perceive the rewards and costs of a single life, and of life with another partner, and weigh them against the rewards and costs of staying in their current relationships. A spouse may perceive that getting a divorce may result in severe economic hardship. Or the person may strongly believe that divorce is morally wrong. In both instances, the person may perceive the costs of the alternative to marriage to be too high, even though the rewards of staying in the marriage may be very low.

Individuals compare the cost–benefit ratios of the options before them. The rewards to the cost of staying in a relationship are evaluated against the alternatives outside the relationship, with a net result promoting a greater or lesser commitment to the relationship. This may in part explain why a spouse would remain in a relationship in which he or she repeatedly experiences physical abuse or infidelity, such as with the case of Wilma, described in the previous chapter. According to the social exchange theory, one may determine that a client is highly dependent on his or her mate, resulting in high tolerance for low rewards in the union. Coupled with this condition, he or she may have a strong view that marital relationships should be maintained at all costs, anticipate great economic hardship after divorce, sense the emotional insecurity of living alone, and consider divorce as destroying his or her family and affecting the children. In essence, the extreme dependence and concomitant expectancy in a relationship, in conjunction with the high cost of leaving (compared to the alternatives), incline a spouse to remain in the relationship despite how unfulfilling or psychologically damaging it may be.

Reciprocity in Relationships

There are two senses in which reciprocity is used in family therapy. The idea stressed by behaviorists, as well as by folk wisdom, is that if you give more, you'll get more—*quid pro quo* (Latin for "this for that"). The other sense, proposed by the systems theorists, is that in a relationship, one family member's behavior is partly a function of the others' (Minuchin & Nichols, 1998 [cited in Dattilio, 1998a]).

The extent to which spouses exercise reciprocity in their exchanges of rewarding and unrewarding behaviors is based in part on the social exchange theory and has received a great deal of attention in the professional literature.

Neil Jacobson and his associates have found that both rewarding and punishing relationship events tend to have an immediate impact on distressed couples (Jacobson, Follette, & McDonald, 1982). In contrast, nondistressed couples appear to possess a nonreactive quality in relation to negative behavior; in such couples, punishing behaviors are absorbed without response. This failure to immediately reciprocate prevents the couple from escalating into a chain of intense negative exchanges. For example, Mary witnessed her husband's failure to take out the trash because he was angry at her, but decided to let it slide rather than respond. Her behavior (i.e., not responding) may have had a positive effect on her husband, who noticed that Mary allowed this behavior to slide without making a comment, and changed his thinking about her jumping on him at every opportunity. Such a nonreactive quality is likely the product of an ongoing high rate of positive exchanges between nondistressed partners. Of course, it is important for spouses to monitor their cognitions about always engaging in such behavior, in order to avoid storing resentment that may be expressed later in a destructive fashion (i.e., passive–aggressive behaviors). John Gottman has described a "bank account" model of marital exchange in which the positive investments made over time sustain the couple through situational nonreciprocity (Gottman, Notarius, Gonso, & Markman, 1976). In essence, negative behaviors, rather than being exchanged, are not reciprocated, presumably as a function of the accumulation of the positive behavioral exchanges. These results serve as a foundation of encouraging couples to increase their rate of positive exchange while decreasing negative behavioral exchange.

The social exchange model has become one of the hallmarks of behavioral marital therapy and has been used with tremendous success. Epstein and Baucom (2002) have suggested that the social exchange model may work optimally when therapists take into account the various rates of behavioral exchange that occur between spouses. Each spouse's subjective appraisal of how desirable or pleasant the partner's behaviors are is important. Each spouse's standard for what constitutes an equitable exchange is vital, along with the attributions about why a partner may never agree to concede during the course of exchange in the relationship. In addition, spouses' expectancies about future exchanges may serve to set the tone for interaction down the road.

Micro-Level versus Macro-Level Interactions in Relationship Exchange

Epstein and Baucom (2002) provide an elaborate chapter that focuses on the micro-level behaviors that occur in a couple's interaction and broader macro-level patterns. In brief, micro-level behavior occurs in specific situations, whereas macro-level behavior involves broader patterns across a number of situations.

The authors' theory of relationship exchange emphasizes the need to focus on couples' macro-level interactions, such as one partner's attempting to maintain power in the couple's relationship. Traditionally, in cognitive-behavioral approaches to couple therapy, the focus has been on micro-level behaviors—that is, the spouses' idiosyncratic appraisals of each other's behavior and how they influence pleasing and displeasing actions (i.e., the degree of togetherness versus autonomy between members of a couple, or degree of intimacy). Specific focus centers on the attributions spouses make about their own behaviors, as well as their spouses' behaviors, and the various interpretations of these interactions made by each.

But recently, more attention has been given to the notion that macro-level behaviors are also significant to a couple's relationship. Systems theorists traditionally understand a couple's relationship as actually a very small social system that is embedded in layers of larger systems (Nichols & Schwartz, 2008). Larger systems, which include the nuclear family, the extended family, neighborhoods, and larger community systems, profoundly influence a couple's relationship. Epstein and Baucom (2002) purport that larger systems may have both positive and negative effects on individual and conjoint needs. In essence, the couple's or family's environment places demands and stresses on its relationships, but also provides positive resources that support them. Therefore, an emphasis is placed on the importance of identifying macro-level behavioral patterns that affect relationships and can be used as guides for identifying specific micro-level behavioral changes that are most likely to enhance relationships.

The following sections discuss some of the micro-level behavioral patterns that can meet individual and communally oriented needs.

Rituals

Rituals are behaviors that hold some valid meaning that a couple or family repeats on a regular basis. For example, Jack and Lupe regularly dine at a little restaurant where they had their first date. This is symbolic in the sense that they recall the emotions that revolved around their budding relationship. They have also developed social relationships with the owners and other patrons that reinforce their position in the community and their status as a happy couple.

Boundary-Defining Behaviors

Couples and families vary in the balance they strike between shared and autonomous behaviors. For example, Helen enjoys her pottery classes one night per week, in which she has developed her own social network; whereas Toby plays poker with his buddies, with whom Helen does not interact regularly. These interactions outside the marriage and the family provide Helen and Toby with outlets for extending their reach as individuals. One of the benefits of this type of outlet is that it helps the individuals to define themselves as a couple socially yet function cohesively among other couples.

Social Support Behaviors and Exchange

Some couples donate their time together for a charity drive, and others team up with other couples who work together for a common purpose. Aside from the gratification derived from doing something good for society, they also share the benefit of social interaction and support.

One of the strengths of identifying micro-level patterns of behavior is that they indicate how spouses address their communal needs, which inadvertently reflects on their individual needs. For example, the spouses above who donate their time to a charity may experience both a sense of fulfillment in the relationship by working together for a good cause and individual satisfaction by giving back to their environment.

3

The Schema Component in Cognitive-Behavioral Therapy

THE CONCEPT OF SCHEMA

The term *schema* has its origin in the Greek root word *scheen* (σχηπα), which means "to have" or "to shape." Additional definitions include "a mental codification of experiences that include a particular organized way of perceiving cognitively and responding to a complex situation or set of stimuli" (Webster's dictionary, 1989). The term *schema* also has various meanings that pertain to a host of other fields (see Young, Klosko, & Weishaar, 2003, for an elaborated explanation).

Aaron Beck suggested that schemas play a central role in accounting for the repetitive themes in free associations, images, and dreams, believing that they may actually be inactive at times, only later to be energized, or deenergized, rapidly as a result of changes in the type of input from the environment (1967, p. 284). In his early work, Beck portrayed a somewhat unrefined concept of the notion of schema that he later went on to expand in subsequent writings (Beck et al., 1979).

Other theorists later expanded on the original concept of schema. For example, Segal (1988) wrote that schemas involve "organized elements of past reactions and experience that form a relatively cohesive and persistent body of knowledge capable of guiding subsequent perception and appraisals" (p. 147). Young (1990) broadened this concept when he introduced his application of a schema-focused approach to personality disorders. Young went on to propose that "although Beck and his associates (1979, p. 304) refer to the importance of schemas in treatment, they have offered very few specific treatment guidelines within their treatment protocols to date" (Young, 1990, p. 9). For this reason, Young went on to expand Beck's model of schema and suggested a four-level theory, which involves (1) early maladaptive schemas, (2) schema maintenance, (3) schema avoidance, and (4) schema compensation. This concept was applied specifically to personality disorders, which was further developed by Young and colleagues in a popular text titled *Schema Therapy: A Practitioners Guide* (Young, Klosko, & Weishaar, 2003). In fact, Young is credited with developing what is referred to in the contemporary literature as *schema therapy* (1990, 1999), which serves as a significant extension of traditional cognitive-behavioral treatments and concepts. Schema therapy, according to Young, blends elements from cognitive-behavioral, attachment, gestalt, object relations, constructivist, and psychoanalytic schools of thought into a rich, unifying conceptual treatment model (Young et al., 2003). However, Young's model is primarily designed as a system of psychotherapy suited for individuals with entrenched chronic psychological disturbances, namely, personality disorders. Whereas it might be said that traditional CBT is quite effective with Axis I disorders (i.e., mood disorders, anxiety, eating disorders, substance abuse, etc.), schema therapy demonstrates more effectiveness with the personality disorders listed in Axis II (Young et al., 2003). In the area of couple and family therapy, however, the focus falls somewhere between CBT and the systems approach owing to the intergenerational nature of relationships.

Although schema-focused therapy with couples and families does involve some attention to individual schemas of self, there is a greater emphasis on the relationship system and the schemas that develop specifically around the self within the relationship. It also explores and makes use of family-of-origin and early life experiences of individual partners and family members.

Young developed schema therapy primarily to treat individuals with chronic characterlogical problems (Young et al., 2003, p. 5). However, nowhere in any of Young's works are there any detailed applications of schema therapy in treating couples or families. Although Young does mention that schema therapy can be used successfully with couples, only recently has some application of schema therapy been addressed in regard to couples and families (Dattilio, 2005b, 2006b).

As applied to couples and families, schema therapy addresses the core themes that reflect the relationship dynamics. By addressing these themes in an analytic and structured fashion, schema therapy helps patients to make sense of conflict, marital gridlock, and dysfunctional interaction patterns that contribute to relationship problems. The use of education and direct confrontation helps couples and family members to become aware of their thinking and behavior and to take effective action toward changing them.

The therapist also works as an agent to identify enabling factors in the spouses or family members that may be serving to keep these behaviors and patterns alive.

As mentioned previously, the concept of schema was initially introduced in the cognitive therapy literature several decades ago in Aaron T. Beck's early work with depressed individuals (Beck, 1967). Beck's theory related primarily to depressed individuals' basic negative beliefs about themselves, their world, and their future. Beck's work drew from earlier cognitive theories in developmental psychology, such as Piaget's discussion of accommodation and assimilation in schema formation (Piaget, 1950). The work of George Kelly regarding cognitive constructs also served to shape Beck's theory of schema (Kelly, 1955), as well as Bowlby's attachment theory (1969). The concept of schema has since become the cornerstone of contemporary cognitive-behavioral therapy. Much as the cardiovascular system is central to the functioning of the human body, Beck proposed that schemas are central to a person's thoughts and perceptions and have an integral influence on emotions and behavior. In essence, schemas are used as a template for an individual's life experiences, as well as how he or she processes information. In addition to Beck, many other researchers and clinicians have done a significant amount of work in the area of schemas and their effect on interpersonal relationships (Baldwin, 1992; Epstein & Baucom, 2002; Epstein & Baucom, 1993; Epstein, Baucom, & Rankin, 1993; Epstein & Baucom, 2003; Dattilio, 1993, 1998a, 2001b, 2002, 2005b, 2006b).

Consistent with systems theory, the cognitive-behavioral approach to families is based on the premise that members of a family simultaneously influence, and are influenced by, each other's thoughts, emotions, and behavior (Dattilio, 2001a; Leslie, 1988). In essence, to know the entire family system is to become familiar with individual parts and how they interact. As each family member observes his or her own cognitions, behavior, and emotions, as well as cues from the responses of other family members, he or she forms assumptions about family dynamics, which then develop into relatively stable schemas or *cognitive structures*. These cognitions, emotions, and behaviors may elicit responses from some members that constitute much of the moment-to-moment interaction with other family members. This interplay stems from the more stable schemas that serve as the foundation for the family's functioning (Dattilio, Epstein, & Baucom, 1998). In other words, the deep cognitive structures that organize precepts exert a powerful influence on how family members interact and, even more important, how they interpret their interactions. When this cycle involves negative content that affects cognitive, emotional, and behavioral responses, the volatility of the family's dynamics tends to escalate, rendering family members vulnerable to a negative spiral of conflict. As the number of family members increases, so does the complexity of the dynamics, adding more fuel and intensity to the escalation process.

Unfortunately, to date, there has been very little empirical research to support this theory of escalation that involves cognitive, emotional, and behavioral components specifically within families. Although the theories of Gerald Patterson and his associates (Patterson & Forgatch, 1985; Forgatch & Patterson, 1998; Patterson & Hops, 1972) has contributed significantly to improving family interaction, these studies focus only on behavioral interventions, giving little or no attention to cognitive processes. The major focus on behavior has extended primarily to research on behavioral family therapy. In contrast, significant research on cognitions has been conducted with couples (Epstein & Baucom, 2002).[1]

Because the dynamics of a couple are so closely aligned with family dynamics, many of the theoretical components in models of couple interaction can also be applied to families and have been described in detail in the professional literature (Dattilio, 1993, 2004a; Epstein et al., 1988; Schwebel & Fine, 1992, 1994). Family members' perceptions of family interactions provide the information that shapes the development of their family schemas, especially when an individual member observes such interaction repeatedly. The pattern that the individual deduces from such observations serves as a basis to form a schema or template that subsequently is used to understand the world of family relationships and to anticipate future events within the family. Family schemas are a subset of a broad range of schemas that individuals develop about many aspects of life experiences.

AUTOMATIC THOUGHTS AND SCHEMAS

Automatic thoughts are another key form of cognition in cognitive-behavioral theory that is sometimes confused with schemas, particularly because there is some overlap between the two. Automatic thoughts were first defined by Beck (1976) as spontaneous cognitions that often occur in a fleeting manner and are mostly conscious and easily accessible. Thus, conscious automatic thoughts provide a pathway to uncover one's underlying beliefs or schemas. So, for example, a mother who has difficulty tolerating expressions of negative emotion by family members might experience the automatic thought, "There's no room for weakness in life," stemming from an underlying belief or schema that a show of weakness can lead to vulnerability. Sometimes cognitions can also occur beyond an individual's conscious

---

[1]Elsewhere, Dattilio (2004) outlines potential reasons why more empirical process research has not been conducted with families.

awareness. Broad underlying schemas are commonly revealed through an individual's automatic thoughts, but not all automatic thoughts are expressions of schemas. For example, many automatic thoughts express an individual's attributions about causes of events that he or she has observed (e.g., "My son didn't call me because his wife and children are much more important to him than I am").

Cognitive therapy, as originally introduced by Beck (1976), places a heavy emphasis on schemas (Beck et al., 1979; DeRubeis & Beck, 1988). Several authors have proposed different versions of schema theory to account for the processing of information in a person's life's life. Most of the theoretical perspectives hold that individuals develop such knowledge structures through interactions with their environment. Epstein et al. (1988) refer to an individual's schemas as "the longstanding and relatively stable basic assumptions that he or she holds about how the world works and his or her place in it" (p. 13). These assumptions about commonly occurring characteristics and processes serve an adaptive function by organizing the individual's experience into meaningful patterns and reducing the complexity of the environment. By selectively limiting, guiding, and organizing the information that an individual has available, his or her schemas make efficient thinking and action possible.

However, in spite of these advantages, schemas have also been found to account for errors, distortions, and omissions that people make in processing information (Baldwin, 1992; Baucom et al., 1989; Epstein, Baucom, & Rankin, 1993). For example, if a child is given love and attention from parents only when he or she exhibits certain desired behaviors, then the child is likely to develop a schema that "love and attention are conditional." The more that belief is reinforced in the environment, the more likely it is to become ingrained, and the more the child may be expected to give and receive love on a conditional basis in any close relationship. The individual may apply this schema to other relationships later in life, such as his or her marital relationship and relationships with offspring. Thus, parent–child relationships are influenced by the relatively long-standing schemas that the parents bring to the family and by each child's schemas that develop on the basis of current family interactions.

Consequently, schemas are very important in the application of CBT with families. They are the long-standing beliefs that people hold about others and their relationships. Schemas are stable cognitive structures, not a fleeting inferences or perceptions. They are differentiated from perceptions (what one notices or overlooks in the environment) and from inferences (attributions and expectancies) that a person draws from the events that he or she notices. Dealing with individual family members' thoughts is central to cognitive-behavioral family therapy (CBFT). Although cognitive-behavioral theory does not suggest that cognitive processes cause all family behavior, it does stress that cognitive appraisal significantly influences family members' behavioral interactions and emotional responses to each other (Epstein et al., 1988; Wright & Beck, 1993). Just as individuals maintain their own basic schemas about themselves, their world, and their future, they also develop schemas about characteristics of their family of origin, which are commonly generalized to some degree to conceptions about other close relationships. Elsewhere, I have suggested that greater emphasis should be placed on examining not only cognitions of individual family members, but also what may be termed the *family schema*—those jointly held beliefs among the family members that have formed as a result of years of integrated interaction within the family unit (Dattilio, 1993).

Although family schemas typically constitute jointly held beliefs about mostly family phenomena, such as day-to-day dilemmas and interactions, they may also pertain to nonfamily phenomena as well, such as cultural, political, or spiritual issues. Most family schemas are shared. Sometimes, however, individual family members deviate from the joint schema.

Individuals maintain two separate sets of schemas about families: (1) a family schema related to the parents' experiences in their families of origin and (2) schemas related to families in general, or what Schwebel and Fine (1994) refer to as a personal theory of family life. As noted previously, each person's experiences and perceptions derived from his or her family of origin contribute to forming part of his or her schema about the current family. This schema is also altered by events that occur in the current family relationships. For example, a man who was raised with the belief that family problems should never be discussed with anyone outside the immediate household is likely to become uncomfortable if his wife shares personal business with some of her family. The issue may be particularly salient if he marries a woman who was raised with the idea that it is OK to share personal business with close friends. Such a difference in outlooks may cause conflict, which may in turn affect the schemas of their children and their beliefs about sharing family business with others. For example, if a man maintains an ingrained schema "a wife should maintain a passive role in the marital relationship," then, when his wife disagrees with him, he is likely to make the negative attribution "She is trying to dominate the relationship." This schema may have developed over the course of his life from previous experiences and now shapes his moment-to-moment thoughts. Consequently, as his children are exposed to such beliefs and interactions between him and his wife, they develop their own beliefs about men and women and relationships, which are strongly influenced by what they were exposed to during their upbringing, as portrayed in Figure 3.1.

Elsewhere, it has been suggested that the family of origin of each partner in a relationship plays a crucial role in the shaping of the current shared family schema (Dattilio, 1993, 1998b, 2001b). The beliefs developed in

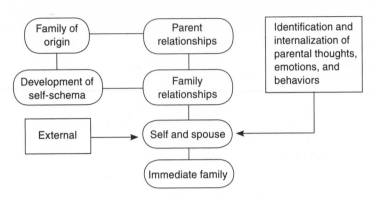

FIGURE 3.1. Schemas in couple and family relationships.

each person's family of origin may be either conscious or beyond awareness, and whether or not they are explicitly expressed, they contribute to the joint family schema. A more detailed example of this process of family schema development is shown in Figure 3.2.

UNDERLYING SCHEMAS
AND COGNITIVE DISTORTIONS

As outlined in Chapters 1 and 2, Baucom et al. (1989) developed a typology of cognitions implicated in relationship distress. Although all of these human cognitions are considered normal, all are susceptible to being distorted (Baucom & Epstein, 1990; Epstein & Baucom, 2002).

Because there is so much information available in any interpersonal situation, some degree of selective attention is inevitable. However, the potential for couples to form biased perceptions of each other must be examined. Inferences involved in attributions and expectancies are also normal aspects of the human information processing involved in understanding other people's behavior and making predictions about others' future behavior. However, errors in these inferences can have negative effects on relationships, especially when an individual attributes another's actions to negative characteristics (e.g., malicious intent) or misjudges how others will react to his or her own actions. Assumptions are adaptive when they are realistic representations of people and relationships. Many standards that individuals hold, such as moral standards about not abusing others, contribute to the quality of couples' relationships. Nevertheless, inaccurate or extreme assumptions and standards can lead individuals to interact inappropriately with others, as when a parent holds the standard that the opinions and feel-

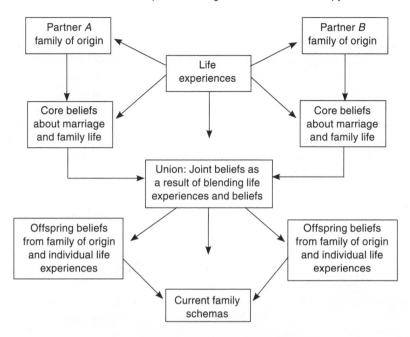

FIGURE 3.2. Development of family schema.

ings of children and adolescents are not to be taken into account as long as they live in the parent's home.

Schemas about relationships are often not articulated clearly in an individual's mind, but exist as vague concepts of what is or should be (Beck, 1988; Epstein & Baucom, 2002). Previously developed schemas influence the way an individual subsequently processes information in new situations. For example, they influence what the person selectively perceives, the inferences he or she makes about causes of others' behavior, and whether the person is pleased or displeased with the relationship. Existing schemas may be difficult to modify, but repeated new experiences with significant others have the potential to change them (Epstein & Baucom, 2002; Johnson & Denton, 2002).

IDENTIFYING SCHEMAS FROM THE FAMILY
OF ORIGIN AND THEIR IMPACT
ON COUPLE AND FAMILY RELATIONSHIPS

Dealing with each partner's individual thoughts is central to working with couples in therapy. Just as individuals maintain their own basic schemas about themselves (self-concept), their world, and their future, they also develop schemas about characteristics of close relationships in general, as well as their own relationships in particular. Ignoring or failing to give adequate attention to underlying schemas can be a grave clinical error. For example, when a therapist failed to take into consideration Sharron's vulnerability schemas about making mistakes and risking failure, he created a major problem when he assigned a homework task to her and her husband in which she was asked to assume the initiative. The homework assignment was too overwhelming to her because she feared failing. The intervention backfired, and Sharron refused to return to therapy.

Schemas are often at the heart of couple and family conflicts (Dattilio, 2005a). It is for this reason that schemas should be addressed during the early phase of treatment, while assessment is still ongoing.

One of the guidelines used for assessing a schema from a family of origin is Richard Stuart's *Family of Origin Inventory* (1995). Stuart's detailed and comprehensive inventory allows spouses to describe how their respective families of origin's experiences influence their lives, marriages, and families. From the information collected in this inventory, the therapist can tailor specific questions for uncovering important schemas regarding couple and family relationships.

Often during the course of couple therapy, rigid schemas held by one or both spouses surface and interfere with progress in modifying negative interaction patterns within the relationship. Although some of these schemas have their origin in experiences that occurred during the course of the present relationship, others are drawn from experiences in prior relationships. For example, a man may hold the belief that his wife tends to cry easily during arguments and therefore anticipates that she will do this each time their arguments become heated. This expectation aligns with his more ingrained global schemas about characteristics of women and emotions in general, based on his previous romantic relationships or what he has learned about women during the course of his life.

Other schemas, however, may be ingrained because they are deeply rooted in experiences from one's family of origin, and these schemas pose a significant challenge in treatment. They are likely to be culturally based and imposed early in one's formative years, making them more resistant to change. Belief systems that hail from one's family of origin usually have been strongly and consistently reinforced and have been internalized during key formative period of life (Dattilio, 2005b, 2006c).

KEEPING THE PEACE: THE CASE OF DAN AND MARIA

Consider the case of Dan, Maria, and their young son, Josh, whose family situation was significantly affected by Dan's experiences during his upbringing, which served to form his schema about arguments. Dan's parents fought constantly, and their battles resulted in Dan's mother leaving the home twice, abandoning him and his father without notice. As a result, Dan developed a deep fear of abandonment and difficulties with attachment. He recalls that his mother left at two critical times in his life, once when he was 12 and later when he was 16. She left the home for good the second time and rarely returned to visit him or his father. As a result, Dan developed feelings of anger and inadequacy and feared rejection and abandonment. In fact, his mother took everything from the house except him and his father. His mother never apologized for her abrupt departure or anything she had done. This left Dan feeling as though he must have done something bad to deserve such abandonment.

What's more important, Dan developed a schema that fighting and arguing leads to separation and divorce, and so one must "do whatever you have to in order to keep the peace." For Dan, this included hiding his feelings and not showing any anger for fear of a negative result. Hiding his feelings created a great deal of difficulty for Dan in his relationship with his wife. Eventually, his emotions would build up inside him and be expressed in an angry outburst. On several occasions, Dan lost control of himself and acted out physically against his wife. She left him and took their son, Josh, with her. Dan recalls feeling that he was not able to express himself until he became overwhelmed and lost his composure. His wife's departure conjured up Dan's childhood feelings of abandonment. This time, both his wife and son were gone.

Unfortunately, this schema was passed on to Josh, who also felt that he needed to be a peacemaker and couldn't express his anger about conflicts in the family. Josh rarely expressed his feelings, which affected his relationships with girlfriends as he grew into adolescence and started dating.

Much of my work with this family focused on Dan's rigid schema that "arguing leads to divorce." I attempted to help him become more assertive and to express his feelings in a more modulated fashion. For example, I had him begin by expressing some of his negative emotions to his wife, Maria. I took the liberty of coaching Maria to be supportive and be a good listener to Dan. This helped to desensitize Dan's fears of rejection and abandonment to a great extent. It also involved teaching him communication skills, as well as developing the concept that there are such things as "good debates and healthy arguing" and that not all arguing and disagreements lead to separation and divorce. This psychoeducational component was conducted in the presence of their son, Josh, so that he could observe his father's transformation.

Schemas from Dan's family of origin had been passed down and had contributed to the erosion of a present relationship. Cognitive-behavioral techniques that involve specific communication skills, assertiveness training, and behavioral exercises, and that address issues of attachment, were vital in helping Dan to change the course of his relationship with his wife, as well as the future of his son's potential relationships with others. It was also important for Dan to make a conscious effort to restructure his schemas about disagreement and abandonment. This involved some cognitive rehearsal in which he would reassure himself that it was OK to have disagreements and that they don't always lead to catastrophic outcomes. Because his son looked up to him, it was important that Dan address these issues, not only for himself and his wife, but for his son as well, and that the entire family be incorporated into the change process.

Parents and other primary caretakers have a powerful influence on the development of children's belief systems, particularly when beliefs are conveyed in the context of strong cultural underpinnings. For example, until recently in Western culture, females were assumed to serve as homemakers and males as primary breadwinners. This became a standard expectation of many as values were transferred from one generation to the next (McGoldrick, Giordano, & Garcia-Preto, 2005). Although this standard has shifted significantly with changes in contemporary societal norms, some individuals of both genders still maintain the schema that a woman's role is to focus on domestic responsibilities, as opposed to being employed outside the home. Similarly, traditional gender role beliefs tend to portray the female parent as being responsible for distributing affection in the household, and the male parent as the disciplinarian. Clearly, such standards would cause significant conflict in many contemporary relationships, particularly if the two spouses held differing schemas. For many couples in their later years who grew up during the post-World War II generation, however, traditional gender role expectations may still be shared by spouses.

Of course, people often have contradictory attitudes about family life, gender roles, and related issues. A woman, for example, may be highly motivated to pursue a professional career, and this goal may be supported by her friends and family. Yet, deep down, something makes her feel that her real job in life is to serve her husband and children. These conflicting attitudes may contribute to a general vulnerability or a feeling of being stuck (i.e., "I need to pursue my career for self-esteem reasons, but feel guilty when my husband and children complain").

Family schemas, such as those mentioned earlier, may be communicated from parents to children in a variety of ways, either directly via specific statements or more subtly through the children's observations of interactions within the family. For example, in some families it has been a tradition passed down from generation to generation for a female to confide in her mother about her sexual activities, particularly during adolescence and early adulthood. Even if a mother has not directly told her daughter that she expects such disclosures, the daughter may easily infer that this is normal mother–daughter conversation because of her mother's matter-of-fact questions about her sexual behavior and the need for parental approval. These exchanges commonly serve to forge a special bond between mother and daughter. When such communications extend into the daughter's adulthood, however, a spouse may become offended because his wife has divulged to her mother what transpires in their bedroom. This discrepancy between the husband's and wife's schemas about boundaries and privacy can have a significant impact on the couple's relationship. The important point here is that married partners generally get their attitudes from their parents.

The pioneering family therapist Virginia Satir (1983) made the statement "The parents are the architects of the family." Satir's work emphasized how role expectations are passed down from one generation to the next. A couple therapist will miss important information if he or she fails to thoroughly explore the belief systems of parents' (or partners') families of origin during the course of assessment and treatment. Obtaining such information helps the therapist gain a better sense of how family-of-origin experiences may influence clients' respective thinking in their current relationship.

Figure 3.3 diagrams the trickle-down effect of schemas from the family of origin. Some of the most notable work in family-of-origin theory was first conducted by Murray Bowen in the 1960s, 1970s, and 1980s (Bowen, 1966, 1978; Kerr & Bowen, 1988). Bowen's theory posits that transgenerational trends in family and relationship functioning reflect orderly and predictable relationship processes that connect the functioning of family members across generations. This heritage may include beliefs, values, and emotions that are transferred from one generation to the next (Kerr & Bowen, 1988; Miller, Anderson, & Kaulana Keala, 2004). Bowen specifically contended that "much of the generational transmission appears to be based on prolonged association" (Kerr & Bowen, 1988, p. 315). By this, Bowen meant that the strength of the transmission often depends on the intensity and length of family relationships.

According to Bowen, "most of it seems to be linked to the deep inclination of human beings to imitate one another" (Kerr & Bowen, 1988, p. 315). In this respect, adult children tend to imitate their parents' interaction in their own marriages and current families. Bowen also cautioned that mere exposure to family functioning does not adequately explain the intergenerational transmission process, emphasizing instead that the actual transmission process was often inconsistent and occurred at an emotional level (Larson & Wilson, 1998). This idea pertains to affect displays without any conscious acknowledgment of underlying thought.

The transmission process involves a level of "differentiation" and patterns of functioning that are transmitted from parents to their offspring via

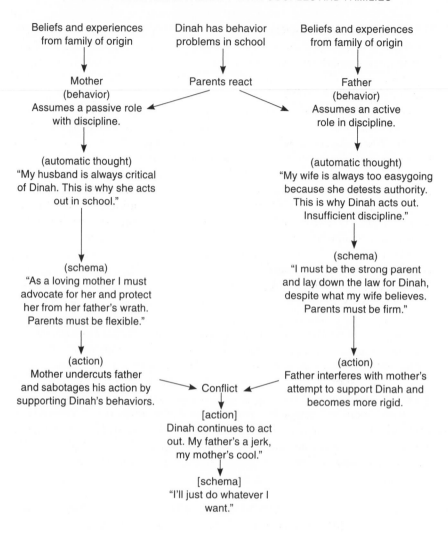

FIGURE 3.3. Family schema.

what Bowen termed the *family projection process* (Kerr & Bowen, 1988). By differentiation, Bowen meant both the individual's ability to function autonomously from others and his or her ability to separate cognition from emotion (i.e., the ability to think logically without undue interference from emotional states such as anxiety). Bowen hypothesized that the degree to which parents and a child have failed to develop a balance between emotional attachment and autonomy on the child's part, as the child grows up, influences how well the offspring functions throughout his or her life. This influence was said to express itself not only through the adult child's individual functioning but also in the functioning of his or her family of origin, having a particularly clear role in dysfunction within the person's spousal relationship (Bowen, 1978).

Neither Bowen nor his colleagues, however, addressed in detail any of the specific cognitions that develop as a result of transgenerational family fusion. The specific manner in which a child incorporates certain family belief systems is not merely a matter of imitation but is more likely due to a deeply ingrained process of internalization, which is refined over years of exposure to family-of-origin experiences that incorporate basic beliefs.

For example, the handling of money is often a point of contention for many couples because of the partners' attitudes acquired from their families of origin. Some families believe that money is something that should be saved and spent only when absolutely necessary. These families value living a frugal life and saving for the future. Other families view money as a tool and as something that should be spent in the here and now. In those families, the expenditure of money is not seen as negative, and there may be less accountability as to how it should be spent.

When spouses have been raised in families that were very different in their philosophies in regard to finances, serious conflict may ensue. An individual who came from a family of origin that stressed the need to save money, and may feel secure in knowing that certain monies are set aside, may have that sense of security shaken if a partner places a different value on its use. However, a partner who comes from a family that believed "you can't take it with you" may feel stifled by a fiscally conservative spouse. The conflict may be compounded when the couple's parents still have a significant influence on how they should spend money in their marriage.

COGNITIONS AND
TRANSGENERATIONAL SCHEMAS

Interestingly, very little has been mentioned in the professional literature regarding specific cognitions and the influence of transgenerational schemas have on the cognitive processes of offspring, particularly on their marital relationship patterns. Until recently, family schemas and how they are transmitted intergenerationally have been given limited attention in the literature on cognitive factors in family relations (Dattilio, 2001a, 2005b, 2006c; Dattilio & Epstein, 2003; Dattilio et al., 1998).

Transgenerational schemas may be positive or negative in content, and they may exist on either a conscious or unconscious level. Clinicians' common experience, indicating that schemas are particularly difficult to change when they have negative content and are associated with negative emotion, is consistent with basic cognitive psychology research findings (Baldwin, 1992). In addition, undesirable schemas are difficult to change when they have strengthened over time, being reinforced repeatedly by life experiences. Furthermore, it is more difficult to modify schemas that are actually not within a person's conscious awareness. For example, if we consider the schema of a young woman who allows herself to be subjected to abuse by her partner because she believes that she is obligated to tolerate such abusive behavior as part of being married, an inquiry into her history may uncover a schema that was shaped by the influence of her family of origin. Perhaps her own parents modeled this type of relationship pattern regarding spousal roles, which had a profound effect on her subliminal belief system. It would not be hard to see how this woman would develop such a schema about marital obligations in light of repeated exposure to the role models in her family of origin (Dattilio, 2006c).

FIGHTING AUTHORITY

I once had a case involving three generations of a Czechoslovakian American family. I saw this family in treatment because of the 10-year-old son's defiant oppositional behavior in school. Upon the initial assessment, I surmised that the child's acting out was, as is true in many cases, related to problems in his family. I asked the parents to come in for family therapy sessions and constructed a genogram, which revealed that both of the child's parents were first-generation Czechoslovakian Americans.

The parents of both the mother and father had been born in Czechoslovakia. Both sets of grandparents were Holocaust survivors, and two of the grandparents had witnessed the direct execution of their own parents, as well as other relatives, by the Nazis during the German occupation in World War II.

The grandparents had eventually been liberated from their respective labor camps and had migrated to the United States. But after witnessing so many atrocities, they had experienced severe depression, which affected them for the rest of their lives. This had inadvertently affected their offspring, who had grown up struggling with their parents' chronic depression and despair. The parents of the 10-year-old told me that, when they were children, they had often become depressed and withdrawn owing to the general emotional atmosphere in their households. They also said they had difficulty trusting others and had experienced a generalized sense of oppression by authority.

This burden had been handed down in an indirect form to their son. Instead of responding with typical depressive symptoms, however, the child had denied his depression and expressed his conflicts via acting-out behaviors in school, which, once again, were a representation of his family's issues with authority. My view of this young boy's behavior was that it was actually an alternative to falling prey to depression. In one way, his alternative of acting out was an improvement over becoming depressed, yet, at the same time, caused trouble for him. My aim in treatment would be to reinforce his avoidance of depression, but to consider other choices of survival in dealing with adversity at school.

Treatment involved family therapy, including family-of-origin sessions in order to address the lineage of depression that had been handed down from one generation to the next. Much of the work involved helping the boy's parents become aware of how an almost 60-year-old trauma had affected several generations of their family and helping the young boy to consider alternate behaviors by which to express himself.

Clearly, a greater emphasis must be placed on examining couples' and family members' schemas that likely are derived from families of origin, particularly those concerning the manner in which relationships should function intellectually, emotionally, and behaviorally. This is particularly important because such schemas involve broad standards that individuals hold regarding their intimate relationships and that commonly contribute to conflict in their relationships. These schemas constitute risk factors for conflict particularly because many of them are not articulated clearly in an individual's mind, but exist as vague concepts of what is or what should be (Beck, 1988; Epstein & Baucom, 2002). When schemas about oneself and one's relationships are ingrained at an early age, they have great potential to operate at a unconscious level and are easily transferred across generations. Schwebel and Fine (1994) liken such cognitions to computer software in that they help family members function in the family setting, shaping their perceptions, thoughts, reactions, feelings, and behavior and guiding them through the challenge of family life (p. 56). When such a schema is pervasive in a family, the members who have internalized it operate according to its tenets without consciously thinking about them.

Tilden and Dattilio (2005) distinguish two major categories of schemas: (1) *the vulnerable core schema* and (2) *the protective coping schema*. The vulnerable core schema refers to those aspects of past experience that are painful and avoided. Welburn, Dagg, Coristine, and Pontefract (2000) also differentiate between schemas according to their places in a hierarchical organization, in which some are determined to have principal importance owing to their connection to basic needs, such as safety and attachment, and others are more peripheral but are related to the principal schemas, such as about being accepted or acknowledged by others.

Vulnerable core schemas are usually established during the early years of an individual's life as a consequence of adult caretakers' failure to validate and confirm the child's feelings and experiences, particularly those associated with his or her core needs, such as attachment (Bowlby, 1982). Such a vulnerable core schema may also be established through traumatic events in adult life. To protect and help him- or herself as much as possible, an individual carrying a core vulnerability schema will need a protective coping schema, or strategies to deal with critical and difficult life situations and events that trigger the vulnerable schema. The use of coping strategies, however, may be maladaptive and cause unwanted consequences. An example of this circumstance follows in the case of André and Iva, whose respective schemas from their families of origin heavily shaped their beliefs about love and intimacy and the need to protect themselves from ongoing vulnerability. Their schemas caused significant dissension in their relationship as conflicts arose between the partners' needs and preferences.

THE CASE OF ANDRÉ AND IVA[2]

André and Iva were in their mid-70s. André, a Romanian-born man with five siblings, worked as a laborer in a steel mill for 40 years. His wife, Iva, was born in the United States to a Polish family and served as a homemaker for most of her married life. André and Iva had three grown children. Their middle child, Rosie, had recently died of a brain tumor. The couple sought treatment with me on the advice of their parish priest because they were struggling with the grieving process over the loss of their daughter, but had also been experiencing marital problems prior to her death. This preexisting tension only exacerbated the impact of the recent loss of their child.

Much of what André and Iva had argued about during their 48-year marriage concerned styles of management in their life together. They differed significantly over how money should be spent and how to discipline their children. André believed that money should be saved and that only "essentials" should be purchased. Iva, on the other hand, believed that money was there to be spent and maintained the attitude "it's no good after you're dead." Iva often recalled a quote from her parents: "The last suit of clothing has no pockets." André believed in physical discipline of the children, whereas Iva was against physical punishment altogether. This difference usually played itself out by Iva's ignoring André's opinions and doing what she felt was best. André would subsequently seek refuge in his sports activities, such as golf. In addition, one of Iva's frequent complaints had to do with the fact that André seemed to care more about sports than he did about her and would show affection to her only in the bedroom when he wanted to have sexual relations. Their problems with intimacy became

---

[2] Adapted with permission from the American Association for Marriage and Family Therapy. Parts of this case first appeared in Dattilio (2005b).

more intense, however, once the children had reached adulthood and moved out of the house. Iva believed that affection should occur outside the bedroom by showing each other kindness and courtesy; this would then serve as a prelude to physical intimacy later, such as hugging or caressing and sometimes sexual relations. André believed that affection consisted only of physical contact, which always occurred behind closed doors. He equated love with sex.

When André and Iva's daughter became ill with the brain tumor, they had difficulty comforting each other. André retreated into his sports activity, playing golf and bowling in a weekly league. In fact, Iva often referred to herself as a "golf widow." During the course of Rosie's illness, Iva escorted her daughter to chemotherapy treatments and tended to her grandchildren and other family members. Because their daughter was a single parent, Iva also helped out by babysitting Rosie's children, tending to meals and other household needs. She often accused André of being selfish and removed from the situation, insinuating that he did not care. André often retorted by saying that Iva just liked to make things worse because of her need to be a "drama queen." Iva also described André as being condescending to her when she failed to show any desire to have sexual relations.

The point of crisis in the couple's relationship came the day when André and Iva buried Rosie. It had been a long day, with the viewing in the early morning, the funeral, and then the family gathering at the home after the funeral. That evening, upon retiring, André had approached Iva with the prospect of being sexually intimate. Iva was absolutely appalled, as most people would be. However, even though this behavior seemed callous, I interpreted it as André's way of expressing his love and deriving comfort for himself. Iva just could not believe that André wanted to have sexual relations on the same day that they had buried their daughter and were still in the grieving process. André reported that Iva "barked" at him, "How selfish and callous you are," and that she became so disgusted that she refused to sleep in the same room with him. André was at a loss as to why Iva would perceive his overtures as being selfish, because he viewed his suggestion of sex as a means of their comforting each other after experiencing such a horrible loss. This event appeared to be the straw that broke the camel's back for Iva, as she subsequently withdrew from André almost completely. At this point, André decided to speak to their parish priest, who referred the couple to me for couple therapy.

Gathering the Background Information

The initial phase of therapy involved gathering background information about the years that André and Iva spent together. We talked about how they met and what attracted them to each other. We also focused on the pervasive issues in the marriage, such as conflicts of opinion as to how money was spent, disciplining of the children, making important decisions, and the significance of emotional and sexual intimacy.

A considerable amount of attention was also given to understanding the belief systems that each spouse had been exposed to during childhood and how such beliefs served to shape their respective schemas about sexual relations, love, and intimacy. More important, we explored André's and Iva's schemas regarding emotional comforting and how each perceived the other's needs for comfort. What was particularly intriguing about this case was that the partners had been married for so many years that their schemas were likely to be extremely ingrained. Yet something needed to change, because they had arrived at a juncture in life at which their relationship was in serious jeopardy if they continued in the same pattern.

André and Iva were seen conjointly in therapy. I decided to assess them together rather than interview them separately because it was important for each to hear the history given by the other. André talked first about his family of origin, stating that his parents were both Romanian and had immigrated to the United States when he was very young. André's mother was said to be of Gypsy blood and to have had a strong influence on the family dynamics. The family was always very close-knit, and, in fact, for many years they all slept in one large bed in their two-room apartment. André had been too young to recall whether he was exposed to any sexual intimacy between his parents, or other family members for that matter, but he recalled that the only time his parents appeared to display any physical affection for each other was at night when they would embrace. They seemed to be disengaged during the daytime hours.

André was close to his mother and described her as somewhat the matriarch of the family. His father was the breadwinner, and, when it came down to "brass tacks," as André called it, "Dad had the final say about everything." In essence then, André's mother was the matriarch only until his father disliked something. Then father would step in and take charge, and mother would acquiesce. The family never had much money, so there was not much to argue about in that area. It was understood, however, that any extra money that they had accumulated from time to time was to be saved. His parents shared this belief, which André adopted and brought to his marriage with Iva. André's father was a foundry worker, and his mother embroidered and made beautiful tablecloths to earn extra income.

Iva described her family of origin as very loving. Her father was strict and her mother compliant, but she could stand up for herself when necessary. The family was the primary focus at home. Iva's father was a postal employee and worked from 7:00 A.M. to 3:00 P.M., Monday through Friday. Her mother worked in a silk mill to supplement the family's income. The family was not wealthy by any means, but there was always sufficient money, and Iva's parents were not afraid to spend what they had. Iva recalled her parents being openly affectionate. She stated, "We could always get a hug from each other when we needed it." Consequently, affection was never a major issue; there was plenty to go around. Iva described the atmosphere in her family of origin as being more relaxed than her impressions of what had existed in André's family. It was also her strong belief that affection between spouses was not something to be restricted to the bedroom, but was to be displayed during the course of the day as well. This was Iva's primary complaint about André, in that she reported that he seemed not to be interested in bothering with her until it was time to have sexual relations behind closed doors. Consequently, Iva often stated, "I feel like a cheap whore; the only time he can show me affection is when he wants to have sex."

As I began to work with this couple and delve into their families of origin, it became very clear to me that André had some experiences while growing up that suggested to him that any affection shown outside the bedroom was shameful. He recalled that on one occasion he and his siblings were encouraging his parents to kiss on their anniversary, but his father made it very clear to them that it was not proper to display affection in public, that it was something to be done only in private. André remembers being ashamed of his feelings. At the same time, he believed that what he was taught by his father was correct etiquette. Consequently, he grew up with the belief that public displays of affection are not proper. In many respects, André grew up suppressing emotions, and he felt that this helped him to be successful in his life in that he had always maintained a level head and never lost control emotionally. Unfortunately, this schema about the experiencing and expression of emotion completely clashed with his wife's beliefs about love and affection, and on many occasions Iva felt starved for affection, as André did when he was a child. But she dealt with it much differently than he had learned to do. Iva's sense of deprivation caused her to become angry and to compensate for feeling deprived by shopping and spending money. This often riled André because of his strong beliefs about what he considered the unnecessary expenditure of money. Consequently, the partners' conflicting beliefs about emotion, affection, and proper use of money were areas in which tension repeatedly surfaced in the relationship, and it was clear that each person's schemas in these areas had their roots in family-of-origin experiences.

Course of Treatment

Initially, much of my work with this couple was exploratory in an educational way. Helping them become aware of each other's life experiences and how these shaped their schemas was a very important step in increasing their understanding that they came from very different family environments. Although this did not necessarily diminish any of the frustration that each spouse experienced currently, it was important for them was to understand that during the vulnerable and impressionable periods during childhood their belief systems about proper roles in couple relationships became ingrained.

The second step in therapy was to have both of them acknowledge that some change was needed, which would mean that each of them would have to depart, to some degree, from the beliefs that had been developed in his or her family of origin. Iva seemed to be more amenable to this than André, particularly because he felt that to change his belief system was to call his parents liars and to ridicule them. As in many cases of couple therapy, more of my restructuring work focused on the schemas of one partner. In this case it was André, because his beliefs were more ingrained. The work with André also served as a model for my work with Iva and laid the groundwork for her to think about how she would go about restructuring her own beliefs. It was important to maintain a balance when addressing both spouses so that one spouse did not feel as though the therapist was biased toward one or the other. Because it was important to start with one spouse and spend sufficient time focusing on his cognitions, I often reminded both of them that I would eventually address the other person in the same fashion. I often cautioned them not to construe this as being picked on, but to consider it as a mode of educating both of them about cognition and behavior.

On several occasions during the course of treatment, I asked André to consider some modifications that he could make to his beliefs about the appropriate expression of love and intimacy. We talked about how his parents likely fashioned their lifestyle around their specific beliefs and that it apparently had worked adequately for them. We also discussed how people differ in their personal needs and that being successful in a relationship requires some flexibility. I began to encourage André to think about how much he would be willing to depart from his initial belief system in order to take into account the fact that Iva's needs for overt affection were different from his. I explained that having a relationship that was satisfying to her, as well as to him, might require some effort on his part to address her needs. He agreed that, because Iva did need some display of affection outside the bedroom, it was something that he could consider. However, he stated that each time he attempted to do this, she would irritate him by spending money unnecessarily and he would recoil and feel as though he wanted to deprive her of any affection because of her "frivolous" spending.

I then discussed with Iva the degree to which she was willing to modify her belief about spending money in order to take into account André's different beliefs about finances, yet at the same time not restricting her spending so much that she would feel deprived. We also discussed how some of her spending might involve passive–aggressive behavior on her part.

The further course of therapy with the couple involved a step-by-step modification of the rigid beliefs that contributed to their marital conflicts, as well as the construction of behavioral change agreements in which they would experiment with new interactions that were consistent with a more flexible approach to meeting each other's needs. We also addressed the issue of acceptance, respecting the fact that it was unrealistic for either partner to expect the other to completely change long-standing beliefs. Therefore, each had to think about how much he or she could accept about the other's beliefs and what was gained by being in a relationship with the other person in spite of their differences. The result was that both partners were willing to work on modifying their thinking sufficiently to make a significant difference in the relationship.

On one occasion, a previous issue resurfaced—how Iva was appalled that André had wanted to have sexual relations on the day they buried their daughter. I had Iva listen closely to André tell her, for the first time, what it meant to him to lose their daughter. André sobbed profusely while talking about the loss. In some respects, he even felt responsible for her death, even though he had nothing to do with causing her illness. He stated that on the night following her burial he was so worn out and defenseless that he felt like a little child, and he needed caressing and holding more than actual intercourse. Not surprisingly, Iva had misunderstood him because of André's typically limited communication about his feelings. She had assumed that because he wanted to be intimate, he was primarily motivated by sexual arousal and automatically wanted intercourse.

Once Iva began to really listen to André, she started to feel bad about the fact that he had needed much of the same thing that she needed at that time, but that she had misperceived his desires and overtures. This challenged a schema that Iva had developed over the years, that André had such a high sex drive that it took precedence over any needs he might have for emotional intimacy and over any consideration of her needs. Iva shifted in her interpretation of what he had needed that night and no longer viewed it as a selfish act, but rather as his way of seeking comfort, attempting to make some sense of the loss of their child, and healing. It was at this point that André and Iva began to realize that because of their early life experiences, they had grossly misunderstood each other.

Therapy went on to address communication skills for expressing feelings and listening to each other empathically, as well *quid pro quo* agreements to exchange behaviors that each desired, which were extremely helpful in increasing the couple's emotional intimacy. We also continued monitoring the partners' interpretations (i.e., attributions) of each other's behaviors. They kept in mind the need to monitor their own thinking and ways that they could slightly change their beliefs from those they learned in their families of origin, in order to accommodate the needs they had in their present relationship. Ironically, this milestone came 48 years after this couple had gotten together and lived a full life, raising three children. At the conclusion of therapy, they both remarked that it was a pity that they had never learned to address these issues decades before, because they might have enjoyed a more fruitful relationship earlier.

With many couples, work must be done to modify each person's schemas from his or her family-of-origin in order to change their linear views that the relationship problems were due to the partner's shortcomings rather than based on contributions from both parties.

4

The Role
of Neurobiological Processes

Recently, there has been a lot of new literature on the role of neurobiological processes in family relationships (Atkinson, 2005; Schore, 2003; Siegel, 1999), which has opened up a new line of thinking about problems involving cognitive and emotional processing with family members. The following case is an example of how sometimes undetected neurobiological impairments may seep into relationships.

FILLING IN THE BLANKS: THE CASE OF MARTY AND LISA

Marty and Lisa had been married for 25 years when they presented for treatment. They had two adult children, one of whom still lived at home. They reported experiencing a great deal of tension in the relationship because of Lisa's belief that Marty just didn't understand her, especially when she tried to express her feelings to him. Marty was a civil engineer who had recently retired, despite being only in his mid-50s. His company had offered an early retirement package that Marty said he "couldn't refuse." Lisa was a teacher who had stopped working outside the home once their children were born. She later returned to teaching after the children reached school age. This is when both spouses claim that the problems in the relationship had started worsening.

There was also tension as a result of Marty's belief that Lisa's career was of greater priority than their relationship. He felt a lack of partnership in the marriage and a severe lack of communication between himself and his wife. As a result, Marty pulled away from Lisa, and the two communicated less and less. Lisa also complained that whatever feelings she expressed to Marty, he would twist into something else, which she found extremely frustrating. Whenever Lisa attempted to clarify her statements, Marty became defensive and retreated behind a wall of silence. Lisa believed that Marty misinterpreted what she said to him in a deliberate attempt to undermine her. Marty insisted that he did understand what Lisa was saying to him, but his subsequent behavior suggested that he didn't understand, and consequently he argued with her. Lisa said, "When Marty doesn't hear me, he just fills in the blanks incorrectly." Moreover, she often felt that she was punished by Marty for expressing her feelings.

As treatment unfolded, the focus was directed toward basic communications training. It soon became clear, however, that there was something wrong with the way in which Marty processed Lisa's verbal statements. Lisa and Marty started to communicate by e-mail because it seemed to work better for them than talking face-to-face.

I noticed more and more that there seemed to be a distinct problem with Marty's auditory processing. He often nodded his head in affirmation when Lisa spoke to him, but later acted as though he had never heard a word she said. It was at that time that I also noticed that Marty sometimes came to the therapy sessions using a cane. Marty explained that, over the years, he had developed a neurological condition known as cerebellar degeneration. This disorder impairs the ability to coordinate body movements.

I also learned (by conducting my own literature review) that a less common symptom of this disease involves difficulty with cognitive processing. Research had demonstrated that spinocerebellar ataxia is inherited and was thought to be the predominant symptom. Some individuals inflicted with this disease also reported experiencing mood disorders, as well as concentration and memory difficulties. In some cases, victims of this disease experienced *alexithymia*, a term coined by the late Harvard psychiatrist Peter Sifneros to describe a condition in which one experiences the inability to recall or to convey emotion in verbal expression. I suggested that Marty consider undergoing neuropsychological testing. He did, and the results yielded evidence of deficits with his auditory processing and sensory integration skills. These results made sense, given what I was witnessing in the interaction during therapy sessions. This new information allowed us to understand that some of the difficulty Marty had in communicating with Lisa was not deliberate, as Lisa had imagined, but a symptom of his cerebral degeneration.

This diagnosis made a world of difference in how Lisa responded to her husband's difficulty. Marty also appeared much less frustrated when this information was revealed. Lisa reminded me, however, that Marty had acted the same way ever since they'd known each other, although, admittedly, the problem had become worse over time. Once this disability was confirmed and explained to them, the next step was for Marty and Lisa to adjust their thinking and reactions to each other within a new framework. This framework allowed them to attribute their problems, in part, to Marty's disorder, which helped to reduce the tension in the relationship.

Sometimes, understanding the brain's chemistry and how it relates to cognition, emotion, and behavior is essential in understanding conflicts that arise in relationships. Although Marty and Lisa's case is an extreme example of deficits, there are other cases that are less extreme and do not involve a deteriorative disease, but reflect a more functional deficit or shortcoming that may still contribute to some dysfunction in the relationship. That is, there may be more subtle deficits that go undetected, of which the etiology is unknown. It is important to understand how profound the neurobiological processes of the human body are in affecting our relationships and how they may limit the change that couples and families make in therapy. How do we determine when someone is struggling with permanent neurobiological deficits? And, more important, what can we do about it? This is not an easy question to answer, and sometimes it may require a referral to a neuropsychologist or neuropsychiatrist for further diagnostic assessment. In some cases, such diagnostic assessments may lead to the need for cognitive rehabilitation, if a particular condition is amenable. The brain's chemistry may affect each of us differently, making it more of a struggle for some than for others to process thought and emotion. Having to separate what is deliberate from what is not can make therapy arduous.

Recently, increasing attention has been paid to the effects of genetics and neurobiology on interpersonal relationships. The emerging field of neuropsychobiology provides us with new insights into how emotional and behavioral patterns develop in intimate relationships (Schore, 1994, 2001, 2003). Some of this work has also been integrated with attachment theory in its application to couple therapy, with an emphasis on dyadic affect regulation (Lewis, Amini, & Lannon, 2002; Goldstein & Thau, 2004). It is possible that, by understanding how each partner's nervous system is affected by "emotional reverberations" triggered in dyadic interactions, couples can work to create greater emotional attunement and establish a more secure base in the relationship (Lewis et al., 2001, p. 131).

Recent research has also supported the hypothesis that romantic relationships may involve a motivational state as fundamental as hunger and thirst. Arthur Aron and colleagues demonstrated through their research that certain dopamine-rich areas light up when we think about our romantic partners, as revealed by functional magnetic resonance imagining (fMRI; Aron, Fisher, Mashek, Strong, & Brown, 2005). Such regions of the brain as the ventral tegmental area (VTA) are known as the motivation and reward system and appear to activate whenever individuals obtain something they deeply desire. Subjects in the Aron et al. study reported a variety of emotions upon gazing at their partners. The brain activity also displayed a diverse array of activation patterns in the amygdala, commonly referred to as the emotional center (p. 335).

In his well-known book *The Developing Mind*, Daniel Siegel (1999) provides an excellent overview of how the brain affects our relationships, and the impact that relationships have on our neurochemistry. Research suggests that the two interact in a way that shapes who we are as human beings. The rest (how we interact), of course, is shaped by our environmental experiences. Siegel focuses considerable attention on the limbic system of the brain, which is centrally located and consists of regions known as the orbital frontal cortex, the anterior cingulate, and the amygdala. These regions play a significant role in coordinating the activities of higher and lower brain structures and are believed to mediate emotions, motivations, and goal-directed behavior. In fact, the limbic brain has sometimes been referred to as the "emotional brain" (Atkinson, 2005). This region also houses neural connections to every part of the neocortex, the more recently evolved part of the brain that regulates, among other functions, perception and behavior. The limbic structures also facilitate the integration of a broad range of primary mental processes that are very important in human functioning, such as in the appraisal of meaning, the processing of social experience, and the regulation of emotions. This information suggests that there is much more that has to do with biochemistry and its impact on relationships than we were previously aware of.

So, why is all of this important to relationships? As we saw with Marty and Lisa, it was a crucial factor that needed to be understood in order to make any headway in treatment. However, what is important to note is that even though our brains are genetically wired to function in a certain manner, they do not act in isolation from our experience. Our neurobiology and life experiences interact in such a way that certain biological tendencies can create characteristic experiences that may greatly contribute to the success of a relationship. Because our minds develop at the interface of neurophysiological processes and interpersonal relationships, specific relationship experiences consequently have a dominant influence on the brain. There is even evidence to suggest that some individuals' limbic systems are genetically structured to develop differently than others. This may explain why some people emote more easily than others. For example, research has suggested that women's limbic systems differ from those of men, which is why they may cry more easily or show emotion differently than men do (Siegel, 1999). Interestingly, however, men have traditionally expressed intolerance toward this attribute of women, which has been recorded throughout the course of time (Coontz, 2005). Hence, such evidence-based information may serve to dispel men's long-held erroneous belief that women cry only to manipulate men in order to get their own way. This is a cognitive distortion that appears to be, in part, erroneously based.

In her recent book *The Female Brain*, Louann Brizendine (2006) cites research conducted at the University of Michigan showing that women use both hemispheres of their brains to respond to emotional experiences, whereas men use only one hemisphere (Wagner & Phan, 2003). It was also determined that the connections between the emotional centers of the brain are more active and extensive in women (Cahill, 2003). This likely explains why women typically remember emotional events, such as arguments, more vividly and retain them longer than men do.

THE ROLE OF THE AMYGDALA

The amygdala is one of the most frequently studied areas of the brain in the professional literature, particularly as it relates to emotion (LeDoux, 1996; Pessoa, 2008). Such subcortical structures as the amygdala are believed to operate quickly and automatically, so that certain triggered features, such as when the whites of our eyes widen in a fearful expression, are relatively unfiltered and always evoke responses, such as flight, that may be important for survival (Whalen, 2004). Such functions that mediate emotion are believed to be more subtle and not always conscious of the stimulus that might have triggered brain responses in an affective brain region (Ohman, 2002; Pessoa, 2005). Studies have examined how the initiation of an appraisal leads to subsequent perceptual biases that reinforce the nature of the initial appraisal. The flow of activation of the brain's circuits begins a process of higher level activations, which subsequently ready the individual, or organism, for a particular response. The amygdala responds to the initial visual representation (i.e., a barking dog) by signaling the same and even earlier layers of the visual processing system and then activating the attentional and perceptual apparatus of the brain (Siegel, 1999). What is particularly interesting is that the amygdala can rapidly bias the perceptual apparatus toward misinterpreting any stimulus (i.e., dangerous vs. safe). All of this occurs in seconds, without any dependence on conscious awareness. So, if a spouse who was raised in a household with an abusive parent becomes the target of frequent physical and psychological abuse by his or her partner, that person may naturally become highly sensitized on a physiological level through the amygdala. Hence, any conflict (i.e., argument) that arises in family situations that resembles the earlier abuse a person sustained as a child, would automatically be activated by the amygdala. This would happen despite cognitive, behavioral, or emotional types of mediational interventions. In fact, depending on the intensity and magnitude of the earlier abuse, the amygdala may have been physiologically groomed or programmed to respond in a "knee-jerk" or "hypersensitive" fashion owing to the priming of body chemistry throughout the years.

Learning to appreciate the biophysiological language of our spouses and family members and how this affects emotion and behavior is very important. For example, consider the visceral reactions that partners and family members show each other in day-to-day interactions. Some nonverbal aspects of communication reflect right hemispheric activity that is responsible for emotion and implicit processing, such as eye contact, tone and volume of voice, and certain body movements, such as facial expressions and posture. Knowledge of this process becomes important when, for example, certain body movements are made by one spouse while thinking about what the other spouse is saying, but are interpreted by the other spouse as being gestures of annoyance—when they are actually a result of right hemispheric processing of the material. Therefore, the negative connotation attached may not be accurate to explain the behavioral display. Educating spouses or family members on how the brain processes certain information and later displays it is a practical tool for bettering relationships.

Likewise, a spouse's or family member's tone of voice that does not match his or her facial expressions of anger may suggest a poor connection with his or her emotions owing to a neurological problem, or that this is a person who is out of touch with his or her feelings. An excellent example of this is portrayed in the following vignette.

In this particular case, a husband and wife came in for a session after they had experienced a very intense argument. The argument had started over the fact that the wife had forgotten to send an acknowledgment (RSVP) that they would both be attending a wedding reception. When they showed up at the wedding reception, there was no table assigned to them, and it became clear that, because the RSVP had never been sent, they were not accounted for on the guest list. This error caused quite a bit of embarrassment, and the husband became irate, stating that his wife was careless and never followed through on things. They became engaged in a heated argument over the notion of the wife's repeated carelessness and inattention to detail.

During the course of this session, as the husband began a tirade about how "fed up and angry" he was about this situation and many others like it, I noticed that his wife's demeanor indicated that she was tense. Her jaw was clenched and she was speaking in a very low tone, saying that she was sorry and that she understood why her husband was upset. At the same time, her behavior told me something different. I noticed that a vein was protruding from her forehead and her face was starting to turn a reddish purple. When asked about whether she was embarrassed, she denied this, but further stated that she understood why her husband was angry and did not blame him. What struck me odd was that this woman's tone of voice did not match her facial expressions and body language. I called her attention to the fact that she was showing all the signs of being furious and ready to jump out of her seat, yet her words were incongruous with her behaviors.

My first thought was, how can I help this woman connect her emotions with her spontaneous thoughts? I decided to give her a hand mirror that I had in my powder room of my office so that she could pay attention to her facial expressions. I also asked her to touch her lower jaw and mandible area, as well as her forehead where the vein was protruding. When I asked her to feel her own face, she was shocked at how tense her body was. I then asked her to attempt to get in touch with how angry she was, as opposed to her expressed sense of feeling sorry. She was eventually able to reveal that she was actually furious at her husband because he rarely took responsibility for such chores as sending RSVPs. She went on to state that it was really hard for her to be angry openly because her husband had always taken a more aggressive stance, which she felt had inhibited her in the past. I explained to her that it was obvious that anger was not an emotion that she allowed herself to experience easily. Instead, she expressed what may be described as a reaction of shame and guilt to her feelings of anger. I also raised the possibility that her absentminded behaviors had continued because she was actually furious with her husband, and her resentment could be fueling a passive–aggressive response.

That dialogue became a reference point that I used when discussing feelings with this couple, which were expressed by the wife nonverbally, particularly with gestures, facial expressions, and visual cues. The concept of being attuned to each other's nonverbal communications was potent in helping them to recognize the incongruence of their verbal expression and behavioral display, and to become aware of the impact of this incongruence on their negative interactions. While learning to value balance and harmony, couples and family members can also learn how to process the pain of their periods of miscommunication, keeping in mind that conflict is a normal part of any couple relationship, a reflection of the differences between the two separate partners (Gottman, 1994).

In the same vein, nonverbal behavior may also have a different meaning from the manner in which it is interpreted. For example, during a family therapy session, parents expressed their anger with their prepubescent daughter because she always rolled her eyes when they interrogated her about an issue. The parents would scold her for "getting a smart-ass look on her face," which the daughter would reportedly deny she was doing. She claimed to be unaware of it and insisted that she wasn't being "smart-assed" at all and that she had done this her entire life. When I explained that the daughter's tendency to "roll her eyes" to the right might indicate that she was using her left hemisphere to process the words being said to her, this action took on an entire new meaning for the family. The daughter's behavior may have been, in part, a "smart reaction," but it was important that the family understood that sometimes reactions can't always be interpreted at face value.

The use of cognitive techniques, such as the *positive sentiment override* suggested by Gottman (1999), involves teaching people to acknowledge the relevance of their amygdala's response to the present situation and a past trauma, as in the aforementioned case of abuse. The initial arousal mechanism is then modified by using a kind of self-talk strategy to reduce the physiological reaction. Such imagery techniques can be useful in having the amygdala "sigh with relief" that it does not have to respond in the way it was programmed. So, even if one's physiological response to a particular stimulus cannot be completely changed, one's response to the initial arousal can be modified to become more flexible. In the earlier case of Marty and Lisa, such cognitive techniques were useful in helping Lisa not to become so "lit up" emotionally, as she liked to put it, when Marty "twisted around" what she said. "I had been viewing his behavior as a way of manipulating me or making me look like some kind of a dope," she said, "but restructuring my thinking seemed to diffuse my anger about it and allowed our communication to flow a little better."

Cognitive techniques may serve to dampen the intensity of the physiological arousal process, as well as to restructure the distribution of neuronal groups. This can affect the reactivation of the cortex, which controls abstract reasoning, which then permits the metacognitive processes of self-reflection and impulse control to occur. Such an intervention can lead to a tolerance of levels of arousal that previously may have been overwhelming. Strengthening the metacognitive cortical capacity can pave the way for greater accessibility to tolerance during emotionally charged situations.

Prolonged periods of the flooding of emotions without an effective mediational process can result in prolonged states of disorganization (Siegel, 1999). A flood of emotions sometimes needs to be understood as a problem with processing, as opposed to a "neurosis" or "manipulation" on one's part. That is, emotions can often overwhelm us in the same way a water main breaks and spews its contents all over the place. Teaching techniques such as ventilation and/or emotional regulation can be vital to couples in distress (see Chapter 2). Deep breathing and progressive muscle relaxation may also help individuals to lower the energy of circuits and the tension in their bodies. In addition, biofeedback can be used to teach couples and family members how to regulate these processes. The majority of these techniques are discussed in Chapter 6.

Metacognition can be used as well, which includes the awareness that emotions influence thought and perception, and that we may be able to experience two seemingly conflictual emotions about the same person or experience (Siegel, 1999).

COGNITION VERSUS EMOTION

An interesting controversy has arisen about how cognition and emotion influence each other. For many years it was assumed that cognition was the primary organizer of human experience in the brain (LeDoux, 2000). In fact, this served as the foundation for many theories of psychology. Cognitive therapy rested on the premise that there is a reciprocal interaction between cognition, mood, and behavior and that thoughts greatly influence mood and behavior (Beck et al., 1979). The early Greek Stoic philosopher Epictetus is often quoted by cognitive therapists as saying, "What disturbs human beings most is not the things themselves, but their conceptions of things" (Epictetus, M5 [undated]). Hence, much of the cognitive revolution focused on the cognitive processes as having a profound effect on a person's mood and behavior.

The cognitive revolution was spurred on by earlier discoveries about the brain and its various areas, particularly the neocortex, which facilitates the ability to think in abstract terms. The neocortex is three times the size of the limbic center (often called the emotional brain). The discovery of the neocortex gave fuel to the assumption that thinking, therefore, must be predominant over emotion and has a major influence on human behavior. The neocortex specifically enables human beings to articulate and engage in symbolic thought, as well as abstract categorical thinking. Hence, it was assumed that this area of the brain was responsible for most of the organization of human experience. Consequently, if this is accurate, one would expect to see many more neural connections from the thinking brain to the emotional brain, as opposed to the reverse (Atkinson, 2005).

However, over the past several decades, neuroscientists have called for a reformulation of this understanding of the neocortex, particularly in light of discoveries suggesting that the emotional brain dominates in the organization of human function. Recent research indicates that neural connections from the emotional systems to the cognitive systems appear to be stronger than the connections from the cognitive to the emotional systems (LeDoux, 1996). LeDoux found that neural projections from the brain's emotional (limbic) systems connect to just about every other part of the brain and influence each stage of cognitive processing. However, not all cognitive processes project to the emotional centers. This would suggest a one-way circuitry, which led LeDoux to the idea that emotion can clearly and primarily influence what individuals focus on via their interpretations of what they perceive. This idea is further supported by the finding that emotions are intrinsically linked to appraisal–arousal mechanisms in both hemispheres of the brain and influence all aspects of cognition, ranging from perception to decision making (Siegel, 1999).

In contrast, many cognitive theories are rooted in the belief that logical thinking is the most effective way to deal with situations, particularly those involving important decisions. Consequently, mediating emotional content that might interfere with rational thinking has always been strongly encouraged by cognitive therapists (Beck, 1967; Beck et al., 1979). However, some researchers, such as Damasio (1999), have found that individuals who were most able to keep their emotions out of the decision-making process and focus on purely rational thought actually made terrible decisions (Damasio, 2001). Damasio contends that the human brain is wired in such a manner that subtle stimuli can often bias cognitive processes without the thinker's awareness, thus creating the possibility that an individual may think he or she is being perfectly rational (Damasio, 1999). This contention is supported in part by studies showing that individuals are often unaware of experiencing emotion, when physiological evidence from a galvanic skin response or other types of physical display demonstrate that they are (LeDoux, 1996; Goleman, 1995). This is contrary to the belief that it is neurologically impossible for emotion to be activated without the individual's awareness. LeDoux (1994, 2000) has taken this finding further to explain how the brain forms memories about emotional events that one experiences in life, referring to it as *emotional memory*. This becomes important in working with couples and families, particularly because emotional memory seems to be at the heart of much of the conflict we see with couples and families.

Cognitive theorists continue to argue, however, that emotions simmer beneath the threshold of awareness, yet are still activated neurologically through conscious thought. Because thoughts are often spontaneous, a person may not immediately recognize the impact of his or her thoughts or emotions (Beck, 1976; Gardner, 1985).

As a result of his studies, Damasio (2001) has suggested that a superior definition of what it means to be rational includes the notion that rationality depends on the ability to experience emotion, both in reaction to present situations and when remembering past situations and visualizing future situations (Atkinson, 2005).

Understanding the neuroscience of emotion is important in the process of family therapy because the brain contributes substantially to an individual's ability to function and the individual's own awareness of his or her internal states. The point is not to give ammunition to family members who want to blame their brain chemistry for their actions. Rather, increasing our awareness about our internal states may, in turn, prompt certain brain functions to become more active and, thereby, modulate reason and emotion. In his book *Emotional Intelligence in Couples Therapy*, Atkinson (2005) suggests that the concept of awareness of internal states might be extremely useful in enabling clients to shift from defensive, isolating brain circuits that generate rage and fear to connect to healing circuits that mediate calm and sorrow. He proposes that giving immediate and thorough attention to clients' defensive neural systems allows a therapist to coach clients through sympathetically and respectfully interactive brain states until they feel safe enough to switch to more vulnerable states (p. 32). Atkinson sees the internal sense of safety as the "linchpin of change for couples." Only when an individual no longer feels threatened by his or her partner will the amygdala shut off. That, in turn, will affect the internal alarm system, freeing the person to authentically shift to an intimacy-promoting neural state.

Cognitive-behavioral strategies are an important part of therapy, particularly in affecting the structure of the brain that houses the prefrontal cortex. The key difference, however, is that some theorists believe that rather than using cognition to harness the limbic brain, it might be more effective to put it to work through the amygdala and gradually relax its defensiveness. Atkinson clearly has a point when he suggests that a broader perspective of the cognitive–emotional interplay in the circuitry of the brain is central to facilitate change. However, for many, accessing such a process may be more practical via cognitive and/or behavioral processes, which are addressed in detail in subsequent chapters of this book. Hopefully, additional research in the future will give clarity to this debate and provide us with new information to use in our work with couples and families.

5

Methods of Clinical Assessment

The issue of marital happiness was one of the earliest topics studied by researchers and continues to be a popular topic of study (Terman, 1938). We know from the research literature that one of the most common complaints reported by couples is problems with communication and lack of emotional affection (Doss et al., 2004). Interestingly, mates often demonstrate little agreement on their reasons for therapy. In fact, their reasons for seeking therapy may be very different from the therapist's impressions of the couple's problem. This has been consistently found in the research literature (Geiss & O'Leary, 1991; Whisman, Dixon, & Johnson, 1997). It is for these reasons that therapists need to assess each partner and family member carefully. Clinicians cannot afford to generalize with their assessment procedures or they may run the risk of missing the real motive for a person's seeking intervention.

Most seasoned and skilled clinicians know that case conceptualization is critical to the initial assessment process and that the success of treatment rests on the accuracy of careful investigation. For this reason, it is important to spend time formulating an accurate conceptualization of a couple's or family's situation. This may prove difficult in certain environments, such as in managed care where the number of sessions slated for assessment is limited. In such cases, the therapist must be creative and rely on a shortened form of assessment, resorting to inventories, which are discussed later in this chapter.

Traditionally, couple and family therapy has been characterized by a noted division between assessment and the actual delivery of therapy

(Cierpka, 2005). Many of the traditional methods of assessment involved basic information gathering and only a superficial understanding of relationship dynamics proceeding to develop a therapeutic relationship that muddies the lines between assessment and treatment (Finn & Tonsager, 1977). This trend appears to be changing, however, with the onset of evidence-based practice and the need to remain systematically mindful of conducting a good solid assessment before embarking on the delivery of treatment.

Individual and joint interviews with the members of a couple or a family, self-report questionnaires, and the therapist's behavioral observation of family interactions are the three main modes of clinical assessment (Epstein & Baucom, 2002; Snyder, Cavell, Heffer, & Mangrum, 1995; Dattilio & Padesky, 1990). The goals of assessment are to (1) identify strengths and problematic characteristics of the individuals, the couple or family, and the environment, (2) place current individual and family functioning in the context of its developmental stage and changes, and (3) identify the cognitive–affective and behavioral aspects of family interaction that could be targeted for intervention. In addition, therapists should also familiarize themselves with the couple's or family members' *dance*, as the systems theorists say, getting a good handle on how the system functions and how power and control are balanced. We want a window into what makes the family members tick, how they deal with crisis and conflict, and, most of all, what causes the system to malfunction.

We should also keep in mind that assessment continues throughout the course of treatment. Even though the initial phase of assessment may appear to be the formal inquiry, assessment should continue even until the end of treatment, inasmuch as the therapist will always discover new information about a couple or family that may change or modify the course of treatment. A good clinician continues to reappraise the case long after treatment is under way.

INITIAL JOINT INTERVIEWS

Joint interviews with a couple or a family are an important source of information about past and current functioning. Not only are they a source of information about the members' memories and opinions concerning characteristics and events in their relationships, conjoint interviews also give the therapist an opportunity to observe the family interactions firsthand. Although a family may alter its usual behavior in front of an outsider who is a stranger, even during the first interview it is common for members to exhibit some aspects of their typical pattern, especially when the therapist engages them in describing the issues that have brought them to therapy. Cognitive-behavioral therapists approach assessment in an empirical manner, using initial impressions to form hypotheses that must be tested by gathering additional information in subsequent sessions.

In the treatment of families, cognitive-behavioral therapists generally begin the assessment process by convening as many family members as are likely to be involved with the presenting concerns. Rather than insisting on everyone's attendance in order to begin therapy, however, the therapist focuses on engaging those members who are motivated to attend and then works with them in engaging absent members. Ideally, all family members are invited; however, at times there may be resistance (Dattilio, 2003). Outlying members can sometimes hold up the entire process, thus thwarting the intervention. Therefore, I try to have every member of a family present, but if this is not possible, I work with those members who are motivated to receive treatment. I rarely leave the decision to the family members or accept their word on who will or will not attend. If certain members refuse to come in, I call them by phone and have them tell me themselves that they are not interested. Often, when I call and reassure them that I need their help, they consent to attend.

Like therapists with other systems-oriented models, cognitive-behavioral therapists assume that the difficulties a family presents may be a sample of a broader problematic family process. Thus, beginning with the initial contact, the therapist is observing the family process and forming hypotheses about patterns that may be contributing to the problems that brought the family to therapy.

Gathering Background Information

During the initial joint interview, the therapist asks each member of the family about his or her reasons for seeking assistance, about each person's perspective on those concerns, and about any changes that each member thinks would make family life more satisfying. The therapist also asks about the family history (e.g., how and when the couple met, what initially attracted the partners to each other, when they married (if relevant), when any children were born, and any events that they believe have influenced them as a family over the years. Applying a stress and coping model of assessment, the therapist systematically explores the demands the couple or the family has experienced, based on characteristics of individual members (e.g., a spouse's residual effects from childhood abuse), relationship dynamics (e.g., unresolved differences in partners' desires for intimacy and autonomy), and their environment (e.g., heavy job demands on a parent's/spouse's time and energy). The therapist also inquires about resources the family has to cope with those demands and any factors that influenced its use of the resources, such as a belief in self-sufficiency that blocks some people from seeking or accepting help from outsiders (Epstein & Baucom, 2002). Throughout the interview, the therapist gathers information about the family members' cognitions, emotional responses, and behavior toward each other. If a husband becomes withdrawn after his wife criticizes his parenting skills, the therapist may draw this to his attention and ask what thoughts and emotions he experienced upon hearing his wife's comments. He might reveal automatic thoughts such as, "She doesn't respect me. This is hopeless," and feelings of both anger and deep sadness.

CONSULTATION WITH PREVIOUS THERAPISTS AND OTHER MENTAL HEALTH PROVIDERS

Couples and families who come for treatment often have been to other treatment providers during their lifetimes for the same or other types of problems. An important question for the therapist is whether to contact these previous providers for information regarding the case. Many therapists believe that they can start from scratch, despite what may have occurred during the course of earlier treatment. Others feel that they may gain vital information from other treatment providers as to what occurred and what was (and was not) effective in their particular approaches. In fact, therapists are often surprised by the information they gain from former treating therapists that the couple or family has failed to convey.

If one of the spouses is currently in individual therapy when a couple comes for family therapy, it can be helpful to consult with his or her therapist. Consider the following case, in which a couple was experiencing difficulty in a 26-year marriage.

THE CASE OF SAM AND JERRI

Sam had a long history of alcohol and cocaine abuse early in his marriage to Jerri. He had discontinued cocaine use years before, but continued with alcohol until 3 years prior to their entering marital therapy. Their relationship was fraught with Jerri's constant frustrations with Sam's alcohol use and her belief that he was hiding money and having extramarital relationships. Despite being an alcoholic, Sam denied ever hiding any money or being deceitful, but his wife simply could not accept that and assumed the worst. Once Sam had attended a rehabilitation center and followed up with AA (Alcoholic Anonymous), he stopped drinking and seemed to straighten up and attend to their family business, as well as to his relationship with his wife. Despite this improvement, however, Jerri continued to suspect that Sam was being deceitful.

Much of the present tension revolved around Sam's feeling that he could never win with his wife and that, no matter what he did, she did not believe he was being honest. At one point, Jerri even urged him to submit to a polygraph test, which Sam agreed to do. Yet he feared that he might fail, owing to the heart condition he had developed because of his earlier cocaine use. Jerri had no history of substance abuse, but displayed many of the characteristics that Sam often said fit the criteria for a borderline personality disorder. Sam reported that he had been online, looking up various disorders, and had come upon a site that listed personality disorders. When he read the criteria for "borderline personality disorder," he felt that this description best fit his wife. She had difficulties with trust, imagined abandonment, and had had a tumultuous upbringing, in which her father was abusive to her.

Many of these issues were addressed in therapy. I relied heavily on the fact that each of the spouses was in individual therapy. During the course of couple therapy, Sam asked whether Jerri's therapist was addressing the issues of her unreasonable suspiciousness and fear of abandonment. He also stated that Jerri would often put him in a double bind (that "he would never do the right thing in her eyes"), which was very stressful and frustrating for him. Sam cited the example of a time when he was on business trip. When he telephoned home, his wife informed him that she had gone to the doctor's office and received some abnormal Pap smear results. Sam voiced his concern and said that he wanted to return home early from the trip in order to be supportive to his wife, but Jerri said that there was no need for him to do so. Sam claims that he said several times, "I want to come home early so I can be with you," and Jerri reassured him that it was not necessary, and insisted that he complete his business trip. Subsequently, Sam continued with the rest of his trip as planned. He claimed that when he arrived home, Jerri berated him, stating that he should have come home anyway, despite her telling him not to, because that was the "right thing to do." Sam said he felt that he was locked in a "damned if you do, damned if you don't" situation. "I can't live with this," he stated. "It drives me crazy, this kind of stuff. It seems like she is playing head games with me and will flip-flop at the drop of a hat." Sam further said that he did not feel that Jerri was telling her therapist about these behaviors and wondered about how therapy services should be coordinated.

I suggested coordinating treatment with the spouses' individual therapists. All parties agreed, and I contacted each of the individual therapists for a three-way telephone conference. Both individual therapists agreed that it would be useful, and it was decided that such conferences would occur at varying intervals during the course of treatment. They occurred every 3 months for 1 year and proved to be extremely helpful in keeping all parties on the same page with treatment. Ultimately, Sam and Jerri made great strides in therapy, and their relationship became warmer and more trusting, thanks in large part to my being able to coordinate with their individual therapists.

Although some mental health professionals may scoff at this idea, it really does make a lot of sense to coordinate treatment. It helps to ensure that the various professionals involved with a couple are not working at cross-purposes, but are headed in the same general direction. Coordinating interventions, obviously, has to be exercised with caution, and all therapists have to agree. However, it can often be very useful and lead to productive results.

INVENTORIES AND QUESTIONNAIRES

Cognitive-behavioral therapists commonly use standardized questionnaires to gather information on family members' views of themselves and their relationships. This is particularly helpful when a therapist's time is limited, such as in managed care situations. A therapist often asks couples and family members to complete questionnaires before the intake interviews, so that he or she can ask for additional information about the questionnaire responses during the initial interviews. Naturally, individuals' reports on questionnaires are subject to bias, such as blaming others for family problems and presenting themselves in a socially desirable way (Snyder et al., 1995). Nevertheless, judicious use of questionnaires can be an efficient means of surveying family members' perceptions of a wide range of issues that might otherwise be overlooked in the intake interview. Issues that are noted on questionnaires can also be explored in greater depth through subsequent interviews and through behavioral observation.

Assigning inventories and questionnaires early in the assessment period may also help determine the motivation of spouses or family members to make changes in their relationships. Motivation to change is one of the best prognostic indicators of successful treatment.

A variety of measures have been developed to provide an overview of key areas of couple and family functioning, such as overall satisfaction, cohesion, communication quality, decision making, values, and level of conflict.[1] Examples include the Dyadic Adjustment Scale (Spanier, 1976), the Marital Satisfaction Inventory—Revised (Snyder & Aikman, 1999), the Family Environment Scale (Moos & Moos, 1986), the Family Assessment Device (Epstein, Baldwin, & Bishop, 1983), and the Self-Report Family Inventory (Beavers, Hampson, & Hulgus, 1985). Because the items on such scales do not provide specific information about each family member's cognitions, emotions, and behavioral responses regarding a relationship problem, the therapist must inquire about these during interviews.

For example, if scores on a questionnaire indicate limited cohesion among family members, the therapist might ask the members about (1) their

---

[1]Discussed here are some representative questionnaires for assessment within a cognitive-behavioral model, even though many were not developed specifically from that perspective. Resources for reviews on a variety of other relevant measures can be found in Touliatos, Perlmutter, and Straus (1990).

personal standards for types and degrees of cohesive behavior, (2) specific instances of behavior among them that did or did not feel cohesive, and (3) positive or negative emotional responses they experience concerning those actions. Thus, questionnaires can be helpful in identifying areas of strength and concern, but a more fine-grained analysis is needed to understand specific types of positive and negative interaction and the factors affecting them.

An advantage of general couple and family functioning inventories is that their subscales provide a profile of areas of strength and deficits within the couple or family. Moreover, some family members are likely to report concerns on questionnaires that they would not mention during joint family interviews.

However, many inventories are long, and therapists must decide whether they can gather comparable information more efficiently through interviews.

A number of questionnaires developed specifically from a cognitive-behavioral perspective can also be helpful in the assessment of couples and families. For example, Eidelson and Epstein's (1982) Relationship Belief Inventory assesses five common unrealistic beliefs that have been associated with relationship distress and communication problems in couples: (1) disagreement is destructive, (2) partners should be able to mind read each other's thoughts and feelings, (3) partners cannot change their relationship, (4) innate gender differences determine relationship problems, and (5) one should be a perfect sexual partner. Baucom et al.'s (1996) Inventory of Specific Relationship Standards assesses the degrees to which individuals hold standards for their couple relationship regarding boundaries (degree of autonomy versus sharing), distribution and exercise of power/control, and investment of time and energy in the relationship.

Roehling and Robin's (1986) Family Beliefs Inventory assesses unrealistic beliefs that adolescents and their parents may hold concerning each other. The parents' form assesses the beliefs that (1) if adolescents are given too much freedom, they will behave in ways that will ruin their future, (2) parents deserve absolute obedience from their children, (3) adolescents' behavior should be perfect, (4) adolescents intentionally behave in malicious ways toward their parents, (5) parents are blameworthy for problems in their children's behavior, and (6) parents must gain the approval of their children for their child-rearing methods. In turn, the adolescents' form includes subscales assessing the beliefs that (1) parents' rules and demands will ruin the adolescent's life, (2) parents' rules are unfair, (3) adolescents should have as much autonomy as they desire, and (4) parents should have to earn their children's approval for their child-rearing methods. In addition, a number of instruments have been developed to assess partners' attributions concerning the causes of events in their couple relationships (e.g., Baucom et al., 1996b; Pretzer et al., 1991).

There are a few self-report questionnaires that provide information about specific types of behavior that partners perceive occurring in their relationship. Christensen's (1988) Communication Patterns Questionnaire is most relevant for a systemic view of couple interaction, because the items ask about the occurrence of dyadic patterns regarding areas of conflict, including mutual attack, demand–withdrawal, and mutual avoidance. In addition, the revised Conflict Tactics Scale (CTS2; Straus, Hamby, Boney-McCoy, & Sugarman, 1996) provides information about a range of verbal and nonverbal forms of abusive behavior in couple relationships that many individuals choose not to reveal during interviews.

To date, no questionnaires are available to assess family members' moment-to-moment or typical emotional responses to each other (except overall level of distress). Therefore, it may be prudent to rely on interviews to track the emotional components of family interaction.

Numerous other self-report questionnaires have been developed to assess aspects of parent–child relationships and general family functioning. Excellent reviews of these measures can be found in the texts by Grotevant and Carlson (1989), Touliatos, Perlmutter, and Strauss (1990), and Jacob and Tennebaum (1988). Some instruments, such as the Family Environment Scale (Moos & Moos, 1986), and the Family Adaptability and Cohesion Evaluation Scales–III (Olson, Portner, & Lavee, 1985), assess family members' global perceptions of such family characteristics as cohesion, problem solving, communication quality, role clarity, emotional expression, and values. Other scales, such as the Family Inventory of Life Events and Changes (McCubbin, Patterson, & Wilson, 1985), Family Crisis-Oriented Personal Evaluation Scales (McCubbin, Larsen, & Olsen, 1985), and the Family of Origin Inventory (Stuart, 1995), provide more specialized assessment of family functioning (e.g., members' perceptions of particular stressors and family coping strategies). Because the family of origin is also an important factor in treatment, as mentioned previously, the Family of origin Scale (Hovestadt, Anderson, Piercy, Cochran, & Fine, 1985) is an excellent tool to measure the self-perceived levels of health in a person's family of origin. In general, these scales do not provide data about specific cognitive, behavioral, and affective variables central to assessment, but they do tap into a variety of important components of family functioning likely to be of interest to family therapists.

A few instruments focus on family members' attitudes about parenting roles and thus are more directly relevant to cognitive assessment. The basic reason for using these inventories in the early stages of the family assessment is to draw on the family members' ability to express themselves nonverbally. Sometimes they are more willing to answer items on inventories than to reveal themselves verbally in the family context. In addition, they allow clinicians to highlight specific areas to focus on and address during individual or family sessions. For example, if several members of a family respond to an issue concerning trusting other family members on the Family Belief Inventory, this is certainly an area to pinpoint during the course of questioning. An affirmative response to the statement, "Our family members don't know how to communicate with each other," is also an area to address.

Although these inventories focus on cognitions and beliefs, they are not always enough to reveal more serious psychopathology, which can indeed cause turbulence in the course of couple or family therapy.

Depending on the extent of a psychopathology, additional psychodiagnostic testing may be required. If the treating clinician is not necessarily trained in clinical psychology, he or she should make a referral for psychodiagnostic assessment to narrow or clarify a specific mental disorder. This is particularly important when the clinical picture becomes mixed and the need to rule out certain disorders becomes critical. For example, differentiating between schizoaffective disorders and bipolar disorders in regard to treatment is often a challenge. Determining whether a psychotic process does exist or a delusional system is intact may make a tremendous difference in the course and outline of treatment. Whenever a therapist suspects that any significant psychopathology exists, I definitely recommend that the therapist refers the individual for a psychodiagnostic assessment, inasmuch as it is extremely important to determine if such diagnoses exist early in the treatment process.

As noted earlier, even though all of these cognitive and behavioral measures are the individuals' subjective reports of their experiences in their relationships, they can provide useful information about aspects of couple and family interaction that are not otherwise observable by the therapist. The measures that are discussed here are very helpful as adjuncts to careful interviewing and assessment. Some of the case examples in Chapter 9 illustrate how I use such measures during the course of treatment.

ADDITIONAL PSYCHOLOGICAL
TESTING AND APPRAISALS

Occasionally, the need may arise for more specific assessment, especially if serious psychopathology is suspected in spouses or family members. The Minnesota Multiphasic Personality Inventory–2 (MMPI-2) and the Millon Clinical Multiaxial Inventory (MCMI) are two of the more popular instruments for determining levels of psychopathy in individuals. Family therapists who are also licensed as psychologists may, if they are comfortable with using these measures, elect to employ personality or projective testing in order to determine if a personality disorder exists with one or more family members that might impede the course of treatment. They may also elect to refer to an independent source for such testing and assessment. It is important to determine whether more serious psychopathology exists in order to plan for an adjustment in the treatment process and/or to alter its course. In cases in which serious psychopathology does exist in one or more family members, a referral for individual treatment may be necessary.

Couple and family therapists who are not licensed as psychologists are cautioned to adhere to their respective state laws regarding qualification in employing psychological tests so as to avoid violating the law (Dattilio, Tresco, & Siegel, 2007).

In any event, more detailed assessment is always recommended in order to optimize the assessment process and render a more effective plan of treatment.

GENOGRAMS

Genogram diagrams of an extended family system have been used frequently by couple and family therapists. Unlike a family tree, which includes only names, dates, and places, a genogram is used both diagnostically and therapeutically to uncover important information about a person's history and family of origin. Genograms include emotional processes, such as triangles, fusion, emotional cutoffs, and deaths. Genogramming has been a significant aspect of family therapy and a frequently used technique almost since the beginning of the family therapy movement. For several decades, its many advantages have contributed to its continued use. Genogramming has been written about extensively in certain texts (McGoldrick, Gerson, & Petry, 2008; Kaslow, 1995).

A genogram relies on the use of symbols to depict family members across generations. This is particularly important when dealing with mental illness and psychopathology in tracing the connecting links to a person's family of origin. The process also helps individuals to depict those relatives who make up their historic past and present and who may have contributed to a specific mental illness. To create a genogram, individuals are asked to draw a family schematic for as far back as they can remember. The family schematic descends, beginning at the top of the page, from the senior progenitors to the youngest children in the group. A chronological diagram emerges, showing how people are related to one another, and may contain information such as dates of birth, marriage, divorce, and death. An area of particular interest is explored by attempting to trace whether any emotional or behavioral problem or clarified mental illness was present in any of the ancestors. Typically, this involves having a patient or a family embark on visiting living members of the family of origin and jog their memories for missing information. The therapist's role is to coach the individual on the specific questions to ask in order to obtain relevant information. Interestingly, in many cases, individuals have unearthed long buried family secrets that clearly affected the course of treatment.

The reason for having individuals produce genograms is also to put them in touch with the intergenerational transmission process, as Bowen (1978) referred to it. Such information shows clear reasons for the way things were done, or how a person's pathology evolved through the generations of family members. This is not an excuse for individuals to blame their problems on ancestors, but a tool to understand how links occur.

Figure 5.1 is a genogram with a key for the symbols used.

Genogramming has also been a very useful process in aiding many to become aware of a family's tendency to triangulate relationships, which is believed by some theorists to be a source of mental illness. Triangulation is a reactive process whereby a third person who is sensitized to the anxiety in a couple or family moves in to offer reassurance or calm things down. A classic example is the teenage daughter who attempts to reduce her parents' intense marital conflict by talking individually to each parent or to the parent with whom she has the most influence. In this respect, her intervention serves to pull the parents together. As her parents grow to be dependent on her intervening, she becomes triangulated, which can often be a very uncomfortable or burdensome role for her. Consequently, such information may help individuals learn how to detriangulate and ultimately develop more healthy and satisfying interpersonal relationships with their own immediate families. For an excellent resource on genograms, see McGoldrick et al. (2008) or Kaslow (1995).

ONGOING ASSESSMENT AND CASE CONCEPTUALIZATION THROUGHOUT THE COURSE OF THERAPY

As stated earlier, case conceptualization is ongoing throughout the entire course of treatment and does not cease after the assessment phase. Although the bulk of the assessment may occur during the intake period, therapists continue to reassess the situation as they gain more knowledge about the couple or family they are treating. It is important that therapists also inform families with whom they work that the assessment process will be ongoing until the end of treatment and that, depending on what surfaces, it may alter or change the course of treatment.

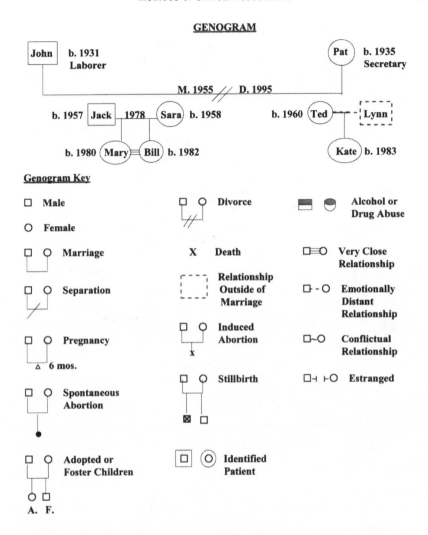

FIGURE 5.1. Genogram.

SPECIFIC DIFFICULTIES
WITH THE ASSESSMENT PROCESS

Certain difficulties can arise during the course of the assessment phase. One has to do with information that is shared during individual sessions with spouses or family members that the person revealing the information requests to be kept in confidence. This often places the therapist in a precarious position, such as when a spouse confesses that he or she has had an extramarital affair, but doesn't want the indiscretion revealed. Once such information is shared, be it in confidence or not, the therapist has already colluded with the revealing spouse, which renders that therapist less objective. Unfortunately, there is little that can be done about this situation. It is best handled in one of two ways. Some therapists choose to take a rigid stance and say, "You must end the affair and confess to your spouse or I will not treat you." This is unrealistic, in my opinion. A therapist is better off reviewing the negative impact that the affair (and secrecy about it) will have on treatment, and allowing the offending spouse to decide whether to disclose it. If that person experiences difficulty in deciding, then it is appropriate to refer him or her for individual therapy. Either way, it is not the role of the therapist to reveal the confidential material to the other spouse. It should be the responsibility of the offending spouse to choose to do so.

The same holds for a family member who reveals in a private session that he or she has committed an act that he or she wants kept secret from the other family members. Sometimes, spouses or family members can become very angry with a therapist when they learn that he or she was aware of certain information and did not reveal it. I usually explain to clients up front the ethical constraints I have as a therapist and why I cannot reveal such information, but do indicate that I have encouraged the offending individual to take responsibility for him- or herself and share this appropriately.

In addition, there are times when confidentiality needs to be broken, such as in reporting elder abuse or the abuse of a child. Moreover, every therapist must adhere to his or her duty to warn the appropriate party in the event that any threats are made against that person.

Family therapists vary widely in the extent to which they conduct formal assessments. Typically, when an individual is interviewed, a structured interviewing schedule, such as the Structured Clinical Interview Schedule for DSM-IV (SCID; Spitzer, Williams, Gibbon, & First, 1994), may be used to render a differential diagnosis. Various psychological tests, including projective techniques and personality inventories, may also be ordered. One thing that seems to be universally agreed upon is that, regardless of the approach in assessment, most therapists probably spend too little time making careful and detailed evaluations of individuals and their families before embarking on treatment.

When involving a family in treatment, an important step is to identify problems that have become entrenched because they are embedded in powerful, but often invisible structures. Thus, becoming aware of and developing a clear understanding about the family structure is extremely important in understanding the development of psychopathology and how the family perpetuates such problems. The ways in which the problem impacts the family and affects that dynamic is also important for a therapist to focus on.

Therapists need to ask about actual functioning subsystems and the nature of the boundaries between partners.

An additional area of importance is the determination of boundaries in couple or family systems, along with the identification of any existing triangles. Triangles are described as a stable relationship structure that involves a third person (Guerin, 2002). Identifying triangles is also a very important part of early assessment. A further understanding of who plays what roles in the family is essential, particularly with matters of power and control. From a cognitive-behavioral standpoint, understanding the schemas and interrelationships that contribute to family dysfunction is key to developing a solid treatment plan.

BEHAVIORAL OBSERVATIONS AND CHANGE

Because of the limitations of self-report inventories, it is extremely important for a clinician to observe samples of a couple's or family members' interactions directly. Careful and detailed observation of behavior and its consequences are crucial in developing an understanding of family dynamics. In my early family therapy training in the 1970s, prior to the era of DVDs, we recorded sessions with an earlier form of videotape known as a Beta Max. There were often problems with the Beta Max in that a picture was visible, but there was no sound, owing to the flaws in the mechanism. I recall that, on one occasion, this serendipitously gave my supervisor the idea of having us watch videotapes of families without the sound in order to simply observe their nonverbal behavior. It was interesting to see how many of us, as students, could make inferences on the basis of nonverbal behavior and later elaborate on them once we had sound to match to the video footage. There is a lot to be said about nonverbal behavior and what can be discerned from it. It is important to note that a verbal exchange sometimes distracts observers from the nonverbal behavior, which is of equal, and sometimes greater, importance.

Opportunities for behavioral observations exist from the first moment a family enters a therapist's office. An experienced couple and family therapist becomes adept at noticing the process of verbal and nonverbal behaviors between family members as they talk to one another and the therapist. Although the topic and the content of the discussions are important, the goal of systematic behavioral observation is to identify specific acts by each individual, and the sequence of acts among family members, that are either constructive and pleasing or destructive and aversive. In particular, those behaviors that may be destructive, aversive, and manipulative should be noted and documented. The observation of family interaction can vary according to the amount of structure the clinician imposes on the interaction, as well as the amount of structure in the clinician's observation criteria or coding system.

Obviously, family members' act differently while in the therapist's office from the way they act at home, but, through interactions, family members can reveal significant patterns that provide insight into issues in the relationships. With disorders such as depression and schizophrenia, there are often dominant themes in the family interaction between parent and child, in which they may cut off or devalue each other in subtle ways. These are clearly areas of note for clinicians. Determining which family members tend to be more spontaneous, as opposed to others who fade into the background, is often very telling. One of the benefits of imposing very little structure in family therapy is the ability to sample a family's communication in a natural way within the office setting. In this manner, the therapist can pinpoint where a significant amount of dysfunction occurs.

STRUCTURED FAMILY INTERACTION

In contrast to allowing a relatively unstructured interaction, clinicians can provide a family with specific topics for discussion, which may be even more revealing in regard to how its members function together. The goals of family members, such as trying to understand one another's thinking patterns and feelings, or to resolve particular relationship issues, may be pertinent. What family members do with each other's emotions is extremely important. This is seen particularly in areas of severe psychopathology. For example, using some of the inventories mentioned previously, such as Spanier's (1976) Dyadic Adjustment Scale, may allow individuals to rate the degree of conflict in which their interaction affects one another. The demonstration of affection, amount of time spent together, and so on, helps the clinician to select specific content area to focus on in treatment. Obviously, as a skilled clinician begins to observe various behaviors, areas of weakness and disturbance will surface, particularly when heated issues arise. A skilled clinician is able to look for coalitions or alliances that are formed among family members and illustrate how they contribute to polarization within a family unit. A detailed list of questionnaires and inventories to use with couples and families appears in Appendix A.

A good way to observe what goes on in a family is to instruct its members to engage in problem-solving discussions during the course of a session. During such discussions, the therapist can actually see the difficulties in communication. This technique is similar to the enactment that Salvador Minuchin and other family therapists have used in treatment (Minuchin, 1974). Depending on the modality of treatment the clinician is using, he or she may choose to become more directive in the process and focus on certain interventions. Family members who fail to define a problem in specific behavioral terms may handicap themselves in developing a feasible solution. Others fail to evaluate advantages and disadvantages of proposed solutions and subsequently become discouraged when they try to carry out a solution and encounter unanticipated obstacles or drawbacks. Hence, the therapist may choose a particular intervention to address the issues in different ways.

How family members deal with frustrations in themselves and others often provides therapists with clues as to what may contribute to anxiety and depression in the family system. By observing family members' discussions during therapy sessions, a clinician can identify specific problematic behaviors and can plan interventions to improve family problem-solving skills and address issues of dysfunction. A clinician's observation of repetitive patterns of thought, emotion, and behavior that may contribute to depression or anxiety is important in uncovering dysfunctional patterns among family members. Using basic principles of functional analysis, a clinician can observe antecedent events and consequences that may be controlling the negative interaction between family members.

For example, parents may complain repeatedly that their child rarely reveals his feelings, but, interestingly, the clinician observes that whenever the child does express his feelings, his parents either turn away or overtly cut him off and deny his feelings by saying, "Well, you shouldn't feel this way" or "No, you shouldn't feel that way, it's foolish." Such circular causal processes in family interactions can be observed when a clinician notes how one individual's behavior prompts the other's withdrawal and vice versa, and the effect that this has on an individual's dynamics. This dynamic can be highlighted in terms of acknowledging destructive patterns that may be contributing to depression and low-self esteem or any one of a number of elements of psychopathology.

ASSESSMENT OF COGNITIONS

Clinical interviews with family members together, or individually, provide opportunities for clinicians to elicit idiosyncratic cognitions and to track influential processes that cannot be assessed by standardized questionnaires. *Socratic questioning* is a method that involves a series of (systematic) questions that are used to chip away at defenses, both during the exploration and assessment phase and at the beginning of treatment, in order to uncover a person's thoughts and underlying beliefs (Dattilio, 2000; Beck, 1995). Socratic questioning may enable a clinician to piece together a chain of thoughts that mediate between events and relationships and each individual's emotional and behavioral responses. An approach that uses Socratic questioning involves a technique known as *downward arrow*, developed by Aaron Beck and associates (1979). This technique was developed to uncover the underlying assumptions of an individual that generate dysfunctional or distorted thoughts. The clinician using the downward-arrow technique identifies the initial thought and then follows it with questions like "If so, then what?"

For example, a therapist treated a family with an adult son who was reluctant to move out because he felt the need to remain attached to his family for "safety." He had become avoidant and withdrew socially, requiring excessive and constant reassurance from his family. The downward-arrow technique yielded the results shown in Figure 5.2.

As this technique revealed, the son's core belief rested on the fear of failure and even death. He believed he was nothing without his family. Interestingly, in reviewing the family dynamics, the therapist found that although the parents wanted very much to see their son go out and be successful with his life, they also had their own doubts about his ability to survive on his own and subtly reinforced his remaining at home. Use of the same technique in examining the parents' cognitions uncovered some of their fears that perhaps their son wasn't capable of functioning on his own, despite the fact

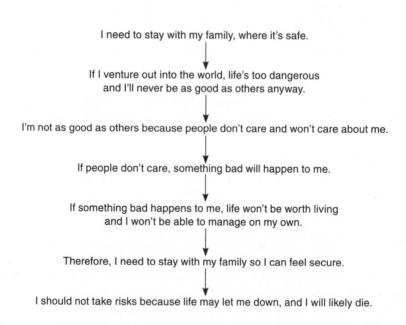

FIGURE 5.2. Downward arrow of avoidant son.

that he was an adult. It also uncovered the hidden aspect of the parents' own counterdependence: "We would be lost without him needing us any more." So, many of his parents' behaviors were subtly reinforcing his dependence and staying at home, when, overtly, they were making statements that they wanted him to move out and become more independent. This type of subtle double-bind situation seemed to create a lot of confusion and dysfunction and caused stuck movement for the son, as well as the family.

Addressing cognitions of this type is very important in family treatment. Restructuring the parents' thinking so that they would become more optimistic, and actually follow through and take the risk of promoting their son's independence, would embolden them to support their son's independence. Any work done with their son in terms of his taking steps to begin to move outward, take risks, and see that maybe he is not as destined to fail as he anticipates, would be of great benefit.

It was also essential to address the parents' own dependence needs, that is, their son remaining dependent on them. The use of the downward arrow technique served to uncover an underlying schema of vulnerability and helplessness, along with the fear of failure, in all family members. The technique allowed each individual to become aware of his or her chain of thoughts, to see how it led to erroneous conclusions and reinforced longstanding assumptions that were not necessarily correct.

INDIVIDUAL INTERVIEWS

Individual interviews with each member of a family are often conducted next (after the initial conjoint session) to gather information about past and current functioning, including life stresses, psychopathology, overall health, coping strengths, and so on. Often family members are more open about describing personal difficulties such as depression, abandonment in a past relationship, and so forth, without other members present. Individual interviews give the clinician an opportunity to assess possible psychopathology that may be influenced by problems in the person's couple or family relationships (and in turn may be affecting family interactions adversely). Given the high co-occurrence of individual psychopathology and relationship problems (L'Abate, 1998), it is crucial that a couple and family therapist be skilled in assessing individual functioning or make referrals to colleagues who can assist in this task. The therapist can then determine whether joint therapy should be supplemented with individual therapy.

As noted earlier, the therapist must set clear guidelines for confidentiality during individual interviews. However, if the therapist learns that an individual is being physically abused and appears to be in danger, the focus shifts toward working with that person to develop plans to maintain safety and to take steps to exit the home and seek shelter elsewhere if the risk of abuse increases.

I have already described how the therapist has opportunities to observe couple and family interaction patterns during the initial joint interview; for example, the style in which, and degree to which, members express their thoughts and emotions to each other; who interrupts whom; and who speaks for whom. In a cognitive-behavioral approach assessment is ongoing throughout therapy, and the therapist observes family processes during each session.

These relatively unstructured behavioral observations are often supplemented by a structured communication task during the initial joint interview (Baucom & Epstein, 1990; Epstein & Baucom, 2002). Drawing from information that the couple or the family provides, the therapist may select a topic that all of the members consider an unresolved issue in their relationship and ask them to spend 10 minutes or so discussing it while the therapist videotapes them. Or the therapist might ask the family members to express their feelings about the issue and respond to each other's expressions in any way they see appropriate, or they might be asked to try to resolve the issue in the allotted time. Typically, to minimize influencing their interactions, the therapist leaves the room. Such taped problem-solving discussions are used routinely in couple and family interaction research (Weiss & Heyman, 1997), even though family members often behave somewhat differently under these conditions than they do at home. Therapists can use behavioral coding systems that were developed for research purposes, such as the Marital Interaction Coding System (MICS-1V; Heyman, Eddy, Weiss, & Vivian, 1995), as guides for identifying frequencies and sequences of family members' positive and negative verbal and nonverbal behaviors (e.g., approve, accept responsibility, positive physical contact, complaint putdown, cross-complaining). As with observations of family interaction during interviews, the cognitive-behavioral therapist considers these data to be interaction samples that might be typical of the family process but that require verification through repeated observations and reports from the family members about interactions that occur at home.

IDENTIFICATION OF MACRO-LEVEL PATTERNS AND CORE RELATIONSHIP ISSUES

The therapist collects information over the course of the joint and individual interviews, plus family members' responses to questionnaires, and looks for broad macro-level patterns and themes that may reflect core relationship issues. Thus, the cognitive-behavioral therapist takes an empirical approach to assessment, using initial observations to form hypotheses but waiting until repetitive patterns emerge before drawing conclusions about a family's central problems and strengths. For example, during the first joint family session, parents may describe setting firm limits on an adolescent daughter's behavior, and the therapist may hypothesize that there is a clear power hierarchy in the family. However, in an individual interview the daughter may reveal that she can easily bend the rules and talk her parents out of imposing punishments, and in other joint family sessions the parents may fail to respond when the daughter repeatedly interrupts them. In this case, evidence accumulates that the parents have relatively little power over the daughter's behaviors.

ASSESSING MOTIVATION TO CHANGE

One of the most important aspects to investigate during the assessment phase is *motivation to change*. This is likely one of the best prognostic indicators that a couple or family will do well in treatment. Hence, asking questions such as, "Who initiated the idea to come for treatment?" or "What brought everyone here?" is extremely important. In addition, assessing the level of discontent and state of unhappiness can indicate how motivated a couple or family may be to make a change. How hopeless spouses or family members are also affects their motivation level. Individual members' cognitions about each other's desire to change, their perception of the therapist's competence in facilitating change, and their level of tolerance for enduring change are all very important factors.

The use of early homework assignments may also serve as a test for determining motivation to change. So, although it is not typical to assign homework during the assessment phase, simply having family members complete questionnaires or do other small tasks may be an early prognostic tool. It is interesting that in a recent study conducted by Dattilio, Kazantzis, Shinkfield, and Carr (in press), couple and family therapists indicated that one of the main reasons for not assigning homework tasks was due to their anticipation of clients' noncompliance. No one gets better in treatment without hard work, and the completion of homework assignments is a good sign that clients are willing to do the work. This also gives a clue as to how they work together and tells us a lot about the family dynamics.

Finally, therapists need to rely on their gut or intuition about how motivated family members are to make a change. According to social exchange theory, if people are sufficiently disenchanted in a relationship, then the motivation level for seeking change may also be high, especially if they believe that real change can be achieved.

FEEDBACK ON THE ASSESSMENT

CBT is a collaborative approach. The cognitive-behavioral therapist continually shares his or her thoughts and impressions with the clients and, together with them, develops interventions designed to address their concerns. After collecting information from interviews, questionnaires, and behavioral observations, the therapist provides the clients a concise summary of the patterns that have emerged, including (1) their strengths, (2) their major presenting concerns, (3) life demands or stressors that have produced adjustment problems for the couple or the family, and (4) constructive and problematic macro-level patterns in their interactions that seem to be influencing their presenting problems.

The therapist and the clients then identify the clients' top priorities for change, as well as some interventions that have potential to alleviate the problems. This is also an important time for the therapist to explore potential barriers to couple or family therapy, such as members' fears of changes that they anticipate will be stressful and difficult for them, and to problem solve with the family regarding steps that could be taken to reduce the stress. It is also important for both the therapist and the clients to assess the potential working relationship between them and determine whether or not it's a good fit. Usually, the assessment period provides ample time for all to determine whether they can work together effectively, although this will continue to be reevaluated as the process of treatment progresses. The therapist should think about whether the clients seem to feel understood and ask how things are going so that he or she obtains a good sense that everyone feels sufficiently comfortable to move forward in treatment. Periodic reevaluations of the therapeutic alliance are important and should be discussed at varying intervals during the course of therapy (Dattilio, Freeman, & Blue, 1998).

IDENTIFYING AUTOMATIC
THOUGHTS AND CORE BELIEFS

A crucial prerequisite to modifying partners' or family members' distorted or extreme cognitions about themselves and each other is to increase their ability to identify their *automatic thoughts*. After introducing the concept of automatic thoughts that spontaneously flash through one's mind, the therapist coaches couple and family members in observing their patterns of thought during sessions that address their negative emotional and behavioral responses to each other. In the cognitive-behavioral model, monitoring one's subjective experiences is a skill that can be developed. In order to improve the skill of identifying their automatic thoughts, clients are typically asked to keep a small notebook handy between sessions and to jot down a brief description of the circumstances in which they feel distressed about the relationship or are engaged in conflict. This log should also include a description of the automatic thoughts that come to mind, as well as the resulting emotional responses and any behavioral responses toward other family members.

I typically use the Dysfunctional Thought Record, a modified version of the Daily Record of Dysfunctional Thoughts (Beck et al., 1979), initially developed for the identification and modification of automatic thoughts in individual cognitive therapy. Through this type of record keeping, the therapist is able to demonstrate to couples and families how their automatic thoughts are linked to emotional and behavioral responses and to help them understand the specific macro-level themes (e.g.. boundary issues) that upset them in their relationships. This procedure also increases family members' awareness that their negative emotional and behavioral responses to each other are potentially controllable through systematic examination of the cognitions associated with them. Thus, the therapist is coaching each individual in taking greater responsibility for his or her own responses. An exercise that often proves quite useful is to have couples and families review their logs individually and indicate the links between thoughts, emotions, and behavior. The therapist then asks each person to explore alternative cognitions that might produce different emotional and behavioral responses to a situation.

An example of examining automatic thoughts involves the following case in which a young South American couple, who were married only 2 years, came to me for therapy.

THE GOOD LOVER: THE CASE OF ROBERTO AND ZARIDA

Roberto and Zarida began experiencing difficulty in their relationship and felt that it was important to address it as early as possible. As a result, they received my name from Zarida's gynecologist. During the initial conjoint session, Zarida said that she felt that Roberto was overcontrolled during their sexual relations, which, over time, caused her to feel that she wasn't sure that he loved her. Yet Roberto had reminded her many times that he loved her more than anyone he had ever been involved with, which is why he chose to marry her. Zarida, however, stated that she just "felt that something wasn't right" and that Roberto seemed to be very inhibited and conservative in his lovemaking, which troubled her. Zarida went on to say that she was particularly upset because she knew that Roberto had had many sexual encounters with women during his single years and often fondly referred to him as a "Casanova." Roberto had clearly had many more sexual relationships than Zarida, who had had only one other boyfriend prior to marrying Roberto. Besides, Zarida also recalled that when she and Roberto first began dating, he was a "tiger" with her sexually and they had had some of the most enjoyable lovemaking she ever experienced.

When I asked why this troubled her so much, Zarida went on to say that she knew Roberto was known as a "good lover," and she remembered hearing from some of the other women whom he had dated that he was a very amorous man. Zarida struggled, however, with the fact that, despite Roberto's claiming how much he was in love with her, he was not very demonstrative during their sexual relations. "Our lovemaking always occurs in the same position and seems to be dull and conservative." When I asked Roberto about this in the conjoint session with Zarida, he had very little to say. I sensed that there was something else going on, at which point, with Zarida's permission, I decided to meet with Roberto alone on a separate occasion in order to explore the issue in more detail.

During the course of my individual session with Roberto, he told me that during his years as a single man, he was with a number of women and was very sexually active. He went on to describe for me in detail how his sexual relations were quite versatile and that he prided himself on being a "good lover." I tried to delve into why he had so much difficulty in being the same way with the woman whom he truly loved and had married, and he explained to me that it had to do with his attitudes and beliefs about women and sexual relations. "I was a good lover to these women because they were only my mistresses. I wasn't in love with any of them, but did lust after them. At best, maybe I was fond of them, but these former relationships consisted more of a physical attraction than a true romantic relationship." Roberto went on to explain to me that he had a dichotomous belief about "having sex with women and making love to the one whom you wed." Roberto explained to me that he didn't want to look at his wife in the same way he looked at his former mistresses, because it would somehow cheapen her. That is, he believed that if he were versatile sexually and tried different activities, such as oral sex, or other avenues of foreplay, this would place his wife in the same category as his mistresses, which was something he wanted to avoid. He said that he had the highest regard for his wife and that he didn't want to devalue their relationship by engaging her in many of the sex play activities he maintained when he was a "wild bachelor."

This conversation sparked further discussion about Roberto's rigid views and the fact that, when one engages in various sexual activities, it doesn't necessarily cheapen the love relationship. Roberto had developed a distortion about this that involved "dichotomous thinking." He derived some of this thinking from his own mother, who drove this notion into his head and always told him, "Men have sex with their girlfriends, but they make love to their wives." Interestingly, Roberto's mother had her own reasons for believing in this concept so strongly. It was her way of dealing with her own father's infidelity. It seems that her father was quite the ladies' man and had many mistresses while married to her mother. So, in order to compartmentalize her feelings in her own mind, she formulated this logic as a coping strategy and passed it on to her son.

Roberto went on to take this belief literally—that lovemaking with one's spouse had to involve a conservative demeanor and could not include any activity that might be considered "perverted" or "loose." It also came out that Roberto had some personal guilt about previously being "so promiscuous." He felt that, somehow, he might have "contaminated his wife" by transforming Zarida into one of the "loose women" he dated prior to marrying.

Much of my work with Roberto helped him see the importance of discussing his attitudes about lovemaking with Zarida. When Zarida heard his reasons, she started to laugh, relieved at the idea that this was the only reason that Roberto had not been more versatile in his sexual activity with her. Therapy then went on to focus on helping Roberto change some of his distorted beliefs about sexuality and its impact on his wife and their marriage.

Through gradual behavioral strategies, such as watching some professionally made sex therapy videos for spouses and reading prescribed materials as a collaborative homework assignment, Roberto and Zarida were able to improve their sexual relations. Roberto gradually learned to become freer with his sexual expression toward his wife without feeling as though he was being disrespectful to her or treating her as one of his former mistresses. This also seemed to help Zarida with her depression and her fears about whether her husband truly loved her.

DIFFERENTIATING CORE BELIEFS FROM SCHEMAS

Very often the terms *core belief* and *schema* are confused with each other. Core beliefs are actually one level of a schema. Schemas are the overall template through which one views the world; core beliefs may be components or a specific layer of a schema. Therefore, schemas may contain numerous core beliefs.

For example, in the case of Roberto and Zarida, Roberto's automatic thought was "I need to be sexually respectful to my wife." When he was questioned further, a core belief was uncovered: "I was a versatile lover with my mistresses because I didn't love them." When more of Roberto's schema about sexual activity and relationships was uncovered, it was clear that his schema was "A wife is special and needs to be treated in the most respectful way." It is clear that this was the primary template for his thinking, which included many automatic thoughts and core beliefs.

NEGATIVE FRAMING AND HOW TO IDENTIFY IT

Negative framing pertains to a particular view that spouses or family members maintain about one another or their situation that colors their perceptions and behavioral interactions. This concept was first introduced by Abrahms and Spring (1989) when they coined the term *flip flop factor*. This pertained to a couple's propensity to view each other in a negative light, sometimes viewing a once positive characteristic in the inverse. A good example might be a husband who was initially attracted to his wife because she appeared to him to be relatively "laid back," but now, during a period of distress, may refer to her as being "lazy" or "unmotivated."

With the therapist's help, spouses can challenge such negative frames by listing the negative characteristics, or the inverse of what were once determined to be positive qualities, and have them challenge the evidence supporting their beliefs (Beck, 1988; Dattilio, 1989; Dattilio & Padesky, 1990). This intervention is suggested as a way to encourage spouses or family members to accept the fact that their distortions might be coloring the way in which they view the other, and actually challenge their perceptions.

THE CASE OF MARTHA AND JIM

The following is an example of a technique that was used during a session with a couple in which the wife, Martha, was irritated with her husband. She was asked to first list the redeeming or positive qualities of Jim that initially attracted her to him. She provided a list of these characteristics: He takes charge, knows what he wants, and is intellectual, steady, and charming. When asked to list his irritating characteristics, she wrote the following: controlling, demanding, stuffy, rigid, and manipulative.

When these attributes were lined up juxtaposed, Martha was asked if some of her negative impressions of Jim might be the inverse of what she once found to be redeeming qualities, but are now just viewed in a negative light.

INITIAL REDEEMING QUALITIES	CURRENT IRRITATING QUALITIES
Takes charge	Controlling
Knows what he wants	Demanding
Intellectual	Stuffy
Steady	Rigid
Charming	Manipulative

Delineating this concept sometimes serves as a powerful intervention to help a person examine his or her own frame of mind about another person and evaluate whether that perception is affected by distortion. Negative frames can be extremely strong and powerful, particularly when a couple or member of a family are gridlocked about an issue that is emotionally charged, such as in the earlier case of Roberto and Zarida.

IDENTIFYING AND LABELING COGNITIVE DISTORTIONS

It is helpful for family members to become adept at identifying the types of cognitive distortions involved in their automatic thoughts. An exercise that is often effective is to have each partner or family member refer to the list of distortions and label any distortions in the automatic thoughts that he or she logged during the previous week (see p. 271). The therapist and the client can discuss the aspects of the thoughts that were inappropriate or extreme and how the distortion contributed to any negative emotions and behavior at the time. Such in-session reviews of written logs over the course of several sessions can increase family members' skills in identifying and evaluating their ongoing thoughts about their relationships.

If the therapist believes that a family member's cognitive distortions are associated with a form of individual psychopathology, such as clinical depression, the therapist must determine whether the psychopathology can be treated within the context of couple or family therapy, or whether the individual may need a referral for individual therapy. Procedures for assessing the psychological functioning of individual family members are beyond the scope of this chapter, but it is important that couple and family therapists be familiar with the evaluation of psychopathology and make referrals to other professionals as needed.

TRANSLATING THOUGHTS, EMOTIONS, AND BEHAVIORS IN THE PROCESS OF CONCEPTUALIZATION

A vital aspect of assessment involves understanding the interplay between thoughts, emotions, and behavior. Consequently, the process of conceptualization is extremely important, particularly when trying to understand how individuals interact in couple and family relationships, as well as how their thoughts, emotions, and behaviors affect each other. One of the initial steps in helping members become aware of their different dynamics is to utilize the Dysfunctional Thought Record. This is a good way to initially have them start to keep track of their emotions and how they affect automatic thoughts and behavior. It is a prime tool for them in understanding how their schemas drive their thoughts and how all of this has an impact on emotion and behavior. It should also be understood that there is a reciprocal dynamic between these three domains, which is best described by Figure 5.3.

ATTRIBUTION AND STANDARDS AND THEIR ROLE IN ASSESSMENT

Attribution and standards are important indicators of problems in relationships. Once individuals begin to outline their thoughts, emotions, and behavior and link them to schemas, it is important for them to determine how attributions and standards have developed as a result of their particular styles of thinking. It should also be stressed that the adherence to attributions and standards subsequently generate additional automatic thoughts, emotions, and behaviors that contribute to the ongoing cyclical

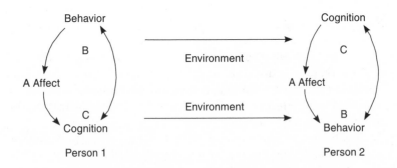

FIGURE 5.3. Reciprocal model of family interaction.

process. All of this becomes important, particularly as individuals begin to make changes in their interactional dynamics and restructure their thinking to affect the rest of their emotions and behaviors. Attributions and standards are certainly subject to change as new information shapes the redevelopment of schemas and the overall interaction between spouses or family members.

TARGETING MALADAPTIVE
BEHAVIORAL PATTERNS

Once automatic thoughts, emotions, behaviors, and the accompanying attributes and standards have been identified, citing specific maladaptive behavioral patterns that contribute to dysfunctional interaction is the next step. As spouses or family members identify these behavior patterns, behavioral prescriptions and exercises may be used as homework assignments to begin to change the course of interactional patterns. These, of course, are also accompanied by testing and reintegrating automatic thoughts on the basis of new information that individuals gather from observation and reconsideration.

TESTING AND REINTERPRETING
AUTOMATIC THOUGHTS

The process of a therapist having a client restructure automatic thoughts involves encouraging the consideration of alternative explanations. In order to accomplish this, the therapist needs to help the client to examine evidence concerning the validity of a thought, its appropriateness for his or her family situation, or both. Identifying a distortion in one's thinking or seeing an alternative way to view relationship events may contribute to the emergence of different emotional and behavioral responses to other family members. Questions such as the following are commonly helpful in guiding each family member in examining his or her thoughts:

- "From your past experiences or the events occurring recently in your family, what evidence exists that supports this thought? How could you get some additional information to help you judge whether your thought is accurate?"
- "What might be on alternative explanation for your partner's behavior? What else might have led your partner to behave that way?"
- "We have reviewed several types of cognitive distortions that can influence a person's views of other family members and can contrib-

ute to that person's getting upset with them. Which cognitive distortions, if any, can you see in the automatic thoughts you have had about...?"

For example, an adolescent who believed that his parents were being unfair in their restrictions on his activities reported the automatic thoughts "They enjoy restricting me. I never get to do anything," which were associated with anger and frustration toward his parents. The therapist coached him in discerning that he was engaging in mind reading and that it would be important to learn more about his parents' thoughts and feelings on the matter. The therapist encouraged him to ask his parents to describe their feelings. Both replied that they felt sad and guilty about having to restrict their son, but that their fears for his well-being, based on his past drug use, were outweighing their urge to let him have more freedom. The son was able to hear that his inference might not be accurate, and the therapist noted to the family members that they probably would benefit from problem-solving discussions to address the issue of what types of restrictions were most appropriate. Similarly, the therapist coached the son in examining his thought "I never get to do anything," which led to the son's recounting several instances in which his parents did allow him some social activities. Thus, the son acknowledged that he had engaged in dichotomous thinking. The therapist discussed with the family the danger of thinking and speaking in extreme terms, because very few events occur "always" or "never."

Thus, gathering and weighing the evidence for one's thoughts are integral parts of CBT. Family members can provide valuable feedback that can help individual members evaluate the validity or appropriateness of their cognitions, as long as they use good communication skills. After individuals challenge their thoughts, they should rate their belief in the alternative explanations and in their original inference or belief, perhaps on a scale from 0 to 100. Revised thoughts should not become assimilated unless they are considered credible.

FORMULATING A PLAN OF TREATMENT

Subsequent to the assessment phase, a clinician may want to establish a structured plan of treatment that can be modified as treatment progresses. By identifying the pertinent targets to address, listing the specific objectives and established interventions may serve as somewhat of a roadmap for the clinician to follow during the course of treatment.

There are many ways to achieve this, but one of the more structured methods is to resort to treatment plan manuals that can be modified to apply on a case-by-case basis. An example of such a manual is *The Couples Psychotherapy Treatment Planner* (O'Leary, Heyman, & Jongsma, 198) and *The Family Therapy Treatment Planner* (Dattilio & Jongsma, 2000). These treatment planners may offer the clinician a specific guideline to address treatment goals, objectives, and interventions with couples and families. It is recommended that the clinician establish some sense of treatment plan in order to serve as a general guideline in the interest of maintaining an evidence-based approach with clients.

Treatment plans also allow for the access of reviewing specific goals of therapy with clients and serve to facilitate collaboration between therapist and clients.

6

Cognitive-Behavioral Techniques

EDUCATING AND SOCIALIZING COUPLES AND FAMILY MEMBERS ABOUT THE COGNITIVE-BEHAVIORAL MODEL

It is important to educate couples and families about the cognitive-behavioral model of treatment. The structure and collaborative nature of the approach necessitates that the couple or family members understand the principles and methods involved. The therapist initially provides a brief didactic overview of the model and periodically refers to specific concepts during therapy. In addition to presenting such "mini-lectures" (Baucom & Epstein, 1990), the therapist often asks the clients to read portions of relevant popular books such as Beck's (1988) *Love Is Never Enough* and Markman et al.'s (1994) *Fighting for Your Marriage*. It is also important to explain to clients that homework assignments will be an essential part of treatment and that bibliotherapy is a type of homework that helps to orient them to the model of treatment. Understanding the model keeps all parties attuned to the process of treatment and reinforces the notion of taking responsibility for their own thoughts and actions.

The therapist also informs the clients that he or she will structure the sessions so as to keep the therapy focused on achieving the goals they agreed to pursue during the assessment process (Epstein & Baucom, 2002; Dattilio, 1994, 1997). Part of the structuring process involves the therapist and the couple or the family setting an explicit agenda at the beginning of each session. Another aspect of structuring sessions involves establishing ground rules for client behavior within and outside sessions; for example, individuals should not tell the therapist secrets that cannot be shared with other family members, all family members should attend each session unless the therapist and the family decide otherwise, and abusive verbal or physical behavior is unacceptable.

At the same time, therapists should not use a hard sell in introducing the therapeutic model. Because everyone is different, not all couples and families will buy into a rigid version of the cognitive-behavioral model, and therapists should be amenable to adapting it to fit a couple's or family's nature and personality. For example, some clients find the cognitive-behavioral model helpful but too demanding, and consequently refuse to complete inventories or homework assignments because they feel that these exercises lock them into a particular course of treatment. A therapist can modify the approach to a great degree without altering the basic tenets or principles of the treatment.

I often like to tell clients that by examining our thinking styles, we can have a significant impact on our emotions and behaviors, and this is one of the things we are going to explore during the course of therapy. Such soft sell is often very effective with couples and families.

IDENTIFYING AUTOMATIC THOUGHTS AND ASSOCIATED EMOTIONS AND BEHAVIOR

A crucial prerequisite to changing family members' distorted or extreme cognitions about themselves and each other is to increase their ability to identify their automatic thoughts. After introducing the concept of automatic thoughts—thoughts that spontaneously flash through one's mind—the therapist coaches the members of a couple or a family in observing their thought patterns during sessions that are associated with their negative emotional and behavioral responses to each other. Then, in order to improve the skill of identifying their automatic thoughts, clients are typically asked to keep a small notebook handy between sessions and to jot down a brief description of the circumstances in which they feel distressed about the relationship or are engaged in conflict. This log should include a description of the automatic thoughts that came to mind, the resulting emotional responses, and any behavioral responses toward other family members. We typically use a modified version of the Daily Record of Dysfunctional Thoughts (Beck et al., 1979), initially developed for the identification and modification of automatic thoughts in individual cognitive therapy. A sample for the modified version, the Dysfunctional Thought Record, can be found in Appendix B.

Through this type of record keeping, the therapist is able to demonstrate to couples and families how their automatic thoughts are linked to emotional and behavioral responses and to help them understand the specific macro-level themes (e.g., boundary issues) that upset them in their relationships. This procedure also increases family members' awareness that their negative emotional and behavioral responses to each other are potentially controllable through systematic examination of the cognitions associated with them. Thus, the therapist coaches each individual in taking greater responsibility for his or her own responses. In future sessions, an exercise that often proves useful is to have the couple or family members review their logs and indicate the links between thoughts, emotions, and behavior. The therapist then asks each person to explore alternative cognitions that might produce different emotional and behavioral responses to a situation.

Figure 6.1 illustrates the *Dysfunctional Thought Record* of Richard, who became angry with his wife, Samantha, when he went to use the SUV and the gas gauge registered empty. You can see how Richard's automatic thought "Samantha left me with no gas again. She doesn't give a damn about anybody but herself" led to his agitated mood. Once Richard was able to determine that he was engaging in the distortions of "all-or-nothing thinking" and "magnification," he was subsequently able to redirect himself to consider a more rational, balanced thought and calm down.

ADDRESSING SCHEMAS
AND SCHEMA RESTRUCTURING

Rigid Schemas

Sometimes couple or family members maintain rigid beliefs or conceptualizations about certain issues. When these are violated by new information that is incongruous with the resisting schema, instead of acquiescing and accommodating or assimilating this material, they may become more rigid and stalwart and utilize rationalization as a defense mechanism instead of incorporating the new information into their schema and adjusting to it. This can happen with couples and family members who are pathologically more rigid in their belief systems.

Changing Family-of-Origin Schemas

Individuals are sometimes reluctant to change their thinking from that of their family of origin because they view it as being disrespectful, or they see it as a sign of allegiance to their parents to maintain such a belief system. This happens despite the fact that sometimes the new thinking is more rational and functional. It's a lot like changing the decor in a home to keep up with the times. Sometimes the old decor has just outlived its purpose and needs repair or restoration. Sometimes an individual's beliefs and thinking

Directions: When you notice your mood getting worse, ask yourself, "What's going through my mind right now?" and as soon as possible jot down the thought or mental image in the automatic thoughts column.

Date Time	Situation	Automatic Thoughts	Emotions(s)	Distortion	Alternative Response	Outcome
	Describe: 1. Actual event leading to unpleasant emotion, or 2. Stream of thoughts, daydreams, or recollection, leading to an unpleasant emotion, or 3. Distressing physical sensations.	1. Write automatic thought(s) that preceded emotions(s). 2. Rate belief in automatic thought(s) 0–100%.	Describe: 1. Specify sad, anxious/ angry, etc. 2. Rate degree of emotion 0–100%.	1. All-or-nothing thinking 2. Overgeneralization 3. Mental filter 4. Disqualifying the positive 5. Jumping to conclusions 6. Magnification or minimization 7. Emotional reasoning 8. Should statements 9. Labeling and mislabeling 10. Personalization	1. Write a rational response to automatic thought(s). 2. Rate belief in alternative response 0–100%.	1. Rerate belief in automatic thought(s) 0–100%. 2. Specify and rate subsequent emotions 0–100%.
	Went out to the SUV in a hurry and noticed the gas gauge read "E."	Samantha left me with no gas again. She doesn't give a damn about anybody but herself.	Pissed off Frustrated Agitated	1. All-or-nothing thinking 6. Magnification	Maybe she was in a hurry and didn't notice. I shouldn't take it so personal. She's a good person and is human. People make mistakes. God knows that I make enough of them.	Somewhat less agitated 50%

Questions to help formulate the ALTERNATIVE RESPONSE: (1) What is the evidence that the automatic thought is true? Not true? (2) Is there an alternative explanation? (3) What's the *worst* that could happen? Could I live through it? What's the *best* that could happen? What's the *most realistic* outcome? (4) What should I do about it? (5) What's the effect of my believing the automatic thought? What could be the effect of changing my thinking? (6) If _____ (person's name) _____ was in this situation and had this thought, what would I tell him/her?

FIGURE 6.1. Richard's Dysfunctional Thought Record.

styles about certain situations need to be restored and revitalized as well. It is unrealistic to expect that an old belief or style of thinking can function without any modification to adapt to a new situation. Life often means change; things evolve.

INSTITUTING ENACTMENT THROUGH REFRAMING AND REHEARSAL

When family members attempt to identify the thoughts, emotions, and behavior that occurred in past incidents, they may have difficulty recalling pertinent information regarding the circumstances and each person's responses, particularly if the family interaction was emotionally charged. Imagery, role playing, or both may be helpful in reviving memories of such situations. In addition, these techniques often rekindle family members' reactions, and what begins as a role play may quickly become an *in vivo* interaction.

Family members can also be coached in switching roles during role-playing exercises to increase empathy for each other's experiences within the family (Epstein & Baucom, 2002). For example, spouses can be asked to play each other's role in recreating an argument they recently had concerning finances. Focusing on the other person's frame of reference and subjective feelings provides new information that can modify one spouse's view of the other. Thus, when a husband played the role of his wife, he was able to better understand her anxiety and conservative behavior concerning spending money, based on her experiences of poverty during childhood.

Often, the members of a distressed couple have developed a very narrow focus on problems in their relationship by the time they seek therapy; therefore, the therapist may ask them to report their recollections of the thoughts, emotions, and behavior that occurred between them during the period when they met, dated, and developed loving feelings toward each other. The therapist can focus on the contrast between past and present feelings and behavior as evidence that the partners were able to relate in a much more satisfying way and may be able to regenerate positive interactions with appropriate effort.

Imagery techniques should be used with caution and skill and probably should be avoided if there is a history of verbal or physical abuse in the relationship. Similarly, role-play techniques should not be used until the therapist feels confident that family members will be able to contain strong emotional responses and refrain from abusive behavior toward each other.

Although the recounting of past events can provide important information, the therapist's ability to assess and intervene with family members' problematic cognitive, affective, and behavioral responses to each other as they occur during sessions affords the best opportunity for changing family patterns (Epstein & Baucom, 2002).

BEHAVIORAL TECHNIQUES

Communication Training

Improving family members' skills for expressing thoughts and emotions, as well as listening effectively to each other, is one of the most common forms of intervention found with various approaches to therapy. In fact, many believe that communication skills are among the main ingredients that make relationships work (McKay, Fanning, & Paleg, 2006). John Gottman (1994), who conducted a substantial amount of research on couples' relationships, reported that studies of couples who remained married have demonstrated the significance of communication, predicting the longitudinal course of relationships, and thereby predicting either divorce or marital satisfaction. In fact, in a longitudinal study with violent couples Gottman and Gottman (1999) made similar predictions, with accuracy, that the likelihood of divorce would remain high. Gottman (1994) found that the core of balance in these relationships involved emotional behavior, cognition, perception, and physiology, all of which the researchers found could be used to accurately predict divorce. Gottman believed that each spouse establishes a balance of positive and negative aspects in these four areas, with the balances determining the ultimate fate of the relationship.

Gottman (1994) found that couples gravitating toward divorce showed more negativity than positivity in their emotional behavior and marital interaction. He went on to designate specific negative interactions—complaint/ criticism, contempt, defensiveness, and stonewalling—as the most predictive of the relationship demise. These terms came to be classically known as "the Four Horsemen of the Apocalypse" (1994, p.10):

1. *Complaint/criticism*: Complaint as an expression of disagreement or anger about specific issues, which may escalate into criticism, becoming more judgmental, global, and blaming after repeated attempts to resolve the issue.
2. *Contempt*: A mockery, insult, sarcasm, or derision of another individual, indicating incompetence or absurdity, (e.g., disapproval, disdain, judgment, put-downs, etc.).
3. *Defensiveness*: An attempt to ward off or protect oneself from a perceived attack. A response may be denial or responsibility for a problem, a counterattack, or a whine.

4. *Stonewalling*: The listener fails to provide any cues to the speaker so that a "stone wall" is placed between the listener and the speaker. Emotionally, the speaker perceives the listener as being detached, smug, hostile, disapproving, cold, or disinterested.

Couples who experience communication problems tend to recast the entire relationship in terms of "the distance and isolation cascade" (Gottman & Gottman, 1999, p. 306). This involves a pattern of (1) viewing the marital problem as severe, (2) believing there is no point in working on the issues with the other spouse, (3) feeling flooded by the other spouses's complaint, (4) arranging lives in parallel fashion so less and less time is spent together, and (5) loneliness.

Another distinction has been made with respect to linear versus circular communication. Linear communication reflects cause–effect thinking and is other (outside of self) focused. When a spouse is engaging in this type of communication, he or she does not talk about or disclose him- or herself, or talks about him- or herself as simply reacting to others. Circular communication reflects a more mature, differentiated, and abstract form of thinking. At this level, spouses can talk about their reciprocal interlocking patterns of relating. For example, a wife may indicate that she is angry because of her husband's nonverbal behavior. She can clarify the meaning of her concern and, perhaps, elaborate in response to his behavioral display. In this way, the partners are able to see how the behavior pattern of each affects the other and to cognitively incorporate this knowledge into their belief systems. Patterns of communication begin to become clearer through this type of discussion.

Content-oriented communication deals with just the specific content issue at hand. In content communication, family members focus only on what they are thinking, not on how they are thinking. Process communication is more mature, differentiated, and abstract. Family members can look outside themselves in order to become their own observers. They may discuss the manner in which they are talking to each other and how they need to change dysfunctional patterns of interaction and communication.

Most traditional communication training programs suggest that therapists facilitate the couple or family members moving from linear to circular communication and from content to process communication in order to promote a healthy exchange. This process may unfold during the course of a therapeutic dialogue in which the therapist can point out specific communication deficits and make suggestions in terms of strategies to improve communication and interaction. One way to do this might be to propose various strategies for both the speaker and the listener, such as those listed in the following sections.

Strategies for the Speaker

The speaker needs to identify the needs of the listener. Speakers may consider the following strategies or guidelines when expressing themselves:

1. *Speak attentively.* The speaker should make an effort to speak in the same manner consistently, maintaining appropriate and direct eye contact, and looking for body signals (facial or postural) that indicate that his or her partner is being receptive to what the speaker is saying. The use of a consistent, even tone, with moderate variation may be best, even when individuals are angry or upset.
2. *Ask meaningful questions.* Maintaining brevity in conversation and cutting to the chase are always desirable; however, sometimes using questions that elicit yes-or-no answers may truncate the conversation and render it unproductive. Instead, a speaker may consider asking questions that lead to fuller responses from the listener because they will help to facilitate more circular communication— communication in which there is equal exchange between speaker and listener.
3. *Do not overspeak.* Speak to the point and avoid drawn-out statements. This often gives the listener a chance to clarify and reflect on what he or she is hearing.
4. *Accept silence.* This allows the listener to digest what is being said and give it some additional thought. Don't interpret silence as resistance. Sometimes the best way to make points is to pause or use periods of silence after speaking.
5. *Avoid cross-examining.* Firing questions at the listener when attempting to learn something during conversation may be very destructive. Diplomacy and respect may be a far better means of helping your listener to hear the message you want to convey.

Strategies for the Listener

Often couples and family members listen to each other, but only on a minimal level. They do not actually hear what is being said. Good listening skills involve clear understanding of what is being said and the ability to respond in circular conversation. Listeners may consider the following guidelines:

1. *Listen attentively.* Attempt to maintain good eye contact with the speaker and acknowledge that you are hearing him or her by displaying goal-directed behavior and affirming responses.
2. *Do not interrupt.* It is often difficult for you to hear when you are talking. It is also often construed as a sign of rudeness and disre-

spect. There are various strategies that may help you contain your-self when you are attempting to listen to content that you do not want to hear, or that may infuriate you (e.g., see "The Pad-and-Pencil Technique" on page 130).

3. *Clarify what you hear.* Attempt to make a clear summary about what you hear at the end of a speaker's statement. This can often help to ensure that you are obtaining the message that is intended. It is also important to admit when you don't understand, or something is not clear, so that it can be restated.

4. *Reflect on what you hear.* This may differ from seeking clarification. Reflection involves conveying to the speaker that you are aware of and understand what is being said. In essence, this is repeating the speaker's statement with some sense of affirmation to indicate that the message is being received.

5. *Summarize.* Both speaker and listener should always attempt to summarize their conversation so that no loose ends are remaining and both have a clear understanding of what has been conveyed. This is probably one of the essentials of circular communication. Summarizing also allows individuals to construct a follow-up and future conversation.

In addition, I sometimes recommend some reading for clients to help them become more attuned to listening to others. An excellent resource for this is *The Lost Art of Listening* by Michael P. Nichols (1995).

Communication training is an essential part of cognitive-behavioral therapy because it can have a positive impact on problematic behavioral interactions, reduce family members' distorted cognitions about each other, and contribute to regulated experience and expressive emotion. Guidelines for speakers also include acknowledging the subjectivity of your own views (not suggesting that others' views are invalid), describing your emotions as well as your thoughts, pointing out positives as well as problems, speaking in specific rather than global terms, being concise so that the listener can absorb and remember your message, and using tact and good timing (e.g., not discussing important topics when your partner is preparing to go to sleep). The guidelines for empathic listening also include exhibiting attentiveness through nonverbal acts (e.g., eye contact, nods) and demonstrating acceptance of the speaker's message (a person's right to have his or her personal feelings). Whether or not you and your partner agree, it is important to attempt to understand or empathize with the other person's perspectives and to reflect your understanding by paraphrasing what the speaker has said.

After training, family members should receive handouts describing communication guidelines that they can utilize and refer to whenever needed during verbal exchanges at home.

Gottman and Gottman (1999) listed 11 goals in their intervention strategies, which, when met, signal the termination of therapy. For instance, the markers of divorce, particularly the "Four Horsemen" mentioned earlier, must be significantly and meaningfully reduced as a couple works out its conflicts. Moreover, the ratio of negativity to positivity must be reduced. The authors feel that a buffer must be established that can facilitate a partner's anger being seen as valuable information rather than a personal attack on the other. They also suggest creating a "love map" to be maintained on a daily basis. This can provide a means for spouses to continue learning about each other's worlds by periodically updating their knowledge. It is also recommended that spouses create a positive sentiment override (POS). Sentiment override is defined as "a discrepancy between insider and outsider perspectives." This involves messages and observations that are usually described as objectively negative or irritable, but are instead viewed as neutral or even positive by the receiver of the messages (Gottman & Gottman, 1999, p. 313). The maintenance of a POS is achieved by turning toward versus turning away, thereby suggesting that the spouses are more emotionally connected and engaged with each other. Much of this connection is nonemotional and occurs in the daily mundane events of marriage and neutral family contexts. Gottman and Gottman (1999) believe that each person needs to accept influence from his or her spouse, especially the husband from the wife, and suggest the following points for spouses to consider:

• Use a soft rather than a harsh start-up when dealing with conflict.
• Effectively repair negative interaction chains.
• Use positive affect for de-escalation.
• Learn how to physiologically soothe your partner and yourself.
• Acquire the tools to make each conversation better than the last without the help of the therapist.

It is also often important for therapists to model good expressive and listening skills. They may use videotape examples, such as those that accompany the Markman et al. (1994) book *Fighting for Your Marriage*. During sessions, the therapist coaches the couple or family members in following the communication guidelines, beginning with discussions of relatively benign topics so that negative emotions will not interfere with constructive skills. As the individuals demonstrate good skills, they are asked to practice them further as homework assignments with increasingly conflictual topics. Following the aforementioned guidelines often increases each individual's perceptions that others are respectful and have goodwill toward them.

Sometimes, despite the rules or guidelines used in communications training, family therapists may find that spouses and family members continue to experience difficulty in refraining from butting in or arguing with others. This can be trying to therapists' clinical patience and make for a lot of wasted time in therapy. Some of the techniques discussed in the following paragraphs may be extremely useful in working with individuals who continue to experience this difficulty.

Conveying Empathy

One of the most common complaints by family members is that others fail to demonstrate any empathy for feelings they have expressed or difficulties they may be going through. Teaching couples and family members to listen and express empathy sometimes requires training and demonstration. Along with listening skills, the demonstration of understanding and the expression of empathy are essential, particularly as they lead to the next issue, which is a sense of validation. Empathy is a prerequisite to intimacy and positive exchange. Several researchers (Guerney, 1977) have developed complete treatment programs focused on the principles for developing empathetic skills. A noted program (Conjugal Relationship Enhancement), as well as one promoted by Barry Ginsberg (1997, 2000) in his Relationship Enhancement Approach, provide effective ways for enhancing relationship satisfaction.

Validation

The concept of validation has appeared in a number of texts on couple and family therapy and has been particularly noted by Gottman, Notarius, Gonso, and Markman (1976) and Markman et al. (1994). Validation should be clearly distinguished from reflection and agreement, in the sense that it is a communication of acknowledgment without necessarily agreeing. Subsequently, family members can be validating in their responses without necessarily giving in to disagreements, which sometimes helps to quell the tension in a negative exchange. The following is an example of validation of feelings without necessarily agreeing.

JACKIE: I can't believe that the Schleagels didn't even look at us when we passed them in the restaurant with the Davises the other night. I felt so ignored.

LUKE: Well, I don't know that they were ignoring us. Maybe they didn't have their glasses on or didn't see us. But I certainly can see how you would feel awkward and unacknowledged.

JACKIE: Well, I did. What does it take to glance at us and acknowledge our presence by waving or something? I know it was crowded and noisy in there, but, even so, it just gives me such a sense of being disregarded.

LUKE: I know. I could see that it was really bothering you while we were there and I felt bad for you, but I didn't take it the same way. I just roll with that kind of stuff. I try not to let little issues like that get to me, it's just not worth it.

Luke did an excellent job of validating his wife's feelings, although, at the same time, not agreeing with her that their friends were disregarding them. It is easy to see how a spouse can be supportive, yet at the same time suggest that maybe his wife needs to take a look at a different perspective and reconsider some alternatives. Luke's response actually served to facilitate some transitional thinking for Jackie and possibly encourage her to consider if she might be engaging in a cognitive distortion or, at the least, an unrealistic expectation.

Validation is extremely important in relationships. It often makes the difference between whether individuals feel isolated or detached in their exchanges with spouses and family members, and whether there is some sense of security in the relationship. Validation is also an excellent response to a spouse or family member when he or she is emotionally upset, as in the preceding exchange. Whether or not the partner's behavior has caused the feelings, validation can serve as a nice mediary. Therapists can incorporate regular validating exercises in their work with couples and coach spouses on how to recognize the need for validation and provide it when it would be helpful.

Techniques for Modifying and Reducing Interruptions in Communication

During the course of their work, family therapists are almost certain to encounter individuals who aggressively interrupt each other as they attempt to tell their own versions of a particular story or express their emotions. This is natural, particularly when emotionally charged topics are discussed. While not all interruptions are necessarily bad, such intrusions frequently create an atmosphere of dissension and, at times, may inhibit the therapeutic process. Every therapist is destined to encounter such situations and will need to rely on numerous strategies to control them. There have been a number of interventions suggested in the professional literature throughout the years that were designed to remedy this problem. For example, (Markman, Stanley, and Blumberg (1994) developed a strategy that involves providing the partners with a piece of linoleum or other type of floor covering, which is held by the individual speaking in order to indicate that he or she "has the floor" and that the partner is to refrain from interrupting or interfering (p. 63). Although this technique has proven effective in some cases, it has been disastrous in others, particularly when impulsive, angry individuals are involved (I was once hit in the face with a flying piece of linoleum). This is especially problematic when the content of a partner's presentation is presumed by the other partner to be inaccurate or is inflammatory (Dattilio, 2001c).

Another technique suggested by Susan Heitler (1995) involves the therapist interrupting the intervening spouse or family member and asking that person to cease the argument, or simply telling him or her to "stop." Again, this technique is sometimes effective, but because it may have to be repeated numerous times, it can take valuable time away from the therapeutic process and become frustrating to the therapist, who winds up functioning more like a referee than a clinician (I once found myself saying "stop" a total of 146 times during a single session with a volatile family) (Dattilio, 2007). Such an intervention can also cut off some of the affective expression that may actually be an important component of the treatment process, thus thwarting the expression of vital material.

The Pad-and-Pencil Technique

Couples and family members have shared with me, on numerous occasions, that one of the main reasons they spontaneously interrupt each other is because of fear that they will not have an opportunity to express their own spontaneous thoughts or emotions. Therefore, it is important to create a mechanism by which individuals will be able to capture their automatic thoughts and emotional responses without interrupting the flow of treatment.

While working with an emotionally charged couple some years ago, I developed an intervention that I found effective in helping couple and family members to contain their impulsive urges to interrupt each other's self-expressions.

One day during a session, I noticed the wife of this couple fidgeting with a pen she was holding while her husband was giving his rendition of an argument they had 2 days before. This argument had led to a physically abusive exchange in which the woman slapped her husband and caused the situation to become quite loud. Both partners were intent upon expressing their renditions of this story. While listening to her husband's view of what occurred, the woman became increasingly anxious and, consequently, fidgeted more and more with the pen in her hand.

The cognitive-behavioral therapist in me wanted to ask her what was going through her mind, but, at the same time, I did not want to interrupt her husband's train of thought. I thought to myself, "If she had an opportunity to write down her own automatic thoughts and the accompanying emotions, she would then be able to direct her attention toward a constructive task and, at the same time, capture some of the intensity of her feelings. She would also feel reassured that her own thought content or emotions would not be lost and that she could refer to them once her husband finished speaking." I asked her to do this and also suggested that her husband engage in the same type of exercise while she spoke. I provided each of them with a pen and a pad of paper so that they could record any thoughts or emotions they experienced while listening to the spouse's rendition of the incident, thus assuring that the content could later be discussed. Much to my delight, this intervention worked extremely well. It kept each spouse occupied and engaged as each silently allowed the partner to speak. Both reported feeling satisfied that none of their thoughts or emotions were left out or ignored.

The actual process of the cognitive-behavioral exercise of writing is not only cathartic, it decreases interruptions, allows spouses and family members to focus their attention, and helps them listen to what is being said while keeping written track of valuable information.

This technique, like many others, does not work in every case. In fact, some individuals find it to be a mechanical intervention and refuse to comply. It may also encourage some spouses not to listen to each other, and they must be reminded to listen as well as write. However, this technique should often be considered when partners or family members continue to interrupt each other. Such behavior may also have to do with issues of boundaries and control, which need to be addressed as well. At the very least, the pad-and-pencil technique is a method that may allow the topic of disruption to be revisited in a new light. One is reminded that necessity is the "mother of invention." Consider using this invention early in the treatment phase, because it is more likely to be effective the sooner it is employed.

Problem-Solving Strategies

It is not surprising that couples and families often experience difficulty with problem solving inasmuch as it rests so heavily on getting along and communicating. When negotiation is involved, it often requires the ability to weigh alternatives in a calm and collected fashion, which has been documented to be the most difficult in areas of disagreement (Bennun, 1985). This is why problem-solving strategies have always been an important part of cognitive-behavioral therapy with couples and families (Dattilio & Van Hout, 2006).

Epstein and Baucom (2002) provided a summary of the findings of a number of investigators, which yielded three important sets of factors in problem solving with couples and may also be applied to families. These factors involve instrumental, task-oriented issues. The authors noted the following:

1. Specific communications, such as accepting responsibility or expressing contempt.
2. Patterns of interaction, or the ways that partners respond to each other, with constructive discussions by both partners indicating more satisfied relationships.
3. Incorporation of the preferences and desires of both individuals into solutions. (Epstein & Baucom, 2002, p. 39)

Cognitive-behavioral therapists also use verbal and written instructions, modeling, and behavioral rehearsal and coaching to facilitate effective problem solving. The major steps in problem solving involve achieving a clear and specific definition of the problem in terms of behaviors that are or are not occurring, generating specific behavioral solutions to the problem without attacking one's own or other family members' ideas, evaluating the advantages and disadvantages of each alternative solution and selecting a solution that appears to be feasible and attractive to all members involved, and agreeing on a trial period for implementing the selected solution and assessing its effectiveness. Homework practice of the skills is important for their acquisition (Dattilio, 2002; Epstein & Baucom, 2002).

The following is a set of steps adapted from Epstein and Schlesinger (1996) that can be used with couples and families as guidelines for problem solving:

• Define the problem in specific behavioral terms. Compare perceptions and arrive at an agreeable description of the problem.
• Generate a possible set of solutions.
• Evaluate the advantages and disadvantages of each solution.
• Select a feasible solution.
• Implement the chosen solution and evaluate its effectiveness.

This is an area that may be strategically assigned as homework on a repeated basis with the therapist reviewing the process and the outcome with the couple or family on a routine basis.

Behavioral Exchange Agreements

Behavioral exchange agreements are an integral part of cognitive-behavioral therapy. Contracts to exchange desired behaviors have an important role in reducing family tensions. However, therapists should try to avoid making one family member's behavioral exchange solely contingent on another's. Therefore, the goal with behavioral exchange agreements is for each person to identify and enact a specific behavior that would involve self-improvement, regardless of what actions the other members take. The major challenge facing the therapist is to encourage family members to avoid "standing on ceremony" by waiting for others to behave positively first. Brief didactic presentations on negative reciprocity in distressed relationships, the fact that one can have control only over one's own actions, and the importance of making a personal commitment to improve the family atmosphere are some interventions that may reduce individuals' reluctance to make the first positive contribution.

The following vignette illustrates a behavioral exchange agreement.

THE CASE OF SALLY AND KURT

Sally complained that Kurt had a bad habit of reading the daily newspaper while in his easy chair and then dropping the used newspaper on the floor in a disorganized pile for the housekeeper to later throw out. Instead, Sally wanted Kurt to place the used newspapers in a paper bag next to his chair and then take them out to the trash at the end of the week. Sally felt that this would look neater than leaving them on the floor in a disorganized fashion. Kurt finally agreed to do this in exchange for Sally's remembering not to place empty clothes hangers on the doorknob of their bedroom, a habit that Kurt said drove him "nuts." Such an exchange agreement seemed to be effective in maintaining the changed behavior for both Kurt and Sally.

Interventions for Deficits and Excesses in Emotional Responses

Although cognitive-behavioral therapy is sometimes characterized as neglecting emotions, this is a misperception. A variety of interventions are used, either to enhance the emotional experiences of inhibited individuals or to moderate extreme responses. For family members who report experiencing little emotion, the therapist can (1) set clear guidelines for behavior within and outside sessions, in which expressing oneself will not lead to recrimination by other members, (2) use downward-arrow questioning to inquire about underlying emotions and cognitions, (3) coach a person in noticing internal cues to his or her emotional states, (4) repeat phrases that have emotional impact on the person, (5) refocus attention on emotionally relevant topics when an individual attempts to change the subject, and (6) engage the individual in role plays concerning important relationship issues to elicit emotional responses. With individuals who experience intense emotions that affect them and significant others adversely, the therapist can (1) help a person to compartmentalize emotional responses by scheduling specific times to discuss distressing topics, (2) coach the individual in self-soothing activities such as relaxation techniques, (3) improve his or her ability to monitor and challenge upsetting automatic thoughts, (4) encourage the person to seek social support from family members and others, (5) develop his or her ability to tolerate distressing feelings, and (6) enhance the person's skills for expressing emotions constructively so that others will pay attention.

Contingency Contracts

This technique was initially developed by Richard Stuart (1969), who believed in focusing on the interpersonal endorsement in which couples and family members responded to one another. It was Stuart's contention that rather than focusing on how an undesirable or disruptive response of a disgruntled spouse or family member could be modified, it was more effective to shift the focus to how the exchange of positive behaviors could be maximized and have spouses actually write up a written contract to do so. This strategy was based on the principle of reciprocity, introduced earlier by Joseph Wolpe (1977). The use of reciprocity was designed to achieve a balance in behavioral exchange. An example is the use of the *quid pro quo*.

The pioneering family therapist Don Daveson (1965) had suggested a similar strategy, using the medical and social analogies of *homeostasis* and *quid pro quo*. The *quid pro quo*, as suggested by Stuart (1969), was aimed at building up the status of a spouse or family member to serve as a mediator of reinforcement in order to influence the behavior of the other spouse or other family members. This was achieved by having one spouse do something that the other wants. Therefore, it is hypothesized that a spouse or a member of a family will be more likely to change his or her behavior in order to please someone who pleased him or her. Likewise, such a person would not be as motivated to change his or her behavior to please someone whose own behavior is not seen as unconditionally rewarding.

The latter attitude is often seen early in couple therapy when spouses are gridlocked and one says to the therapist, "I'm not going to make the first overture toward change. Why should I? He (or she) never takes the first step." This type of power struggle or gridlock is exactly what *quid pro quo* is designed to stop. Stuart suggested taking the initiative of intervention away from the couple or family by developing a setting in which the frequency and intensity of mutual positive reinforcement can be maximized. So, in a situation in which spouses are gridlocked, rather than focus on why, a therapist might instruct them to simultaneously search for positive qualities of one another rather than focus on the undesirable aspects. Stuart outlined a four-step process of employing this strategy:

1. Identify a rationale for mutual change.
2. Have each spouse or family member initiate changes in his or her own behavior first.
3. Record the frequency of the targeted behavior on a chart.
4. Have each spouse or family member sign a written contract for a series of exchanges of desired behaviors.

Certain symbols, such as tokens or quarters, can be used as rewards. In this way, an individual can build up a credit balance, which can later be exchanged when he or she is the recipient of rewarding behaviors from others. (Tokens are not typically well received by contemporary family members; hence, written contracts are mostly used.)

Assertiveness Training

A form of social skills training often used in family therapy is assertiveness training. The often shy and intimidated behaviors that are observed with family members that cause them to avoid speaking up for themselves, or in some cases, coming off as being too aggressive, may be one of the areas that cause great difficulties in relationships. When it becomes a prominent issue with interaction, there may be a need for formal training in identifying the difference between aggressive and assertive responses. Having spouses and family members practice all three types of responses—nonassertive, assertive, aggressive—with each other may be helpful in aiding them to realize that assertive behavior benefits them by achieving salubrious interaction.

The therapist can use role play during the course of the sessions, refer individuals to training programs, or assign the viewing of assertiveness training tapes, particularly those involving the context of a couple or family. Allowing spouses to observe same-gender models within their relative age range can be very helpful in showing them the difference between assertive behavior and nonassertive or aggressive behaviors.

Cultural issues must also be kept in mind when suggesting assertiveness training, particularly with couples and families of various origins, such as those who hail from cultures that discourage women from speaking up to their husbands. Homework assignments involving the practice of assertive behavior, or bibliotherapy assignments to read books, such as *Your Perfect Right* by Alberti and Emmons (2001), may also be used.

Paradoxical Techniques and Interventions

Paradoxical techniques and interventions have been around for a long time (Dowd & Swobodoa, 1984). Initially proposed by humanistic existentialists (Frankl, 1960) and subsequently by behavior therapists (Ascher, 1980, 1984), their principles have been applied to human psychological change.

As used by couple and family therapists, paradoxical techniques and interventions, which have been better known by the term *prescribing symptoms* (Watzalawick, Weakland, & Fisch, 1974), date from the mid-1960s, when Watzalawick, Beavin, and Daveson (1967) recommended their use in couple and family therapy.

There are several types of paradoxical techniques (Weeks & L'Abate, 1979). Specific goals are essential to paradoxical interventions, which have also been referred to in the professional literature as "pragmatic paradox" (Weeks & L'Abate, 1982). In this respect, paradoxical intention places the individual, couple, or even family, in somewhat of a double- bind situation in which there is no real choice, or what would amount to a "no-lose" situation in the case of a therapeutic paradox. The basic concept is to produce a second-order change in the structure of a system.

As early as 1928, Dunlap (1932) began applying a technique that he referred to at the time as *negative practice* to various problems, which included nail biting, enuresis, and stammering. Dunlap would direct the individual to practice a symptom under prescribed conditions with the anticipation of extinguishing the habit. Paradoxical prescriptions are most commonly divided into those directed toward the encouragement of symptomatic behaviors and those directed toward the rules that govern and are peculiar to a particular couple or family (Weeks & L'Abate, 1979). Paradoxical methods have further included those that utilize prescription, such as (1) encouraging a patient to enact his or her symptomatic behavior, (2) giving permission to couples and family members to experience these symptoms, and (3) practice, which involves encouraging the refinement of the symptomatic behavior, and prediction, which involves suggesting that the couple or family members deliberately relax (Bornstein, Krueger, & Cogswell, 1989). Paradoxical methods can be tricky and the therapist needs to be cautious of how and when to use them. The therapist must conceptualize the problems systematically, considering all factors involved with the problem at hand.

Weeks and L'Abate (1982) are well known for their basic principles of paradoxical psychotherapy used with couples and families. They delineated five principles to be followed. The first principle utilizes the symptom as an ally. The symptomatic behavior of the couple or family is not considered in negative terms, but, rather, is viewed as a vehicle for change. This approach is based on the idea that the function of the symptom has been to preclude change in the family system to begin with. Principle two, which is to identify the specific symptom, is applicable to symptoms that occur within a social context and is, therefore, crucial when dealing with couples and families. Principle three places the symptom under conscious control. If the therapist is working with an individual, the paradox may be constructed consciously through enactment and can magnify the symptom. When the symptom occurs within a system of interaction, such as in a couple or a family, all members of the system should be included. One strategy to accomplish this may involve having other members of the family help the identified individual to actually experience the symptom. The second strategy may involve having another member(s) assume a paradoxical role(s). The classic example that Weeks and L'Abate cited is as follows:

> Assume the symptom is a daughter's acting-out and taking charge in the single parent family. The daughter is told to exaggerate her taking charge of her mother. At the same time, the mother is told to assume the paradoxical role of the child. She is instructed to give up her position of authority and to be a helpless child. (1982, p. 91)

Weeks and L'Abate went on to elaborate their fourth principle, which involves blocking the appearance of the symptom. This is to be accomplished by predicting or prescribing an actual relapse. Finally, principle five serves to ensure the client's involvement. This is achieved through several techniques, such as instructing the individual to have the symptom. Alternately, a paradoxical message may be put in writing to be read on a regular basis by the individual (e.g., "I must keep acting out against my parents' wishes").

One of the most commonly utilized paradoxical strategies is the implementation of prescriptions. Essentially, this technique involves instructing family members to exaggerate the symptom they are complaining about. Therefore, if they say that the family atmosphere is characterized by frequent fighting, they may be encouraged to learn a more effective manner of fighting. They may be requested to set aside specific times during which they must fight. DeShazer (1978, p. 21) illustrated an example in which he had a couple deliberately start a fight and had them toss a coin to decide who was to go first. He then instructed the partners to take turns yelling and screaming at each other for 10-minute intervals. Each of the partners took a turn as a yeller and nonresponsive listener, subsequently alternating their positions. It was DeShazer's intention to have this couple fight "in order to stop fighting." In essence, this was a systemic symptom description designed to shift the negatives so as to obtain a positive outcome. This is often the essence of paradoxical intention (Dattilio, 1987).

Duncan (1989) outlines two types of general interventions. One is restraining, in which the therapist discourages change and may even deny that change is possible. There are reportedly many types of restraining interventions, which can be used at varying intervals in the therapeutic process to help facilitate change or maintain changes that have already been made.

The second is therapist-style interventions, which involve the manner in which the therapist approaches the client and the method by which the client's beliefs and values are incorporated and respected by the therapist. See Duncan (1989) for a more complete description of these techniques.

There are several rules of thumb that should be followed when using paradoxical strategies. Weeks and L'Abate (1982) outlined five basic principles that are applicable with individuals, couples, and families and are different from the prescriptions outlined on page 136: (1) positively reframe the symptoms, (2) link the symptoms to all members of the system in the couple or family, (3) reverse the symptoms vector, (4) prescribe and sequence paradoxical intervention over time, (5) utilize a paradoxical intervention that can ensure that family members will act on the task in some manner.

It should also be understood that paradoxical strategies may be more appropriate for certain types of cases than others. It is usually chronic, severe, or long-term problems that respond best to paradoxical interventions. Birchler (1983) further outlines this system for using paradoxical methods and suggests that paradoxical interventions should be employed only after a family member has learned and successfully employed basic communication and problem-solving skills. This is to ensure that family members will feel relatively confident that they can overcome any problems that arise as a result of this fairly complex intervention. Birchler also advises a complete review of the case to ensure that other, more straightforward approaches would not be effective and to rule out the use of other measures before resorting to paradoxical interventions.

Paradoxical interventions are probably best used for families that are legitimately stuck in a gridlock or resistant to other therapeutic interventions. As stated previously, Birchler (1983) stresses that the crucial criterion of a successful intervention be based on a strong functional analysis of the system prior to implementation. Paradoxical interventions are relatively complex and difficult to employ, and therefore a solid understanding of the interactional system within the couple or family is imperative. It is also important that a paradoxical assignment be explained to families in a matter that underscores its necessity in view of previous failures or barriers to change and after more conventional techniques have been exhausted. Some cognitive-behaviorists have also suggested, in the past, that the use of paradoxical measures as a general strategy in couple therapy might be inconsistent with the behavioral perspective (Jacobson & Margolin, 1979). Although such interventions can be helpful at times, depending on the circumstances, there may be a problem in that paradoxical strategies involve a measure of deceit, which may also raise ethical concerns. All of these factors must be taken into consideration carefully prior to implementing paradoxical interventions.

Deescalation and Time Out

Teaching family members to deescalate potentially volatile situations is not easy and, often, many members find themselves in the throes of an emotionally charged situation in which they act out behaviorally before they have time to intervene.

THE CASE OF CURTIS AND MARGO

In a therapy session, Curtis and Margo described an event that was typical for them, one that created a lot of friction. Margo embarked on her rendition of the story: "We were down at the shore for a week. Things were tense all week because we had been fighting a lot before we even went on vacation. I thought that maybe this would be a break for us, but, obviously, things didn't really change. In any event, my parents had the kids and Curtis said that we should probably go get gas in the car before the next day, which was when we were to return home. With all of the people leaving the seashore on the weekend, the lines at the gas station are often backed up, so we decided to take advantage of the break and go fuel up a day ahead of time. There were also some things I wanted to get at the store.

"So I drove and Curtis was in the passenger seat. We were driving down the causeway and I guess I wasn't going fast enough for him. He kept needling me about going too slow and we got into an argument about his 'backseat driving'. At that point, I just got pissed off because we were on vacation and he had to start with his shit. We started to argue about how we were on vacation and I was tired of rushing all the time and … anyway, one thing led to another and I just pushed the accelerator to the floor. I said to him, 'There, is that fast enough for you?' With that, wouldn't you know— a damn cop pulled me over and then the next thing I know, I'm getting a ticket. And this asshole sits there and laughs at me because I'm the one getting the ticket. I was so pissed!"

At that point, I intervened by using the following strategy.

DATTILIO: All right, let's back up a minute and take a look at what has happened here. Obviously, Margo, you were agitated long before you accelerated the car, right?

MARGO: Yeah, sure. I was agitated all week.

DATTILIO: First of all, you know that if you're agitated and you place yourself in a position where you're riding in the car with Curtis, there is a strong likelihood that things will escalate.

MARGO: Yeah, I guess so.

DATTILIO: All right, first of all, you both need to take responsibility and keep in mind that when there is tension between you, either on both ends or on one end, that's the time for you to be aware of the fact that the situation can quickly escalate, particularly with the two of you, which seems to happen very often.

MARGO: Yeah, but everything would have been OK if he wasn't such a pain in the ass.

DATTILIO: Well, that's the problem here. Until we get some of this straightened out, you need to be consciously aware of when you are in tight situations because things are likely to escalate quickly. You both must take responsibility for your respective behaviors.

MARGO: OK, so what should I have done? Should I have pulled over and just gotten out of the car?

DATTILIO: No, but I think that, at that point, if you are starting to feel agitated early on, maybe pulling over to the side of the road and saying, "Hey, look, I don't know that I want to drive if we are going to have this conversation. Maybe you need to drive or do something different." Give yourself a chance to deescalate.

MARGO: Well, we've done that before. I've tried that before and he just says, "No, no, just shut up."

DATTILIO: Yes, but you have a choice. If you sense that things are going to get out of hand, you need to take responsibility and say, "No, I don't want to drive under these conditions," and, if worse comes to worse, you park the car for a while until things settle down. The fact of the matter is, you really could have hurt somebody or gotten hurt yourself by doing what you did and, quite frankly, it was irrational!

MARGO: Yes, I know that it was irrational. It was just a spontaneous reaction at the moment.

DATTILIO: Well, this is where we want to intervene. The best time to intervene is before it becomes emotionally charged, and that means that both of you have to take responsibility to head it off at the pass. Also, pulling the car over would have given Curtis a clear message that you're not going to drive under those conditions. Curtis, what was going through your mind during this event?

CURTIS: Well, she was going ridiculously slow. I know that she is not used to driving in that area, but—I mean—I got the impression that she was just going overly slow to piss me off.

DATTILIO: Is that true, Margo?

MARGO: No, no, I wasn't doing that. I didn't want to bang up the car because there was traffic all over the place and I didn't know where I was going. I wasn't sure where a gas station was located. I don't do that kind of stuff just to irk him.

DATTILIO: So, Curtis, maybe you misinterpreted that and that made things worse.

CURTIS: Yeah, probably.

DATTILIO: Again, we need to be mindful of these kinds of things and the messages that we say to ourselves because they are very powerful, and, if things are going to change, you need to start to change your thinking. This, obviously, will have a significant impact on your emotions as well.

I further suggested to the partners that they could use deep breathing techniques and restructuring exercises as a means of inoculating themselves against future outbursts. Time-out procedures can be very effective when family members are all in agreement. I often have them make the sign of a "T" with both hands to indicate, "I need time out." They also agreed, in advance, that no one will exploit the use of time out, but will use it when they legitimately need a reprieve period. This helps to break up the momentum of an agitated exchange.

Behavioral Rehearsal

After skills training and feedback from the therapist, couples and family members often need to rehearse the specific skills. This can initially occur through verbal coaching and modeling during the therapy process. Such practice sessions have traditionally been referred to as *behavioral rehearsal*, which starts in the therapy session and gradually generalizes to the individuals' environment. A behavioral rehearsal is one of the most essential parts of the treatment sequence because it provides feedback to the therapist regarding the extent to which couples and family members have understood what they have learned and can demonstrate how it should be implemented. In addition, the actual practice is what galvanizes the change and contributes to its becoming a permanent fixture. Behavioral rehearsal can be considered, in a way, a "shaping process," in which both the therapist and spouses or family members learn to adopt a new way of interaction.

The initial rehearsal segment occurs in the therapy session, where feedback is provided on what has been demonstrated and recommendations are made collaboratively on how refinement can occur and be applied to the situation. Consider the following example.

THE CASE OF JOHN AND MARY

John and Mary had difficulty in keeping their arguments from escalating into a shouting match. Part of the initial task was to bring up touchy issues in the therapy session and practice talking about them to the point at which either spouse began to feel uncomfortable or become emotionally upset. At that point, they were instructed to ask for time out and disengage from the conversation to give each other some space within the dialogue to deescalate. This exercise involved the therapist as a coach, intervening or supporting the partners and monitoring their emotional levels and thoughts that contributed to periods of agitation. The repeated rehearsal of monitoring and being able to voice the need to stop became quite a task, but eventually proved to be very helpful. They were subsequently sent home to attempt to do this on their own and then report back at the next session, when each would discuss some of the difficulties in achieving the objective and whether or not they had experienced failure. This practice was repeatedly rehearsed for several visits, at which point John and Mary began to experience some success.

DATTILIO: So, how did your week go?

JOHN: We screwed up. I started to get into a conversation about what needed to be done around the house as spring rolled around, and right away Mary harped on me about getting all these chores done in a week or two. I started to get heated about it but I didn't say anything. It eventually ended up leading into a major blowup between us.

DATTILIO: All right, so what do you feel you did wrong?

JOHN: Well, I didn't speak up soon enough, I guess. It's just a bad habit and something I really need to remind myself of. I tend to tune Mary out because she gets into this mode of nagging at me, and it's just a bad habit.

DATTILIO: Well, that may be, but it is also important that you monitor your thinking about it because this is an essential part of facilitating change.

MARY: I noticed that John got quiet and I realized, uh-oh, something is going on in his head. That's when I decided to stop, but it was a little bit too late and he got pissed off.

DATTILIO: OK, let's go back and try it again. It is going to take us some time to straighten this out because this is a long-standing pattern with the two of you. Such patterns don't go away overnight, but this is part of what behavioral rehearsal is all about.

JOHN: I know, it's just discouraging sometimes.

DATTILIO: Sure, but we'll get there. Let's try it again. Maybe you want to think about some other ways to cue in to this, or perhaps Mary can serve as a cue for you in a less "nagging" fashion to remind you before you get rolling.

MARY: I wouldn't mind doing that just as long as he doesn't take offense to it.

DATTILIO: Well, let's understand that now—before we try—that any attempts that the other makes to remind you of what you are trying to accomplish are OK, so that it's not taken negatively.

JOHN and MARY: OK, we'll give it a shot.

DATTILIO: Good, so let's try the homework again. Look for a topic to discuss and keep track of how you feel you did with it, and then we can discuss it a bit more in the next session.

In the preceding example, it is easy to see that sometimes helping clients to examine their cognitions and behaviors involves very tedious work. Again, this is much of what therapy boils down to—a lot of behavioral rehearsal and encouragement, as well as effort, in reshaping behaviors and behavioral patterns. Change does not occur without a lot of hard work, and much of the therapy process is devoted to reinforcing and encouraging clients to invest time and energy into changing their interactional dynamics.

Role Reversal

In their comprehensive book on marital therapy, Jacobson and Margolin (1979) accentuated the importance of role reversal. This is a role-playing technique that is often used with couples and families to get them to see another's perspective. Jacobson and Margolin suggested that spouses be asked to reverse roles and discuss a problem as it is usually discussed at home, with each person taking the opposite spouse's role. They believed that both the therapist and the partners could become more sensitive to each partner's misperception of their behaviors. Because each of the spouses has a tendency to respond at least as much to the perceptions of the other's behaviors as they do to the actual behaviors, it was the authors' belief that role reversal can clarify the nature of these misperceptions and the therapist, as an objective third party, can then correct them. Assuming the role of the other partner broadens each person's perspective in much the same way that videotape feedback does. By focusing on the other, rather than on him- or herself, a partner, often for the first time, empathically experiences the other individual's position. As a result, this experience can change the way the person thinks about the entire exchange. It also gives a spouse an opportunity to imitate the types of behaviors and demeanor he or she would like to see in the partner, while enacting the role of the partner. This is also a fun exercise and it sometimes gets laughs, which can be a much needed respite during the course of treatment. Through this type of role play, the therapist can also take an instrumental role in shaping positive behaviors and providing feedback.

This technique may be a little more difficult to orchestrate with a large family, and the role play should be performed between two members of a family at a time.

Acquiring Relationship Skills

Much of the cognitive-behavioral approach with families involves the direct teaching of skills for dealing with problems and differences. In this respect, the therapist may be like a coach. The therapist oversees the development and acquisition of skills that the clients will use in the therapy process and when future conflicts arise. In general, this means teaching the couple or family new ways to communicate, solve problems, and deal with change in the system.

Many of the systems-oriented and structural theorists rely on subtle, indirect suggestions and directives, which are seldom explicitly defined in treatment. CBT is more didactic and directive. Therefore, whereas someone like Salvador Minuchin would describe himself as a *reflective* instrument of change, cognitive-behaviorists would regard themselves as *directive* instruments of change. Behavioral rehearsal and guided practice are important in the treatment process, which resembles Guerney's (1977) training model, as well as that which was proposed for marital therapy based on social learning and behavioral exchange principles by Jacobson and Margolin (1979).

Of course, one of the potential problems inherent in the more didactic and directive approach offered by CBT is that clients may form a dependence on the therapist to the point where they fail to do these assignments on their own. This is part of why CBT endorses a collaborative approach in which clients take responsibility for change. One way to reinforce independent functioning in a client is for the client and therapist to collaboratively develop homework assignments that the client can do to implement what he or she has learned. Homework assignments are discussed in greater detail in the following section.

Homework Assignments

An expanded section on homework assignments is provided here because homework is such an important and integral aspect of the cognitive-behavioral approach. It is often regarded as one of the most powerful agents of change (Kazantzis, Deane, & Ronan, 2000; Kazantzis, Whittington, & Dattilio, in press).

The use of homework, or *out-of-session assignments*, is not a new development in the field of psychotherapy. During some of the earliest days of treatment, Freud (1952) suggested that his phobic patients venture out into society and face their fears once they had worked through their conflicts in analysis.

Years later, therapists emphasized the importance of homework assignments, touting them as critical adjunctive components of treatment (Dunlap, 1932). Clearly, cognitive-behavioral therapists are recognized more prominently for emphasizing homework assignments as a key aspect of treatment for a broad spectrum of disorders. George Kelly (1955) was one of the first theorists to introduce the use of homework as an integral component of his fixed-role therapy. Homework was also utilized in short-term approaches to a variety of disorders in an attempt to facilitate treatment gains (Kazantzis et al., 2000). It was the cognitive therapists who found that patients who completed more homework assignments developed a more positive outcome in treatment (Bryant, Simons, & Thase, 1999).

Homework assignments, in my opinion, are a major part of the armamentaria of therapeutic techniques. In fact, in a text on family therapy that I edited, 75% of the authors in more than 16 different orientations indicated that they used homework assignments regularly in their work (Dattilio, 1998a). Cognitive-behavioral family therapists have touted homework assignments as being a cornerstone of treatment (Dattilio, 1998, 2002; Dattilio & Padesky, 1990).

In a recent survey of members of the American Association for Marriage and Family Therapy (AAMFT), it was cited that the majority of clinicians reported using homework in their therapy more so with couples than with families (Dattilio, Kazantzis, Shinkfield, & Carr, in press). It was further reported that three-fourths of responders in this study assign three or more different types of homework assignments during the first ten sessions with clients. The majority of clinicians recommend one to two homework assignments per session.

Homework has also been endorsed by systemic, structural, psychodynamic, integrative, and postmodern approaches. An example is the late family therapist Jay Haley (1976), who had great credence in homework assignments in his work. It appears that homework should be a standard, inasmuch as so much is predicated on what occurs between therapy sessions.

L'Abate (1985) discusses the use of what he calls systematic homework assignments (SHWA). The author assigns a minimum of three homework assignments per session.

There are a number of benefits to using homework assignments (Dattilio, 2005a; Dattilio, L'Abate, & Deane, 2005). First, no situation is more volatile than that of a couple or family in crisis, and the use of homework assignments carries the therapeutic process beyond the therapy sessions. Most of a patient's time is spent outside the sessions, in the home environment where most problems occur. Therefore, homework serves to keep the therapy sessions alive during the interim periods and promotes a transfer from the therapy sessions to day-to-day living.

Homework also helps to move families into active involvement (Prochaska, DiClemente, & Norcross, 1992). An assignment may also be used early in the assessment phase in order to test motivation for change. Homework assignments can also be extremely effective in dealing with resistance from a couple or family throughout the course of treatment.

Another benefit of homework is that the assignments provide individuals with an opportunity to implement and evaluate insights for coping behaviors that have been discussed during the treatment process. Practice serves to heighten awareness of various issues that have unfolded in treatment. Furthermore, homework can increase the expectations for clients to follow through with making changes rather than simply discussing change during the therapy sessions. Exercises usually require participation, which can create a sense that the patient is taking active steps toward change. Alternatively, homework can also set the stage for trial experiences. Such experiences can be reintroduced in the next session for further processing. Modications can be made to thoughts, feelings, or behaviors as the homework is processed in the therapy sessions.

Occasionally, treatment processes can become vague and abstract, particularly in the area of family therapy. By adding focus and structure, homework assignments can reenergize treatment. Moreover, homework can increase clients' motivation to change because it provides them with something specific to work on.

An additional benefit includes the increased involvement of significant others. This is accomplished by way of assignments that call for the participation of others.

Homework strategies are modeled initially when family members interact in a therapy session. They are then instructed to modify their interaction outside the session. In all cases, it is important for the clinician to take into account the couple's or family's ability, tolerance, and motivation to maximize the potential for successful completion of specific homework tasks.

There are various types of homework assignments used with families.

Some of the more common are discussed in the following paragraphs. It should be noted that some assignments may be more suitable earlier in the treatment process (i.e., bibliotherapy, self-monitoring, etc.) and that others should be introduced later in the treatment phase (i.e., action-oriented assignments, cognitive restructuring, etc.).

Bibliotherapy Assignments

Bibliotherapy is important because it helps to reinforce the issues covered during therapy sessions and keeps the client active between sessions. Assigned readings are usually germane to the content receiving focus in the course of treatment. Some of the bibliotherapy assignments may involve having a couple read books such as *Fighting for Your Marriage* by Markman et al. (1994). Families may also benefit from homework assignments such as those found in the *Brief Family Therapy Treatment Planner* by Bevilacqua and Dattilio (2001). Despite our attempts to impress certain concepts on clients during the course of therapy, sometimes having them read about such ideas has a profound effect on their thinking about these concepts.

Audiotaping or Videotaping Interactions at Home

Audiotaping or videotaping conversations and nonverbal behaviors outside the session affords the therapist and the family members a review of some of the interaction that occurs more spontaneously in natural environments. This provides an opportunity to review important new ideas as well as the content that is discussed in sessions. During the in-session review of a tape, clinicians can ask individuals for their retrospective opinions and thoughts about their behaviors and discuss alternative coping strategies or interactions. For example, members can videotape a family meeting, or even a heated argument, so that interactional dynamics can be observed and the breakdown of communication can be identified. Videotaping has an advantage over audiotaping, in that nonverbal behaviors and body language can he observed.

Activity Scheduling

The use of activity scheduling—with emphasis on communication, interaction skills, and problem-solving skills—is extremely important for couples and families. Activity scheduling is intended to diagnose dysfunction as well as to learn new behaviors. For example, a family can try a new activity together (e.g., skiing) and observe how each member reacts to an unfamiliar situation and how individuals assist each other. Do they stick together or go off on their own? A number of manuals introduced into the professional literature capitalize on the specific use of activity scheduling in homework assignments and various out-of-session assignments with both couples and families (Bevilacqua & Dattilio, 2001).

Activity schedules can also be used to help families keep track of their activities on a regular basis. If there are negative interactions or symptoms within the relationship, couples and families may benefit from less demanding forms of activity, such as maintaining a list of activities achieved during the day or talking about tasks that were done. Activity schedules should include a subjective rating of activities that indicates the level of achievement or pleasure they provide.

Clients can use scales to rate activities from 0 (no sense of pleasure or mastery) to 10 (a total sense of pleasure or mastery). The activity schedules and rating scales combined usually encourage individuals to focus on activities that provide a sense of achievement and pleasure. Both are also designed to develop and enhance cohesiveness between spouses and among family members.

Self-Monitoring

In traditional cognitive-behavioral therapies, individuals are usually asked to complete thought or mood assessments between sessions. Monitoring exercises are designed to provide the clinician with accurate information about spouses' or family members' areas of difficulties. The clients are also asked to concentrate on the automatic thoughts and beliefs they experience during the course of these exercises and activities. The rationale for self-monitoring involves helping individuals to get in touch with exactly how they think, feel, and behave and how this impacts their individual dynamics. An example is the use of the Daily Dysfunctional Thought Sheet (Beck, Rush, Shaw, & Emery, 1979), in which individuals are asked to record their thoughts during arguments and make the connection of how they affect their moods and behaviors.

Behavioral Task Assignments

As mentioned earlier, an important part of treatment with couples and families often involves behavioral task assignments. Behavioral assignments may include having individuals use restructured self-talk to search for alternative explanations. Individuals can use this technique by themselves or with a spouse or family members in order to modify certain behaviors. Such behavioral assignments may also involve individuals' locating common bonds between them.

Behavioral task assignments are often most effective when family members are involved in their design and planning. Such planning may include the timing of the assignment, who will be involved, how frequently it will be conducted, and the length of time required to complete it.

Behavioral task assignments should be scheduled for review upon completion, with a discussion of any difficulties the couple or family members had in completing it. If the assignment cannot be completed, an attempt should he made to analyze the roadblocks so that future difficulties can be identified and effectively dealt with in treatment.

Some of the more popular behavioral task assignments include the use of pleasing behaviors, behavioral rehearsal, assertiveness exercises, and role reversal.

Cognitive Restructuring of Dysfunctional Thoughts

Family members sometimes experience difficulty in moving forward and may benefit from structured exercises that allow them to weigh alternative styles of thinking and identify distorted beliefs. The use of the Daily Record of Dysfunctional Thoughts developed by Beck et al. (1979) is one method for reevaluating their thinking styles.

Developing and Implementing Homework Assignments

Sometimes clinicians are guilty of randomly assigning homework simply for the sake of being able to issue an assignment. Giving random assignments runs the risk of angering clients because it can give them the impression that the therapist believes that fixing their problems is simple—"just do the fairly obvious task and your troubles will be over." Strategically selecting homework assignments that are germane to the family and the therapy is a key objective (Kazantzis & Dattilio, in press). Designing specific assignments is crucial, and therefore the should be selected carefully.

A good example of the use of strategic homework assignments is demonstrated in the case of Matt and Elizabeth in the section "Emotional Intensity and Emotional Focus", in which we all agreed that having them both write down exactly what they need from each other when they were being comforted was essential to their problem. This exercise proved to be very effective in their particular case.

Yet had I simply suggested a random exercise for developing emotional intimacy that didn't fit their specific problem, it might have actually backfired, causing more tension between the two of them.

Nelson and Trepper (1993, 1998) have produced two volumes of family therapy interventions, many of which include homework assignments that can be used during treatment. Choosing the timing of an assignment so that it is not too early in the treatment process is essential to maximizing treatment benefits.

I suggest that when incorporating homework assignments, clinicians think specifically about how they wish to use assignments during the course of treatment and what point in the treatment may be an appropriate time to intervene. They also need to think about what they desire to accomplish in assigning homework. In utilizing a specific homework assignment, it may be prudent to use your own style in approaching spouses or family members. Take time to explain and review each assignment with the spouses or family members so that they understand exactly what the assignment objective is and, more important, know exactly what they are to do and why. Often, clients nod their heads, acknowledging that they understand a homework assignment when in fact they are confused about the specific request but are reluctant to speak up.

Homework Compliance

Recent research has supported the importance of inquiring about homework assignments. Bryant et al. (1999) rated therapy tapes regarding homework assignments and compliance. The strongest predictor of homework compliance in their study was therapists' behavior in reviewing assigned homework tasks. General therapeutic skills also predicted homework compliance in this study. These general skills included cooperation in establishing the homework and providing positive reinforcement in the form of encouragement and praise for efforts. The research, though conducted on individual clients, is significant for couple and family therapy as well.

During the process of securing an agreement from each couple or family member to try an assignment, the clinician may encounter a situation in which a certain individual may think that the assignment is silly or simply not a good idea. Such issues need to be addressed up front. The more agreement that is achieved between spouses or among family members about attempting the homework, the more likely the assignment is to be successful.

Follow-Up

Following up on the results of homework assignments is obviously very important. It is strongly recommended that this be considered an agenda for the subsequent visit, unless of course the couple or family members request more time to complete the task. Ensuring follow-up on the results can also provide an indirect message to the couple or family that these assignments are crucial and are not administered simply to fill therapy session time or to give them something to occupy their time outside the session.

Resistance to Completing Homework Assignments

One of the most common difficulties with homework therapy is spousal or family members' resistance to completing homework assignments. This may often occur despite the couple's or family's agreeing to the assignment and acknowledging that it would be helpful. Such resistance may have its roots in more complicated dynamics of the family or couple, or it may be simply that the assignments are being referred to as "homework," which carries a negative connotation for some. Clinicians may chose to consider changing the term *homework* to either *task* or *experiment*. Homework assignments are better received when the therapist suggests, "Suppose we try an experiment." Usually there is something intriguing about the term *experiment*, and for many, its use is less threatening or dictatorial than the term *homework assignment*.

Tactful handling of resistance to completing homework assignments is essential. Couples and family members who avoid completing homework assignments may be providing the clinician with important information about the effect that change may have on them. This may include difficulties with communication, in working as a unit, or simply the awkwardness about experiencing a change in the relationship. Regardless of the reason, it is important to explore the dynamics behind resistance and the alternatives that may be used in dealing with it. Upon discussing this issue in detail, the therapist may decide to reassign the same exercise, to assign a different exercise, or to defer the idea completely until another time.

Testing Predictions with Behavioral Experiments

Although an individual may use logical analysis to successfully reduce his or her negative expectancies concerning events that will occur in family interactions, firsthand evidence is often needed. Cognitive-behavioral therapists often guide family members in devising *behavioral experiments* in which they test their predictions that particular actions will lead to certain responses from other members. For example, a man who expects his wife and children to resist including him in their leisure activities when he gets home from work can make plans to try to engage with the family when he arrives home during the next few days and see what happens. When such plans are devised during joint family therapy sessions, the therapist can ask family members to predict what each person's responses will be during the experiment. The family members can also anticipate potential obstacles to the success of the experiment and make appropriate adjustments. In addition, the family members' public commitments to cooperation with the experiment often increase the likelihood of its success.

An example of a behavioral experiment involves a couple I saw for therapy several years ago and is detailed in the following vignette.

"DON'T TAKE CARE OF ME": THE CASE OF LACY AND STEVE

Lacy and Steve were a middle-aged couple who sought marital therapy because they were experiencing tension in their relationship and were bickering more than usual. The problems seemed to arise after Lacy had broken her ankle and was dependent on Steve to take care of her. Lacy explained that she had always been self-sufficient and the notion of being the least bit dependent on anyone was unacceptable for her. This attitude was creating problems between her and Steve because Steve felt that she was rejecting his help. Steve complained, "I need to feel like I have some worth in this relationship, and Lacy seldom allows me help her because she feels that she needs to take care of everything on her own." Lacy believed that she had always been self-sufficient and, now, when she needed to be taken care of, she had difficulty letting Steve care for her.

I suspected that there was more to Lacy's resistance than simply wanting to be self-sufficient. It was at this point that I began to use a brief version of the downward-arrow technique to try to get to the cognitive distortion beneath her attitude. I asked her to explain to me what it meant to be dependent on Steve.

LACY: It means that I am not capable.

DATTILIO: Lacy, let's just take this initial notion of "I am not capable." What does that mean to you?

LACY: It makes me a child. I am a failure as an adult.

DATTILIO: Just because you need to rely on somebody else doesn't mean that you are a total failure, does it?

Lacy explained that she realized that the difficulty was not a matter of simply being a failure as much as it was Steve's being in control of everything. This all-or-nothing distortion that Lacy developed is not unusual with couples. I explained to her a little about the notion of how these distortions sometimes develop as the result of erroneous thinking. Lacy went on to explain, "I have always prided myself on being an independent person, and now I have to be dependent and that troubles me." We discussed Lacy's propensity to look at things in all-or-nothing terms. I pointed out to her that when she does that, she boxes herself into a corner. It was clear that I needed to help Lacy begin to look at being more flexible in her thinking. When we discussed her family of origin, I learned that both of her parents were extremely rigid in their thinking and that Lacy had come to look at life in all-or-nothing terms. She explained to me that because she was an accountant, her life revolved around black-and-white and dichotomizing things. Lacy went on to explain that she much preferred this way of thinking because it was easier in dealing with life events. I pointed out to her that at this point however, it had now become difficult for her because of her real life change. Lacy's breaking her ankle actually opened the door to a more serious and chronic problem that existed in the relationship, and it was the event of her injury that revealed this deeper issue.

I worked with Lacy on this issue in the presence of her husband so that he could have an opportunity to see how his wife's rigid thinking contributed to the polarization in the relationship. I was able to link Lacy's rigid thinking to difficulties in the relationship and to explain that giving Steve some responsibility for caring for her was an example of what we aspire to in healthy relationships. We also discussed the notion of relationships involving a "give and take" exchange and that when a relationship is lopsided (i.e., one person has all the control and all the duties and responsibilities in the relationship), it creates a skew in the system.

I suggested to Lacy that she take small steps in terms of relinquishing some control to Steve by first letting him do certain chores and then dealing with her thoughts in regard to relinquishing control. I had to help her restructure the thought involving the catastrophe she anticipated, that this was going to give Steve complete control and that she would be completely dominated. Much of this problem had to do with Lacy's previous marriage, in which her husband controlled everything. He was abusive and intolerant and she had very little autonomy in the relationship. I had to remind Lacy that this was not the same relationship and that sharing some of the control and being a little dependent on her husband was not such a terrible thing. This concept also proved to be somewhat of an adjustment for Steve, inasmuch as he was not used to stepping into the role of caretaker. I had to ease him into this via behavioral exercises and help him deal with the frustration that his wife experienced during the course of her relinquishing some control to him step-by-step.

Lacy had always prided herself on being an independent person, and part of being dependent on others was a matter of losing her sense of self. We talked about relinquishing control—with the understanding and balance that everyone needs to be dependent, as well as independent—and about good balance being a healthy thing. I had Lacy test the prediction that she would feel like a failure if she relinquished some control to Steve and allowed him to take care of her. Once Lacy took the risk and allowed Steve to take care of her, she began to see that she didn't feel as bad as she had initially anticipated. This provided her with a measure of reassurance, and she didn't feel like a failure. We continued with a number of successful steps in which Lacy predicted how she would feel, and over time she was able to ease into being more dependent in the relationship without feeling unduly controlled by her husband. Small experiments such as this are often essential to facilitating change in relationships.

This case example is a very important one because it illustrates how CBT is not just a simplistic, quick-fix intervention that involved telling Lacy, "There's nothing wrong with depending on your husband—just do it." The notion of exploring with her the roots of her feelings and beliefs and uncovering some of her fears is much more involved and departs from the common misperception that CBT means giving banal advice.

Behavioral Techniques and Parental Control

Some of the earliest writings in behavioral family therapy focused on parenting behaviors and parental control. The work of Gerald Patterson and colleagues particularly was noted for effectiveness in this area and is still highly regarded among cognitive and behavioral therapists in dealing with parent–child issues (Patterson et al., 1967; Forgatch & Patterson, 1998). The interventions are typically based on operant techniques but also combine other techniques, as demonstrated in the following case example in which I worked with a mother and her son in addressing the son's chronic headache complaints.

"I HAVE A HEADACHE": THE CASE OF CLAY

Clay, a 12-year-old boy, came to therapy as a result of chronic headache pain. Clay's mother reported that he had been complaining of headaches (in the frontal lobe area) on a daily basis for about 8 months prior to treatment. He received an extensive physical and neurological examination, including a sleep EEG (electroencephalogram) and MRI (Magnetic Resonance Imaging), which yielded negative results. At this point behavioral counseling was recommended.

Clay's first mention of his chronic headache pain came shortly after his parents were separated, at which time Clay's mother started spending less time with him because she became busier at work.

Clay's headaches usually occurred in the morning prior to his going to school and again in the evening at bedtime. He described his headache pain as always occurring in the frontal lobe area. The average duration of his headaches was 1½ to 2 hours, during which Clay would cry and complain about the pain until he was attended to by his mother. His mother usually responded by administering Tylenol and spending time with him until the pain gradually faded. Clay's headaches also involved his missing half-days of school.

The primary goal of therapy was to reduce Clay's headache pain so that he could resume his daily activities and increase his school attendance.

It was decided to first implement the use of positive reinforcement for days when headache pain was not reported and to ignore all suspected reports of *nonlegitimate* headache pain. It was only when reports of headache pain were accompanied by an elevation in body temperature that any attention was given. Headaches that were accompanied by an elevated body temperature were designated as *legitimate headaches*. Treatment consisted of administering Tylenol and confining Clay to his bed with no additional verbal attention.

The treatment involved a simple reinforcement schedule, with positive rewards consisting of increased verbal praise and a specific one-to-one interaction between Clay and his mother. The verbal praise and one-to-one interaction, which consisted of playing a game or simply talking, was implemented only when there was an absence of headache reports. Clay was instructed by the therapist to continue to report to his mother each day if his headache pain occurred; she would keep a written record of his headache episodes. The mother was also instructed to ignore Clay's headache reports to the extent of not giving him any type of attention that might be misperceived as reinforcement for having a headache. When a day had passed in which no headaches were reported, mother would reward Clay through the use of verbal praise and acknowledgment. This was something that Clay considered very meaningful and proved to be an excellent means of reinforcement for him.

This simple procedure yielded successful results in a relatively short period of time. Clay responded well to the positive reinforcement and learned that he could obtain his mother's attention in a more constructive and appropriate fashion than through reporting headache pain.

Figure 6.2 depicts the decrease in complaints of headache pain during the period of treatment. A "headache complaint" was defined as the verbal expression of the presence of headache pain that did not accompany an elevation in temperature.

Within 12 weeks of the treatment, the headache pain rapidly decreased through the use of positive reinforcement to the point where psychosomatic headache pain was totally eliminated.

Positive reinforcement is the most widely used technique for changing behavior in the treatment of both children and adults. It can be applied to decrease undesirable behavior, as well as to increase desirable behavior. A prerequisite to developing a successful treatment design is for the therapist to conduct a detailed behavioral analysis to enable him or her to select an

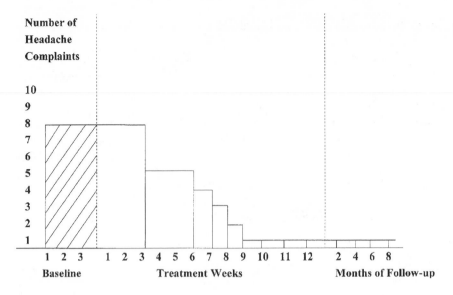

FIGURE 6.2. Number of Clay's headache complaints through treatment and follow-up.

effective reinforcer and increase the frequency of the desired behavior. It also allows the therapist to identify the antecedent of the undesired behavior and plan for the prevention of similar behaviors (Dattilio, 1983).

In this case, as headache pain was attenuated with the use of positive reinforcement, it became apparent that Clay's headaches were a means of manipulating his mother into devoting her undivided attention to him. Following the regular treatment program, informal instructions were given to Clay on ways in which he could gain attention from his mother in a more appropriate fashion.

A 12-month follow-up revealed no occurrence of headache pains that were unaccompanied by additional symptoms. In addition, Clay achieved perfect school attendance during the course of the follow-up period and claimed to enjoy the relationship with his mother much more than he had previously.

ADDRESSING THE POTENTIAL FOR RELAPSE

The potential for relapse with any couple or family is always present, particularly if the problem at hand has been chronic. There are a number of points to keep in mind when working with couples and families. First and foremost, the work is difficult, particularly when we face a situation in which there is more than one set of personality dynamics. This is one of the reasons that couple and family work is so challenging. Second, depending on how long the problem has existed and how deeply ingrained it is, the more likely relapse will occur. If psychopathology—such as depression, anxiety, major personality disorder, or addiction—is present, the likelihood of regression is even greater.

There are a number of steps that can help to ensure against relapse. Much of the program for relapse prevention with marital couples suffering from alcohol abuse proposed by O'Farrell (1993) can also be used with any couple or family members. Family members need to realize that relapse is likely, and individuals need to accept this. This is not to say that it gives them permission to backslide, however. Family members must be mindful that the triggers that contribute to a relapse also contribute to the deterioration of the relationship.

O'Farrell (1993) suggests providing a framework for discussing relapse for family members to follow. The first step is to develop a list of concerns for each member to discuss when he or she feels that the relationship is beginning to deteriorate. Such a discussion should specify high-risk situations and early warning signs of relapse to deteriorative behaviors.

The second step is to develop a plan of action that all family members agree to as a measure to prevent steps toward regression. This can be done at the outset of any indication that things are beginning to deteriorate.

The third step is to discuss the behaviors that should be utilized. Finally, a further individual treatment plan for dealing with cognitions that contribute to anger escalation and deteriorative behaviors should be put in place.

A relapse plan is written and rehearsed on a case-by-case basis to reflect the common deteriorative patterns in a specific relationship. Every relationship is different and, therefore, just as problems differ, the patterns of deterioration differ as well.

All of the interventions to be used are discussed in advance, almost in a choreographic fashion, in the same way that a family may plan for how to exit the home in the event of a fire or another type of disaster. I often inform couples and families that just as cruise lines have evacuation drills, or certain buildings conduct fire drills, family members need to routinely discuss how to deal, in advance, with escalating conflict that may be disastrous. In this manner, they will be prepared for dealing effectively with deterioration. At the same time, this also urges them to monitor their interaction so that, as long as communication is kept up and they are attuned to the nuances of their relationship, they will always be in good shape to avoid deterioration.

HANDLING ROADBLOCKS
AND RESISTANCE TO CHANGE

Roadblocks and resistance to change comes in various forms. Sometimes resistance appears to be next to impossible to overcome, and it can become a real challenge for a therapist to continue with a resisting client.

Sometimes resistance occurs because of one family member refusing to attend therapy. There are various ways to deal with such a situation. Some therapists take the position that no effort should be made to encourage spouses or family members to attend treatment if they don't want to. However, sometimes therapists need to be creative in order to help the therapy process along.

In the particular case of a family that I treated, a young adolescent female resisted her parents' request to come to family therapy because, she contended, they were the ones with the problem, not she. After meeting the parents for the initial session and learning of their daughter's stance on the matter, I asked permission to contact the daughter myself. I called her and informed her that her parents had apprised me of her stance on attending therapy and that I respected her wishes. However, I did ask her if she would be willing to help me help her parents. I proceeded to explain to her that after meeting with her parents, I tended to agree with her that they were the ones who had a problem, and that I needed to work with them on a number of issues, namely, some of their unreasonable demands and their intrusiveness in her life. I said that I could make faster headway if she would share with me some of her perceptions of her parents and help me to better orchestrate treatment. In essence, this took the pressure off the young girl, who agreed to meet with me. I suggested that we meet at a nearby Starbucks so that she would feel more comfortable and less as though she was coming to therapy.

Once we met, I was able to interest her in sharing what she had to say to her parents directly, and she consequently agreed to visit my office with her parents for the next session. This eventually led to her returning for several family visits. What appeared to be this young girl's staunch desire to avoid therapy was actually her fear of being put in a situation where she would be out of control. Once I had reassured her that I could serve as a neutral and objective third party, she felt better about coming to therapy.

PARTNERS' NEGATIVITY
AND HOPELESSNESS ABOUT CHANGE

Often, family members who seek treatment have vivid memories of events in their relationship that override the current positive behaviors that they are currently attempting to pursue. Weiss (1980) referred to this in the literature as *sentiment override*. Such memories often need to be addressed, and couples need to utilize the techniques that help to take away the power of these vivid negative memories.

Negative schemas about the characteristics of the relationship need to be addressed by having the clients test the validity of their fixed views and consider information that suggests that such views can be changed. Coaching the respective spouses to keep track of situational variations in each other's behaviors is a technique in which they note how the behaviors differ from one situation to another (Epstein & Baucom, 2002). Epstein and Baucom suggest that this exercise counteracts the idea of an invariant trait, and it opens the door for exploring the conditions that tend to elicit the other's positive or negative responses. The idea is to weaken the hold of negative memories by demonstrating other patterns in interaction. Thus, the therapist's challenge is to help couples notice and give credit for each small positive change they make, with each spouse taking personal responsibility for making specific changes and overriding old negative memories with new positive experiences. It may also be important for spouses to express regret for their past actions that upset each other, even if they were unintentional.

Reducing spouses' hopelessness about the potential for improvement in their relationship depends on the therapist's ability to coach the partners in behaving more constructively with each other. Having spouses observe and monitor their negative interactions as they decrease, and behave in more positive ways, is the essential goal.

DIFFERENCES IN AGENDAS

It is also important for the therapist to consider the possibility that family members often have different agendas for being in therapy. It is not uncommon for therapists to see that one spouse is more motivated than the other to participate in treatment. It is also possible that one partner is there to heal the relationship, whereas the other is there for help with ending the relationship. Sometimes one spouse may be completely opposed to the idea of conjoint therapy. It is therefore important to discuss what each individual hopes to gain from treatment. The roadblock of conflicting agendas in therapy can be a window into a struggle that the couple is currently experiencing in their relationship as a whole.

For example, therapists might point out how one spouse may be under pressure to participate in therapy, and that the other's resistance to participate seems to reflect a broader demand–withdrawal pattern in the couple's relationship. This is why the issue of standards in relationships, discussed in earlier chapters, becomes so important. The therapist may consider guiding the withdrawing partner to think about the validity of his or her standards and challenge some of the belief systems that underlie them. It is also important for the therapist to point out to each of the spouses how their behaviors contribute to the circular process of their demand–withdrawal pattern, and stress that the best opportunity for change may involve each person's making an effort in modifying his or her behavior.

A good example of this approach might be Diane changing her request that Nick spend all of his free time with her and conceding to accept just a portion of his time. In turn, Nick may initiate a joint activity with his wife from time to time, as well as agreeing to join her in some of the activities that she proposes.

But what happens when it is clear that one spouse wants to continue the relationship and the other wants to end it? It is at this point that the therapist may need to help the couple redefine the goals for therapy, or the conflicting goals will be a roadblock to further work together. The partners may then focus on the shared goal of determining how they can relate in constructive, rather than destructive, ways in dealing with their different individual goals for their relationship. Managing negative emotions, such as anger or resentment, and collaborating in finding reasonable solutions to the important issues of the relationship are essential.

ANXIETY ABOUT CHANGING
EXISTING PATTERNS IN THE RELATIONSHIP

It is not uncommon for family members to experience discomfort or anxiety with changing patterns of the relationship. Such feelings may arise with one or more family members. Change often touches on self-protective strategies that family members have developed in order to avoid being hurt or vulnerable. Often, spouses complain that they feel threatened by the fact that therapy could promote change that will expose an area of personal vulnerability.

This issue has been addressed in the professional literature, particularly as it relates to vulnerability schemas (Tilden & Dattilio, 2005). The therapist needs to explore each partner's thoughts and emotions about proposed changes in the couple's interactions and to probe for underlying concerns when one or both members of the couple experience anxiety about what change involves. Easing them into new behaviors and discussing how the situation will be different are important steps. It is also important to go slowly when making changes in the relationship, because a threat to the homeostasis of a relationship often causes problems. Often, discussing this issue and suggesting techniques for reducing anxiety, both cognitively and behaviorally, are important. Moreover, during the course of the therapy sessions, it is important that there is lots of discussion about what the new behavior will look like and what the difference in the emotional climate of the relationship will be after a change does occur.

RELINQUISHING PERCEIVED POWER AND CONTROL

Another area in which anxiety develops is the potential loss of power and control in the relationship when any type of change is made. It is important that the therapist appreciates the existing distribution of power and control in any given relationship, even when it appears to be dysfunctional. Any precipitous challenge to a family's existing structure is likely to create anxiety and to be met with resistance. This is particularly the case with the spouse who holds more power and perceives the threat of change as being disruptive and debilitating to him or her.

Addressing each of the family members' cognitions or schemas about power and control in their lives, as well as their relationship, is an avenue to be pursued. Again, this may also address issues of their respective families of origin and what their belief systems are concerning power and control. It is important to examine the degree of balance in this area, particularly for establishing a healthy relationship. Any perception of bias or lack of balance needs to be discussed. Strategies should be agreed upon for maintaining or striking a healthy balance. This will also require that the spouses view the therapist as being fair-minded and supportive as they move toward restructuring some of their beliefs.

ISSUES OF TAKING RESPONSIBILITY FOR CHANGE

As could be seen earlier with Margo and Curtis, taking responsibility for existing behaviors, as well as for change, is an essential part of dealing with resistance and roadblocks in a relationship. Family members, particularly couples, are notorious for blaming each other, instead of themselves, for relationship problems (Baucom & Epstein, 1990; Bradbury & Fincham, 1990; Epstein & Baucom, 2002). Obviously, blaming the other partner may involve self-protection, bolstering self-esteem, and taking the pressure to make changes off oneself. It always seems easier to notice the other person's behavior rather than one's own. Individuals commonly think about events in their relationship in linear-causal terms, rather than with circular-causal concepts that involve the two individuals influencing each other.

Because spouses may be too defensive to accept feedback from each other about the effects of their behavior, feedback from a therapist whom the individuals believe has no vested interest in proving that anyone is at fault, may be an effective mechanism for change.

Often, a spouse may need his or her partner to change and may exhibit ingratiating or seductive behaviors toward the therapist, to enlist the therapist as an ally in this mission. Here is one of the therapist's major challenges—to maintain balance and neutrality as a facilitator for change. In this respect, the therapist must absolutely avoid taking sides and help each of the partners to find ways of getting along better and resolving issues in their relationship. It is also important to establish guidelines so that each spouse agrees to take 50% of the responsibility in making change. This helps to avoid any uneven attribution of blame that may surface. I make it a habit to repeatedly remind clients about taking responsibility for their own behaviors and engaging in less blaming behavior with a spouse.

For a more detailed discussion of resistance and roadblocks in couple therapy, see the excellent chapter by Epstein and Baucom (2003).

Many of the types of resistance and roadblocks found in couples are often seen in families as well. Therapists will undoubtedly encounter endless roadblocks and resistance in their treatment of clients, which often becomes more intense with families because of the increase in the dynamics involved. It's important to simply accept the notion that overcoming resistance and roadblocks is a necessary part of the therapeutic process and an important challenge, particularly with difficult cases. The case of the Shim family, which follows, is illustrative.

THE CASE OF THE SHIMS

The Shims were an inner-city family who were ordered to treatment by the court. A major problem from the beginning was that they detested the sentence. The family members, including several of the teenagers, were dressed in a slovenly manner, with poor hygiene. Most of them had rotted or missing teeth. They all showed up for the initial visit, albeit begrudgingly. I had to wonder who was being sentenced, they or I.

Mr. Shim, the father and "head of household," often arrived for therapy with the smell of alcohol on his breath and his silver whiskers corkscrewing in different directions. He usually sat through the sessions with a sardonic smile on his face, saying very little. His wife compensated for his indifference and the children's recalcitrance by talking incessantly. The rest of the family sat disengaged and completely uninterested in what was going on in the room, unless, of course, one of the kids belched or passed gas, thus setting off an avalanche of laughter among the others. I dreaded working with this family. They made no bones about sharing their disdain for me. Certainly, this was not a good therapeutic fit. The roadblocks were not *between* us, they *were* us. But the Shims had little choice and neither did I, as they had been remanded and I was specifically appointed by a high-powered judge to work with them as a favor to the court.

The family had been sentenced in response to charges of theft and receiving stolen property. It was said that the entire family was involved in a theft ring, something the Shims vehemently denied.

Aside from our mutual disenchantment, there were plenty of other barriers to treatment with the Shims, obstacles that gave the term *roadblock* new meaning. There was the father's alcoholism and unemployment and what appeared to be an underlying depression and possible early onset of dementia. Cannabis abuse was rampant among the children. And then there was the mother's denial of everything, particularly of her teenage son's criminal behavior and of her husband's chronic substance abuse. To complete the picture, this family was functioning at a very low intellectual level, probably in the borderline retarded range. Needless to say, all of this made me uncertain about whether I could really do anything for the Shims.

Unfortunately, for therapists who work with families who are forced into treatment, these challenges are not unusual. The major focus in this kind of work is to effect change through restructuring thoughts and modifying behaviors—that is, if change is possible.

ROADBLOCKS

The term *roadblock* is defined by *Webster's New World Dictionary* as a barricade or anything that interferes with progress. In family therapy, as in any form of treatment, roadblocks may occur on both sides of the therapist's desk, as is so poignantly portrayed in the case of the Shims. That is, blocks occur on the part of the therapist as well as the client, a situation that can seriously impede the progress of treatment and sometimes bring therapy to a halt. In the case of the "Shims," I realized that it wasn't just this family that was holding up progress in treatment, but that I had a hand in it myself.

In his more recent work, Leahy (2001) discusses the concept of resistance in cognitive therapy and essentially defines it as anything that impedes the treatment process by either the patient or the therapist. The next section highlights several roadblocks that can often impede the progress of family therapy from both standpoints. Certain steps are discussed regarding what may be done to counteract such roadblocks.

Therapist Roadblocks

Many roadblocks originate with the therapist in working with particularly difficult families. These blocks may include the therapist's own resistance or defense mechanisms that may surface during the course of treatment. The aforementioned case is an excellent example of how resistance occurred on both sides of the fence, particularly with the therapist's reaction to the family's behavior. Sometimes it is not even necessary for a case to be as difficult as the one mentioned here in order for roadblocks to develop.

The therapist's failure to work through his or her own issues derived from his or her family of origin is one of the less recognized roadblocks that occur in family therapy. A perfect example of this situation is the therapist who never worked through conflict with his or her own parents and who may be blinded against recognizing the extent to which a youth is engaging in distortions in his thinking regarding his parents. Because of the therapist's own unresolved conflicts, the course of treatment may be affected. In addition, the situation may become further diluted and transferences may occur.

Another type of roadblock can occur when the therapist feels overwhelmed or helpless in the face of a difficult case because of insufficient training or supervision. Such an impediment can often segue into failure. It may also contribute to burnout or stalled movement, thus hindering the therapeutic process. In working with the Shims, it was essential for me to reevaluate my own cognitions about working with such a difficult situation and to address my own distortions regarding my effectiveness as a therapist.

I later realized that I had been sabotaging myself, even before beginning treatment, by engaging in catastrophic thoughts about what a disaster therapy with this family would be. In a sense, I was resisting having to deal with what I erroneously perceived as "the bottom of the barrel" after having the luxury of dealing with educated, high-functioning families in the past. What is more, I was personalizing the Shims's dysfunction and viewing it as a "failure waiting to happen."

Such catastrophic thinking is usually an indication that the therapist may have lost his or her objectivity and needs to regain some sense of balance. When this happens, it is recommended that the therapist seek peer review or consultation, or even supervision, during periods in which such conflicts arise. In the case of the Shims, I felt the need to confer with a colleague who had worked with families of similar socioeconomic backgrounds. This particular mentor was very skillful in helping me reframe my thinking by suggesting that I not take offense at this family's behavior and recalcitrance. In short, I learned to distance myself appropriately and to view the family members' behavior as a result of their problems. I had to face the fact that I myself was engaging in the cognitive distortion of personalizing and pressuring myself to be successful in a very difficult situation. This family presented with such a daunting front that I viewed myself as being destined to fail. Restructuring my thinking and belief system about success in treatment was an important issue for me; at the same time, getting back on track and dealing with this damaged family system was the best thing I could do. Once I was able to overcome this roadblock for myself, I was able to advance and be more successful in helping this family through its own roadblocks in the treatment process.

Unrealistic Expectations

Setting realistic expectations is a very important part of family therapy, or of any type of treatment for that matter. Being overoptimistic about what one is able to accomplish in treatment is a common pitfall for novice therapists. It can cause stress for the therapist and may set up the therapist and the family for failure. For example, attempting to aid in Mr. Shim's rehabilitation from his alcohol dependence without inpatient detoxification and family support might be considered *magical thinking*. Such an ingrained pattern would certainly not change unless a number of key dynamics in the family changed. A good outcome would require time and much prodding and may not have been very viable, particularly with a family such as this one. The ability to size up a family situation is essential for all parties involved so that realistic expectations can be set. Sometimes, expectations may even need to be reset throughout the course of therapy. Therefore, one way of overcoming the obstacle is to be as realistic and flexible as possible as to what can be accomplished in treatment, and when.

There were a myriad of issues to be addressed with the Shims, and it was unlikely that the majority of the objectives would ever be achieved. I knew somewhere in my mind that the family would not likely remain in treatment. Therefore, to establish a realistic expectation of getting them to show up for therapy was a major accomplishment and obviously a first step.

Cultural Obstacles

Cultural issues are certainly an aspect of treatment that needs to be considered when working with families. Currently, the United States has experienced the greatest influx of immigrants since the early 19th century. It is estimated that more than 1 million legal and undocumented immigrants arrive annually (McGoldrick, Giordano, & Pearce, 1996; McGoldrick et al., 2005).

Although many immigrant families in the United States become acculturated, households may still honor certain customs based on their cultural heritage. Many of these cultural and environmental traditions can be deeply ingrained in the family, which may be perceived by someone unfamiliar with the particular culture as deliberate resistance to change. A classic example involves a Polish family that I worked with several years ago while teaching in Krakow. Upon introducing a homework assignment for which I requested family members to gather information, I perceived the father's noncompliance as a major resistance to treatment. It was not until speaking with a colleague, a Polish psychiatrist, that I learned that such resistance was not uncommon among Polish males, particularly those who were products of the former Soviet rule. He explained to me that, as a result of the Nazi occupation in Poland and the subsequent presence of Communism, many individuals, particularly males, had difficulty with being told what to do. This was not only a cultural characteristic but also a remnant of years of oppression. Once I understood this collective concept more clearly, I was able to restructure my approach and implement it in a more collaborative vein, making it appealing to the father of this family. I essentially asked the father for permission to work through him, which he willingly granted. This example is not unusual, particularly with offspring of families that have been subjected to oppression in various nations (Dattilio, 2001b).

Clinicians conducting family therapy should familiarize themselves with various cultural aspects in the literature, as well as with the environments from which individuals hail, in order to avoid roadblocks. An excellent and comprehensive text on this topic is the book *Ethnicity and Family Therapy* (McGoldrick et al., 2005). This work offers family therapists a great deal of insight into how families of various cultures operate. It may also provide therapists with enough information to determine whether a family is operating from a rigidly held belief due to its culture or whether it is more reflective of a personality trait, or possibly both.

Racial Issues

Sometimes the fact that a family therapist is of a different race or culture from that of the family he or she is working with can become a problem. In the aforementioned case, the fact that I was of a different socioeconomic status surfaced as an issue later in treatment with the Shims, when the topic of dealing with racial issues among families was discussed. Many of the Shim children had difficulty understanding how I, having been reared in an upper-middle-class white neighborhood, could possibly comprehend the struggles they faced. This was clearly an issue that I needed to sort out. I had to decide whether this objection was a smoke screen, allowing them to sidestep the salient issues in therapy. I decided to confront them on this matter and induce them to consider that even though I was not African American and did not live in a lower-socioeconomic environment, I was willing to listen and try to learn to expand my knowledge of their struggles.

Environmental Forces

Another roadblock to treatment may involve families that are exposed to environments that inhibit or impede the changes achieved during the course of therapy. (Obviously, for a family that meets in therapy for 90 minutes each week, returning to an environment that lures them away from the direction of treatment will no doubt be counterproductive in maintaining everything achieved during the course of therapy.) In this particular case with the Shims, therapeutic interventions had very little power against the strong environmental forces that created a need for them to survive via a life of crime and, sometimes, violence. From a behavioral standpoint, the constant reinforcement in the home environment was a great antagonist to any therapeutic change, unless, of course, the family was willing to adopt wholeheartedly the desire to change and therefore make their best attempt to change in the face of those environmental forces. Unfortunately, the goal of changing a person's motivation is sometimes very difficult to achieve and involves the earlier issue of setting realistic expectations. Sometimes, changing behaviors entails changing the environmental surroundings, if possible. I was successful with the Shims in inducing them eventually to consider relocating in order to make a fresh start with their lives.

Psychopathology

Psychopathology is clearly one of the major hurdles in treatment with families, particularly when there is significant psychopathology in one or more family members.

Axis II disorders typically raise challenging roadblocks during the course of treatment, particularly when they exist in one of the parents. Certain personality disorders may impede the process to the point at which progress comes to a screeching halt. In most cases, individuals with severe Axis II disorders resist being referred for individual therapy; however, when the disorder is less severe, certain aspects may be addressed directly in the family therapy process. This, of course, depends largely on the cooperation of the family member diagnosed with the disorder. For example, in the aforementioned case, it was determined during the course of treatment that Mr. Shim had a substantial amount of narcissism with strong passive–aggressive features. However, his heavy substance abuse made it extremely difficult to address his personality issues. The fact that he was also nonverbal during the course of treatment was a major problem, particularly because his wife tended to compensate by speaking incessantly, making it easier for him to remain taciturn and to keep his individual issues covert.

In this particular case, I requested that the parents sit next to each other and I addressed them as a united front. I then attempted to accentuate the mother's power in the hope that it might draw the father's feelings to the surface. I viewed him as being the one who actually had the real power in the family, even though he seldom spoke. He operated behind the scenes; his wife was the front person. In essence, I tried to capitalize on the father's narcissism. Unfortunately, this blew up in my face when Mr. Shim failed to show up for several appointments because of "fatigue." I then decided to switch gears and stroke him by telling him that I needed him to help me address important issues in the family and that I could not do it without him. Taking him off the hot seat and putting his wife in the spotlight was appealing to him. This seemed to pique his interest, and he began to cooperate and show up for visits more regularly, albeit still slightly intoxicated. It would be much later in treatment that I would gradually work my way to addressing his personal issues.

Other psychopathology that may be less severe than Axis II disorders, but just as challenging, are some of the Axis I disorders. For example, in cases in which a parent may be agoraphobic, this diagnosis may have a profound effect on rerouting the distribution of power in the family. There are cases in which children are "parentified," which can also be a major obstacle that must be addressed, not only in family therapy, but also individually.

Low Intellectual and Cognitive Functioning

Insight is one of the important aspects of CBT. Historically, it has been stated that when individuals lack significant insight, they may respond more favorably to pure behavioral interventions. This was certainly the case with the Shim family, who were all functioning at a very low intellectual level. In contrast, however, all family members were very high functioning when it came to "street smarts" and, in many respects, I was no match for them. I did use metaphors as much as possible to help them to expand their thinking. They seemed to respond well to concrete metaphors, as well as to straight behavioral interventions. For example, I had them make a list of the qualities that contributed to their working cohesively in their circles of crime. Even though the behavioral acts were not condoned, I stressed the concept of cohesiveness and how the family pulled together to engage in such covert acts as unlawfully entering a home. We then talked about how some of these same skills could be turned around to be used in a productive fashion that would not get them involved with the law. During the course of these discussions, we used language that they were familiar with, such as "staying thick" and not "ratting each other out," and so forth. I then attempted to transfer this measure of cohesion by urging them to support each other in the same fashion in order to remain clean and abide by the law. We brainstormed about ways to earn money and how to deal with conflicts with the authorities. In essence, we began to include a change of behavior by restructuring schemas indirectly.

Effects of Previous Treatment

Progress in family therapy may be impeded by experiences that the family may have had with previous therapists. In this particular case, the Shims had never set foot in a therapist's office previously, and, as far as they were concerned, they "wouldn't be caught dead with a shrink." In other cases, however, a specific roadblock may involve treatment with previous therapists who work differently and who may have had a negative effect on the family's ability to benefit from treatment. Trust is one of the important factors in therapy. Consequently, if a family came to distrust a previous therapist, establishing a line of trust will require a longer period of time and cause the therapist to proceed cautiously.

Sometimes previous therapy may have been halted by a family because the therapist was being effective or touched on a sensitive issue. The family may tend to use the former therapist as a scapegoat and "trash" him or her. It is essential that a therapist not play into or support the denigration of a previous therapist, but instead direct his or her energy toward exploring alternative ways to help the family.

Applying Pressure at the Wrong Time

It has been my experience that you sometimes have to push during the course of therapy in order to facilitate change. At times, when movement is stalled, you need to nudge a family to elicit change.

For example, at one point in therapy with the Shims, the children had ganged up on the mother about her incessant nagging. The father refused to take a stand, and I decided to nudge him to respond.

DATTILIO: What do you think about what's going on between your wife and kids right now?

FATHER: Don't know. What do you want me to say?

DATTILIO: Say what you think or what you feel.

FATHER: Don't feel anything.

DATTILIO: Well, you must feel or think something.

FATHER: Nope, nottin'.

DATTILIO: Why not?

FATHER: I don't know, I don't much listen I guess.

DATTILIO: So you tune them out?

FATHER: I guess.

This transaction was clearly stalled, particularly because the father did not want to commit himself. My suspicion was that he had lots of thoughts and feelings about what was going on, but that he maintained a certain power in his neutrality. I decided to step in and help the mother deal with her children's criticism by exploring alternatives with her. I then asked the father to deliberately side with the kids against the mother, to join them in criticizing her nagging. He did not like this at all.

DATTILIO: Don't you want to bash your wife for nagging all the time?

FATHER: You're trying to make a fool of me, ain't ya?

DATTILIO: A fool? Why no, what gives you that impression?

FATHER: Bullshit—you's psychiatrizing with me.

DATTILIO: No, I am just trying to get you to 'fess up to your feelings, that's all.

FATHER: Bull ...

DATTILIO: Try to understand that when you sit there all quiet and stuff, you give everyone in the family a very powerful message.

FATHER: What.... what message?

DATTILIO: A silent message that you support them.

FATHER: So, what if I do?

DATTILIO: Then be a man and say so.

FATHER: Up yours!

DATTILIO: Whatever—think about it.

I heard more from this father during this exchange than I had in the previous six sessions. Even though the conversation at this point was rather negative and heated, it produced some movement and got us "unstuck" from our gridlock. From this point in treatment, we were able to move in a direction toward change. That fact that the father was now verbalizing his thoughts and feelings shifted the dynamics of treatment.

As stated earlier, homework assignments are an extremely important aspect of treatment and are often an integral part of a therapist's leverage in overcoming roadblocks (Dattilio, 2002). In the particular case of the Shims, I needed to develop a homework strategy that would facilitate their joint participation and would encourage a positive cohesiveness and some empirical coping strategies. For homework, I decided to assign the task of having them—together, as a family unit—look for new housing. They all agreed that part of their problem was their living environment, so I urged them to each take a part in gathering information on a new home location. This facilitated them in working cohesively toward a common cause that was productive. It was the first step toward working in a positive vein. It also served as a new activity for the Shims to try out together. I also had them tack on a pleasure task of going out to eat afterward—something they had avoided for years.

In our subsequent visit, we discussed everyone's feelings about the experience.

Inoculation against Backsliding

Another very common roadblock in treatment is backsliding. It is easy to fall back into previous behaviors, particularly when the propensity is strong. Therefore, an effective strategy may involve the therapist inoculating both him- or herself and the family against the propensity to backslide and discussing how this should be handled. For example, it was obvious that the Shims might be extremely tempted to again become involved with theft or receiving stolen property. We discussed a mechanism for them to use to cope with the temptation of taking something that did not belong to them. This procedure included following a number of steps to break the cycle of regression.

1. They were advised that if a friend called who was notorious for trouble, they should not accept the telephone call right away but call him or her back. In the interim, they should think about what to say if this person proposed something illegal. They should think about the choices they had at their disposal and the power to choose. Because power was one of the major issues in this family, we spoke about how to exercise their strength by successfully avoiding trouble. (I also suggested that the family members might be afraid to ask each other for support.)

2. Two of the triggers that led to stealing were boredom and anger. Some of the kids reported that they usually committed a theft during periods when they were bored and had little to do or when they were angry about something. Therefore, we developed a list of alternative behaviors for them to consider, which involved more productive activities and facilitative methods for expressing their anger.

3. Avoiding the pitfall of negative self-image was another area to highlight in order to prevent backsliding. Whenever family members got down on themselves, they tended to backslide into old patterns. This pattern is typical. Consequently, the Shims were prompted to monitor each other's negative or unflattering self-talk as a means to promote morale.

4. Restructuring their thoughts about the need to act on impulse provided another major coping skill. Teaching family members to delay acting

on their impulses via thought stopping or diversion of activity was extremely effective.

Conducting any type of psychotherapy is often difficult, regardless of the client's culture. If it were not for the existence of roadblocks in treatment, self-help would occur more successfully, and the need for this book would be nonexistent. Therapists will encounter endless roadblocks during the course of their careers in working with individuals, couples, and families. Learning to use various tools and techniques and to maintain a steady stream of patience is probably the greatest asset any therapist can acquire. In overcoming roadblocks, therapists must first accept the reality that roadblocks are a necessary part of the therapeutic process and an eternal challenge to endure.

7

Special Topics

DIVORCE

Sometimes, despite our best efforts to salvage distressed marriages, couples end up facing divorce.

Despite the traumatic effects associated with the onset of terrorism in this country, divorce continues to rank as the second most severe form of distress that one can undergo, next to losing a child or a spouse to death (Granvold, 2000). Divorce can have a profound impact on individuals and families and clearly needs to be addressed within a therapeutic milieu. Even if an individual desires the divorce, the attendant changes and adaptations have both positive and negative outcomes. Although the positive consequences of these life-changing events may be predominant, some negative outcomes may reach crisis proportions.

Even when divorce seems like a reasonable resolution to an intolerable situation, it is almost always traumatic, to some extent, for everyone involved, even the therapist. The divorce of a couple, after a significant amount of time in therapy, may feel like a failure to a therapist who gave his or her best effort. Sometimes, as healers, we attempt to keep couples from divorcing rather than allowing them to decide for themselves. I know that I have done that at times, and it hasn't always been for the best. Instead, therapists might need to consider helping couples cope with what is imminent, as opposed to trying to force fit something that can't work.

Epstein and Baucom (2002) introduced an enhanced CBT approach that integrates aspects of family stress and coping theory (e.g., McCubbin & McCubbin, 1989) with traditional cognitive-behavioral principles. A couple or family is often faced with a variety of demands to which they must adapt, and the quality of their coping efforts is likely to affect their satisfaction and the stability of their relationships. Demands on the couple or family usually come from three major sources:

1. *Characteristics of the individual members.* For example, a family may have to cope with a member's clinical depression.
2. *Relationship dynamics.* For example, members of a couple may have to resolve or adapt to differences in the two partners' needs, as when one is achievement and career oriented and the other is focused on togetherness and intimacy.
3. *Characteristics of the interpersonal or physical environment.* For example, needy relatives or a demanding boss may stress one parent, whereas the other may see neighborhood violence as a major threat to their well-being.

Divorce is undoubtedly a major stressor. Cognitive-behavioral therapists assess the *number, severity, and cumulative impact of various demands* that the members of a couple or family are experiencing during the course of a divorce, as well as their available *resources and skills for coping* with those demands. Consistent with a stress and coping model, the risk of couple or family dysfunction increases with the level of demands and deficits in resources. Given that the family members' *perceptions* of demands and their ability to cope also play a prominent role in the stress and coping model, cognitive-behavioral therapists' skills in assessing and modifying distorted or inappropriate cognition can be very effective in improving families' coping strategies.

CBT is highly relevant to individuals facing divorce, particularly because maladaptive or dysfunctional self-schemas that have remained dormant may become activated as a consequence of the stress demands of the process (Granvold, 2000). A perfect example can be seen in individuals who experience low self-esteem or feel unlovable and fear rejection. They may come to engage in the strong belief "I am not worthy of anyone's love and, therefore, will never he able to remain married." Therefore, an individual who experiences the extreme emotional pain of rejection may construe his spouse's quest for a divorce as being just another reaffirming measure that he or she is worthless. The intensity of the feeling of rejection and the pervasive consequences of a divorce are capable of providing a state of crisis.

The notion of a divorce may also facilitate a crisis because it violates some of the ingrained schemas that individuals hold about marital relationships. For example, one of the typical areas of conflict is the notion that "once married, one must remain married no matter what." Therefore, if individuals divorce, they fall from grace with others and thus view themselves as "failures" and as marked individuals. Such beliefs may spawn all sorts of catastrophic thought content, such as "I'll never be able to maintain another relationship if I divorce," "I can't stand life without the love of a spouse," "People won't respect me," "I'll never be a good parent," and so on.

The role of CBT is specifically designed to address ingrained beliefs that individuals maintain on the basis of distorted information and the inability to adapt to a situation they may view as being out of their control. Helping individuals to restructure their thinking is a main thrust of CBT approaches.

An example of spouses who were, unfortunately, unable to salvage their marriage is presented in the following vignette. The husband could not get over his wife's infidelity, nor her sexual preference, and the couple eventually decided to end the marital relationship. Consequently, these partners needed help with how to let go of the marriage and reclaim their lives separately from each other. In time, this actually resulted in being a positive outcome for both, as well as for the children.

IT JUST FELT RIGHT TO ME: THE CASE OF SID AND JULIE

Sid and Julie were a young couple in their early to mid-30s, married 10 years, with two children, a 7-year-old girl and a 5-year-old boy. They were referred for marital counseling by a friend because of an infidelity that had occurred in their relationship. Sid recently learned that Julie had been involved in an extramarital affair with a female coworker. He had learned of this when Julie broke down one night and divulged that she was bisexual and had had an indiscretion with a woman at work. Sid's emotional reaction of anxiety and depression required him to see the family physician the next day for medication to help him sleep. Although he had suspected that his wife might be bisexual, he was shocked that she would cheat on him. In revealing the affair, Julie also admitted that she had had a brief lesbian affair with another person earlier in the marriage. This news, Sid stated, simply "blew my mind ... I had no idea, no clue. I thought I was dreaming."

During the initial evaluation, Sid confessed that he was initially in a state of shock. He subsequently began to manifest many symptoms similar to those of posttraumatic stress disorder (PTSD). Even though extramarital affairs do not formally constitute enough criteria for a diagnosis of PTSD, this was nonetheless an acute stress reaction (Dattilio, 2004b). Sid stated that he became obsessed with the idea of his wife's being with another woman and what this meant to his masculinity. He experienced recurrent, intrusive, and distressing thoughts on a regular basis. For example, he often said to himself that his wife became drawn to women because he didn't satisfy her as a man. "I'm not man enough or she would have never looked to women for fulfillment."

During my initial interview with Julie, she made it clear to me that it was not her intention to become involved in an extramarital affair, but she felt that she was living a lie, remaining married to Sid. There was a great deal of tension in Julie's marriage because Sid was always very critical of her. She claimed that she felt good while she was involved in the affair. "It just felt right to me," exclaimed Julie. She admitted, however, that she did experience guilt once Sid began to suspect that something was going on.

During the course of treatment, the focus was on helping both individuals to understand the dynamics that contributed to the violations in the relationship, as well as to process Julie's sexual preference. This focus included areas in which one or both spouses felt unfulfilled. Interestingly, Sid eventually admitted that, at times, he had thought about ending the marriage because he simply was not satisfied with his wife. "She always seemed to have her mind somewhere else, even during sexual relations." However, a great deal of Sid's distress was the result of his feeling inadequate, owing to the fact that his wife went behind his back and became involved with a woman. In addition, when Sid learned that there had been other affairs, he felt like a "fool," and at the same time, he felt bad for Julie, who struggled with her sexuality.

In this case, reconciliation was unsuccessful. Neither Sid nor Julie could surmount their differences. After much work and contemplation, they decided that it would simply be best if they filed for divorce and went their separate ways. So maybe, in a sense, the intervention was successful in that it allowed Sid and Julie to clarify their situation and figure out what could be changed and what could not. They did attempt to remain cordial for the sake of the children. However, this was hard for them in the beginning, particularly because both struggled with introducing Julie's sexual preference to the children.

The divorce therapy phase began when Sid and Julie were able to forgive each other. The idea was to accentuate those aspects of the relationship that were compatible and congenial and for the spouses to help each other to understand Julie's sexual orientation. Therapy also focused on the idea that the dissolution of their marriage was a relief to both parties and allowed them to move on with their lives. Discontent and sexual preference had contributed to Julie's venturing outside the relationship, which ultimately ended their marriage. Interestingly, as we began to discuss this matter, Sid stated that in many ways he now believed that he may have set his wife up to be unfaithful. He admitted that, because of his discontent with her, he didn't give his wife as much attention as he should have and never addressed her disinterest in him. Once the two of them were able to accept the fact that there was not enough in their relationship to sustain it, and that they were operating their relationship on some false pretenses, the tension reduced. Both agreed that it was a relief to let it go. Sid and Julie also recognized that they had some irreconcilable differences in their personalities that really did not make them very compatible with each other. Eventually they both admitted that they would probably have separated long before had they not had children.

Most of the cognitive-behavioral interventions involved helping Sid and Julie to restructure distorted beliefs about force-fitting this relationship into something that just couldn't be. Much of our work also helped them to reconsider the guilt and shame they experienced about the divorce and Julie's sexual preference. This involved telling their respective families, especially their parents, who were somewhat conservative. We also included the children in some of the family therapy sessions to help orient them to their parents' new relationship. Overall, the children handled the situation quite well because Sid and Julie were civil with each other in their divorce proceedings and together explained things as clearly as possible to the children.

Once these individuals had an opportunity to restructure their thinking and consider some of the distorted thoughts in which they had both become embroiled over the years, the tension was reduced and they actually developed a fairly good friendship. Each went on to pursue a new life for him- or herself.

Divorce Mediation

CALLING A SPADE A SPADE: THE CASE OF ART AND MARIETTA

Sometimes, depending on the circumstances, divorce can be a good recommendation (Dattilio, 2006b). I recall seeing a couple in their late 70s who had been married about a year. Art and Marietta had previously been married for 40 plus years to individuals who were also friends. The four of them often got together to play cards, went out socially, and went on trips together. When Art's wife died, Marietta and her husband consoled him for approximately a year. It was at about that point that Marietta's husband died of a sudden heart attack, which left Art and Marietta as the surviving spouses. The two consoled each other over the loss of their former spouses and maintained a friendship for a year or so. Then, because neither wanted to go out with anyone else, they decided that it would be a good idea for them to marry. They felt that this was ideal because they had known each other for many years and were comfortable with each other.

The difficulties started after they were married for 1 year. I worked with them for a year and a half, attempting to address the issues of communication and tolerance, with each one dealing with the other's particular resentment about the current spouse not being like the former spouse. For example, Marietta was angry with Art because he was not as tolerant as her previous husband had been. He had a different temperament and had particular preoccupations, which drove her "nuts." Art, on the other hand, felt that Marietta was insensitive and nothing like his former wife, Helen, who was very understanding.

When, after a year and a half, they simply could not change their ways, it was a mutual decision that, perhaps, it was not the best idea for them to remain married. Moreover, both had readily admitted that although they cared for each other, they were not in love with each other, and that maybe this was what was absent in their efforts to sustain any further relationship. At this particular juncture, the two decided it might be better to dissolve their marriage and just remain friends, which they went on to do quite well.

Sometimes calling a spade a spade is what is needed in a marital situation. Not everyone can salvage a marriage, and sometimes a marriage shouldn't be saved, particularly if it is based on an empty premise or the wrong reasons.[1]

CULTURAL SENSITIVITY

One of the most important requirements of working with couples and families is to remain sensitive to cultural differences. In this age of a diverse society, it is not uncommon for therapists to encounter relationships between people of every possible mixture of nationalities and cultures. Cultural awareness is essential in attempting to work effectively with couples and families.

I've been fortunate to be invited to lecture in more than fifty countries, and many of these lectures involved my participation in live demonstrations of treating couples and families from cultures much different from my own. Some of the issues that have been raised have had to do with a Western influence on one spouse that goes against the grain of his or her culture. For example, a Moroccan couple, who were practicing Muslims in Casablanca, struggled over the young wife's desire to go to parties with her girlfriends. Her husband refused to permit this, yet felt justifiably entitled to attend these parties himself. This became a bit of a conflict when his young wife challenged him. The husband, who was 15 years his wife's senior, took exception to her bold requests and attributed them to the influence of her close girlfriend, who had spent a decade living in the United States. Helping this couple find a common ground was no easy feat. The husband, who was

---

[1]Refer to Dattilio (2006b) for additional coverage on this topic.

close to my age, attempted to ally with me on the basis of age and gender and attempted to pit me against his wife, whom he felt I should scold into submission.

Unfamiliarity with a particular culture and operating on the basis of Western values can easily land a therapist in trouble quickly. This is often the case with many people who hail from patriarchal societies, such as Asian and Mideastern cultures. Sometimes when couples marry cross-culturally, they inherit certain beliefs that may appear silly to one spouse, but carry weight with the other spouse.

I once saw a couple in which the husband was born and raised in the United States, but married a Chinese woman from a remote area of the Himalayas who maintained a lot of old world rituals. One of their arguments had to do with the fact that the wife repeatedly stored brooms and mops upside down in the closet, which the husband felt was silly and unsanitary, because the dirty part of the instrument was up against the wall when it belonged on the floor. When I spoke with the wife, she informed me that she was raised by her grandmother who always drilled into her thinking that people who did wrong in their lifetimes lived under the earth and swept the floors of hell. That is why in this world we need to turn the sweeping brushes and mops upside down when we put them away. This was a ritual that she had practiced since childhood, which continued through to her adulthood in order to honor her grandmother, as well as to honor the "old world" belief about not having contact with those who have done wrong on this earth. This was a particular area of difficulty with this couple, because the husband would become annoyed and could not understand the foolishness of the activity, yet it is very much rooted in the Himalayan culture and the husband failed to be sensitive to this issue.

As a couple and family therapist, it has always been important for me to remain consciously aware of the nuances of the various cultures of the people I was treating. This issue became especially clear to me when I was working with a Korean family in which the parents were recent immigrants.

Chae-myun is the Korean term for "face saving," a concept that is familiar to many Asians. Making a good impression is very important to Koreans in all of their relationships outside the immediate family. Consequently, maintaining chae-myun protects the dignity, honor, and self-respect of the individual and the family. Any therapist should anticipate that clients will be reluctant to reveal vital information if this will cause a loss of chae-myun. Therefore, therapists must be cautious not to make any gestures or comments that might be misconstrued as criticisms or condescension, or it will likely result in a couple or family not returning for treatment.

The Korean culture, as well as many Asian cultures, generally values collectivism and *we-ness*. Forming close relationships with others has a special meaning that is extended to become *we-self*. The mentality operating in a close relationship is characterized by a strong sense of bonding, unconditional friendship, mutual altruism, and exclusive favoritism (Choi, 1998). Family bonding is especially strong, and family members are very protective and appear defensive to others outside the family. Another characteristic of Asian culture is *cheong*, which consists of personal care and attentive, empathetic, helpful, and supportive actions and behavior (Choi, 1998). Once Asians feel a close relationship to others, they then show strong *cheong* to them. Asians are also taught to show respect to their parents and to elderly people.

When therapists try to conduct family therapy, including children and their parents, in this culture, they have to be extra cautious in consideration of the Korean family atmosphere. For example, authoritative Korean parents may view the therapist as someone who is trying to make their children rebellious against them. They will feel offended and as though they are "losing face" in front of a stranger unless the therapist has established a strong rapport with them (Chae & Kwon, 2006). It is important for the family therapist to have an individual session with the parents to discuss the children's problems privately. The therapist can explain how family therapy will be conducted and why the children should speak for themselves in front of their parents. The therapist should also coach the children not to use words that are too strong to describe their opinions and feelings. When working with Korean families, for example, a cooperative and strong relationship with the parents is imperative (Chae, 2008).

It is often difficult to know what or what not to say and what might offend people of certain cultures. Therapists need to be sensitive to the philosophies of certain cultures regarding marriage and separation. For example, on the tiny European island of Malta, in the southern Mediterranean, the notion of divorce doesn't exist, owing to the predominance of Catholicism on the island. Yet in Montreal, Canada, and in Iceland, it is very common for couples to live together and raise families without ever formally marrying.

Other issues have to do with what behaviors or actions may bring dishonor to the family, particularly among offspring who are raised in Western society. A classic example is the following case, in which a young East Indian teenager desired to assert her independence, creating a major conflict in the course of family therapy.[2]

---

[2]Parts of this case first appeared in Dattilio (2005c). Adapted with permission from Springer Science and Business Media.

"YOU MAKE A JERK OUT OF ME": THE CASE OF GOLDIE

Goldie was an attractive 15-year-old Indian girl, who appeared more physically mature than her stated age. Goldie and her family had moved to the northeastern part of the United States from Madras, India, when she was 4. The family had two younger sons, ages 11 and 8. Goldie's father worked as a chemical engineer for a local gas company; her mother was a homemaker, having previously been an English teacher in her native India. The family informed me that the problems began when Goldie reached the age of 14 and started to demand more freedom and to deviate from some of the family's cultural rituals. For example, she insisted that her parents allow her to use heavy makeup, despite their parents' desire for her to bare her face naturally. There was also the issue of her friends, many of whom her parents did not care for. "They don't like them because they are not Indian," Goldie cried, as she glared directly at her father. Both parents sat in silence during the initial family session.

Typically, the father is the most powerful member in the Indian family. Goldie, who was the only female child, would traditionally have the least amount of power in the family. However, Goldie's father sometimes chose to empower her by allowing her certain freedoms. Hence, she began to expect more power in her freedom to choose her friends in social settings, expecting her father to show her tolerance.

Because girls are prepared for marriage at such a young age in the Indian culture, mothers tend to treat their adolescent daughters like adults. This mixed message further contributed to an emotional short circuit for Goldie, which began to be manifested in her acting-out behaviors. She would repeatedly stay out late beyond her curfew, despite her parents wishes. Goldie also felt that her curfew of 10:00 P.M., which was set by her father, was ridiculous. "You make a jerk out of me in front of my friends, saying 'ten o'clock, now don't forget.' Do you have any idea how this makes me feel?" cried Goldie, "especially when all of my friends have curfews of 11:30." But Goldie's parents calmly explained the rules of the house and felt that they did not need to be compared with other households.

As a family therapist, I may have initially reacted to having the father examine his thoughts and beliefs about what it meant for his rules to be challenged. Furthermore, I was curious about what effect relaxing his rules and compromising may have had on his power in the family. However, because it was important that I remain sensitive to this family's culture, it was essential for me not to assume a position in favor of independence for the child so quickly, but rather to seek some type of solution within this family's framework of autonomy and interconnectedness. Thus, my role as a culturally sensitive family therapist was to help Goldie's parents better understand that the process of maturing in this country made it natural for a teenage girl to want to gravitate away from family and closer to independence and autonomy for herself. An aspect that the parents in this situation seemed to overlook was how difficult it was for this young girl to establish a happy medium between her parents' cultural demands and the demands of her American adolescent society. We discussed Goldie's anxiety about being limited in her social activities and her need to adhere to earlier curfews than her friends, which brought forward Goldie's fear of rejection and low sense of self-worth. She feared rejection by her peers, which her parents interpreted as a failure on their part, reasoning that if they had raised their daughter with a solid sense of values, she would not be struggling with issues of self-esteem.

Course of Treatment

In this case, my role as a therapist shifted to using interventions that helped the parents to begin to restructure their thinking. I suggested that they reconsider the struggle that their daughter might be facing in light of social demands. The parents had trouble with restructuring their thinking, particularly the father, who said that his family would lose sight of their traditional Indian values if he changed his thinking. It was his impression that his daughter was beginning to do this by maintaining fewer and fewer Indian friends. It seemed to me that Goldie wanted to move away from the family and that this was a threat to the parents, as well as to the integrity of their culture.

Upon probing a bit more with the parents as to why they decided to relocate to the United States, they explained that, at that time, the job opportunities where they lived in India were not good. As opportunities in the United States abounded, one of the father's friends called and invited him to work in this country. The family decided that it would be a good idea and a good experience for their children to have access to an American education. What emerged was that the parents never anticipated that they would have to adjust culturally, particularly with their children. They had no idea that the children would be pressured by a different culture that would conflict with their own.

It was a challenging task to help this family understand how they might be engaging in some distortions that would affect them in their adjustment to the new cultural situation. After I oriented the family to the cognitive-behavioral model, addressing the difficult task of adapting to their new culture was the next step. I often find that if I can strike the cord of reasoning with the family, they will guide me as to how their culture will fit into the model. For example, during one of the subsequent sessions, I asked each family member to describe for me one aspect of his or her their thinking that might be considered unreasonable for the situation at hand. The following dialogue unfolded:

DATTILIO: With the overview of the CBT model in mind, you can see how, at times, when family members become emotionally charged over issues like the one we are facing, their thoughts and perceptions can become prey to distortions, which is part of the human condition. So let me ask each of you, how might you personally be engaging in distorted thinking in regard to this entire issue? [*Note*: Interestingly, the mother chose to begin talking first. I viewed this as her way of letting her husband and child off the hook—something not unusual in the Indian culture.]

MOTHER: Well, I know that sometimes I tend to worry too much about Goldie and fear that she will either be a part of our family or leave us all completely!

DATTILIO: OK, good. So if you review some of the distortions that we discussed earlier, can you identify the category this falls into?

MOTHER: (*looking at the father for approval*) Well, maybe a couple of them, like "dichotomous thinking" or "overgeneralization."

[The father did not say anything, but I inferred from his silence that he was in agreement. Because the mother had elected to do the talking for both parents, I read this as a way of the father's saving face. I also knew that it would be a major mistake to confront the father and put him on the spot. Consequently, I talked to the father through the mother, which was successful.]

DATTILIO: Good, I agree. And again, you know that when emotions run high, especially when we are talking about family, we tend to engage in distortions. [I then turned to Goldie and asked for her opinion about these distortions.] Goldie, can you see where you might be engaging in the same type of behavior?

GOLDIE: I guess. But I don't think that I'm as bad as they are.

DATTILIO: Well, maybe not in your eyes, but certainly in your parents' eyes you may be. Let's look at some of you own thoughts and behaviors and see if we can link them to any distortions. For example, your statement about your parents treating you as though you are a child—might that be blown out of proportion?

GOLDIE: Maybe—well, yeah—it's just that I get so upset with them all the time.

DATTILIO: Well, let's examine some of the thoughts that go through your mind. For example, what kinds of things do you tell yourself about your parents?

GOLDIE: I don't know. I feel sort of on the spot to say it here, plus I'm not sure. I need to think about it.

DATTILIO: OK, let's try this. How about recording your thoughts on a form such as this one? [At this point I took the opportunity to introduce the family to the Dysfunctional Thought Record (see Appendix B).] Cognitive therapy utilizes a great deal of homework assignments. The basic theory contends that you must practice challenging negative self-statements, or what we call automatic thoughts, just as much as you have been using them in the past. One way to do this is by writing out the corrected statement each time you experience a negative self-statement or, in this case, a cognitive distortion. So I'd like you to use the following form as situations arise. Then each time a situation occurs in which you have a negative automatic thought, write it down. Starting with the left-hand column, record the situation or event in which you had the thought, and in the next column put exactly what the thought was. Next, attempt to identify the type of distortion you are engaging in and the emotional response that accompanies it. Then try to challenge that thought or belief by weighing the evidence that exists in favor of it. After that, write down an alternative response, using any new information you may have gathered. Does that make sense to you?

GOLDIE: Yes, but could we run through it once so that I'm sure I have it right?

DATTILIO: Certainly. Let's try an example.

FATHER: Something happened last week with Goldie when she came in a little past her curfew and I said something about her being 5 minutes late. She started to, well, what I call stand up to my authority by attempting to minimize what she had done, saying it had only been 5 minutes and it was no big deal.

DATTILIO: So let's get everything down on paper. (*They fill in the Dysfunctional Thought Record as a group.*) That's excellent. Do you all see how we attempted to restructure some of our thinking and how that may aid in defusing an otherwise volatile situation?

MOTHER: But what if Goldie was really defying us? I mean, how do we know that's correct?

DATTILIO: Good question! We gather information to support our alternative beliefs, and one of the things you could do is, as your husband indicated on the sheet, talk to Goldie about what her intentions were in arriving home late. This can be applied to all of you at one time or the other as you recognize yourselves engaging in distorted thinking. We want to begin to examine your mode of thought and really question the validity of what you tell yourselves. This may make a monumental difference in how you interact and your emotional exchange.

From this point, the therapist begins to monitor the family members in challenging their belief statements in the fashion demonstrated here. During this process, feelings and emotions, as well as communication skills and problem-solving strategies, are addressed. Regular homework assignments are also employed to aid family members in learning to challenge their distorted thoughts more spontaneously. Eventually, the therapist walks each family member through this specific technique to ensure its correct use. In addition, the use of behavioral techniques, such as the reassignment of family members' roles and responsibilities, became an integral part of the treatment regime in this particular case. The underlying general concept is that, with the change and modification of dysfunctional thinking and behaviors, there will be less family conflict.

The key to working with people from other cultures is to remain mindful of the larger cultural beliefs, as well as the specific family's context, and adapt the approach accordingly. With this family, for example, it could involve expanding the roles of the younger brothers, who would soon be coming into their adolescence. Increasing the responsibilities of the younger brothers could be viewed as culturally appropriate for the family and could serve to decrease the pressure on Goldie and allow her space to individuate as much as the family would permit.

In this particular case, the cognitive-behavioral approach enabled the family members to restructure their thinking in a manner that served to reduce tension. When the father was able to reassure himself that Goldie's need to assert her independence and fit in with her peers was not necessarily an indication that she was abandoning her cultural values, the family relaxed and the tension subsided. Goldie, for her part, was also able to focus more on her relationship to her family and on how to strike a balance between family ties and time with her peers.

The issues of power and control were also addressed, particularly as they related to the parents' role in the family and maintaining the respect of their children. Examining the family schemas about rules and standards helped in restructuring them slightly so that they allowed for some flexibility. In the last session the family reported that the situation was getting much better.

In summary, working with families from any culture that significantly varies from the culture of the therapist requires not only cultural awareness, but a collaborative approach that allows for the individual family's cultural beliefs to inform the treatment goals and process. The cognitive-behavioral approach is ideal for such a collaborative process because the material is generated by the client's own automatic thoughts, not some predetermined ideology. Furthermore, the rational responses are also created by the client, so that they are consistent and believable for the family. Rational responses can include spiritual or religious beliefs that are consistent with the desired behavioral change, which, for Asian Indian families, can include aspects of reducing anger/resentment by accepting one's "dharma," or duty, in life, or being able to overcome challenges by maintaining a religious belief in a higher power. The incorporation of spiritual beliefs and cultural norms is vital to the cross-cultural application of CBT techniques and makes this a highly versatile and universally responsible treatment approach.

DEPRESSION, PERSONALITY DISORDER, AND OTHER MENTAL ILLNESSES

During the course of treating families, it is not uncommon to encounter one or more members of a family who are suffering from a mental disorder. One of the more common disorders covered extensively in the professional literature is depression. There has been additional recognition of depression in relationship problems that frequently occur. As early as the 1970s, it was demonstrated that women who experienced depression reported problems in their marriages, with a direct connection between depression and intimate relationships (Weissman & Paykel, 1974; Brown & Harris, 1978). There are several reviews in the literature that support the correlation between depression and marital functioning, most of which is underscored in an edited text by Beach (2001). Weissman (1987, p. 445) further determined that being in an "unhappy marriage" was one of the risk factors for major depression. Whisman (2001) embarked on a meta-analysis that spanned 26 studies, involving more than 3,700 women and 2,700 men. Marital dissatisfaction was indicated to account for approximately 18% of the variance in wives depressive symptoms and 14% of the variance in husbands' depressive symptoms. The results suggested a strong association between depressive symptoms and marital dissatisfaction.

Further studies examined the impact of major depressive illness on spouses of depressed patients. The results indicated that men and women living with depressed partners experience depression differently and varied in their perceptions of the quality of the marital relationship and in their thinking patterns. Wives of depressed husbands tended to withdraw from social life and to experience guilt, fear, anxiety, and loneliness more than husbands of depressed wives (Fadden, Bebbington, & Kuipers, 1987). Additional studies indicate that there are more depressive thinking styles among women who live with depressed men (Dudek et al., 2001). The study by Dudek et al. (2001) indicated that a man's depressive illness and associated difficulties in relating to his situation strike an issue of upmost priority for a woman (household and intimacy partnership). When a man finds himself in a similar situation, he copes by immersing himself in activities outside the home (e.g., career, friends, sports), drawing satisfaction from these external outlets. In addition, a husband's approach to problem solving may be different and more constructive so that the act draws attention away from marital concerns (Katz & Bertelson, 1993). A woman, however, may be more prone to concentrate on the experience of the negative events, focusing attention more on her emotions and internal coping skills, thus causing her to be more negatively affected by the events (Nolen-Hoeksema, 1987).

Most treatment regimes suggest that therapy may provide members of a couple or family with an understanding of the nature of depression and its role in their relationship, and may assist them in negotiating their relationship to deal more effectively with the problems posed by the depression (Coyne & Benazon, 2001). Coyne and Benazon (2001) further suggest that, providing the depressed individual in a couple or family with a "limited sick role," as is routinely done in interpersonal therapy for depression, can be of particular benefit in CBT. This involves helping couples or family members to lower expectations and renegotiate responsibilities in the relationship, with the coexistence of individual therapy for the person who is depressed. Traditional CBT for depression is recommended, along with the routine of cognitive restructuring and readjusting the expectations and attributions for the remaining spouse and family members in therapy.

Family members should work on their relationships as a way of assisting in the recovery of the depressed individual. There should be a focus on the intensity of their conflict, the impairment of the depressed individual, and the frustration of the spouse or other family members. Sometimes this may be best handled via separate meetings with the family members or having a spouse cojoin the partner in his or her own individual therapy for depression. Family members can benefit from learning special coping skills required to live effectively and humanely with a depressed individual. Family members must also take responsibility for their own roles in the difficulties in the relationship, apart from those that the depression itself has created.

EXTRAMARITAL AFFAIRS

Unfortunately, therapists are often confronted with couple or family situations in which one or both partners have become involved in an extramarital affair. In many ways, this may constitute a crisis, depending on when and under what circumstances that couple/family comes into treatment. Several of the case vignettes used earlier in this book involve situations of infidelity.

Therapists who encounter families in which infidelity has become the main issue often need to address the situation immediately. National studies have found that nearly one-quarter of husbands and more than 1 in 10 wives have had extramarital affairs during their marriages (Laumann, Gagnon, Michael, & Michaels, 1994; Smith, 1994). Extramarital affairs are considered to be among the most frequent problems brought to couple therapy, and they are seen as the second most damaging to relationships. Only physical abuse has a more negative effect than extramarital affairs. Obviously, when both problems exist, physical abuse is the more profound of the two.

Although estimates vary, affairs are reported to lead to divorces at twice the rate of any other problem (Whisman et al., 1997). Several researchers have investigated the effects of and types of interventions in the recovery process following an extramarital affair (Glass, 2000, 2002, 2003; Gordon & Baucom, 1998, 1999; Olson, Russell, Higgins-Kessler, & Miller, 2002). Glass has specifically written about the traumatic effects of marital infidelity on both partners and about the fact that the stress of an affair can be manifested in a variety of symptoms. This is particularly relevant when symptoms involve avoidance of affective expression or of intimacy, which have long been linked to diminished relationship satisfaction (Gottman & Levenson, 1986).

Through in-depth interviews with individuals who have experienced marital infidelity, Olson et al., (2002) have found that there is a three-stage process following disclosure of an affair, beginning with the emotional "roller coaster" and proceeding through a moratorium before efforts at trust building are recognized. It is in the initial roller coaster period that many of the posttraumatic stress symptoms are likely to first be observed. Immediate responses to a partner's disclosure of infidelity, or of an indiscretion, were often found to be intensely emotionally charged, and it is during this phase that many of the negative outcomes of the affair are most apparent. In the period following the disclosure, the partner may confront the offending spouse and express anger, as well as attempt to manage conflicting feelings. The response to betrayal includes strong emotions and behaviors, many of which must be addressed initially in the therapeutic phase. Several excellent texts have appeared in the literature that address infidelity in relationships, such as *After the Affair* by Janice Abram-Spring (1996), along with the sequel, *How Can I Forgive You* by Janice Abram-Spring (2004). Another superb book is *Getting Past the Affair: A Program to Help You Cope, Heal and Move On—Together or Apart* by Snyder, Baucom, and Gordon (2009).

A moratorium stage usually follows, in which there is less emotional reaction and fewer attempts to make meaning of the infidelity. This is typically characterized by a period of calm and acceptance, which is often the point at which some of the cognitive-behavioral interventions may be utilized.

It is important, as part of treatment, always to acknowledge and remain sensitive to the effect that an extramarital affair has had on the offended spouse. At the same time, it is important to underscore the idea that the affair is a symptom of a much greater issue that underlies the relationship and needs to be addressed. Such an understanding may help in the process of moving forward and not dwelling on the symptom. This is often the balance that therapists have to strike between the spouses, particularly because the one who has been offended may tend to perceive the therapist as minimizing the effects of the affair and going on. Therefore, behavioral contracts are often helpful to structure how recurrent hurts or injury may be addressed so that the terms of the contract do not preclude progress and treatment.

Sometimes the effects of an extramarital affair on one spouse may be devastating—contributing to severe symptoms, as demonstrated in the case of Sid and Julie on p. 175. In fact, I have written on the subject of whether an extramarital affair may almost create PTSD-like symptoms (Dattilio, 2004b).

It should also be noted that, in keeping with the theme that an extramarital affair is often a symptom of a much deeper issue, many of the classic cognitive-behavioral techniques for couple therapy are often utilized. In situations that involve families, family therapy may also be utilized in helping the other family members, mainly the offspring, heal in the wake of the infidelity. Although the details of the affair may not be shared with other family members, certainly the fallout of the infidelity needs to be addressed, along with the children's feelings and thoughts about the issues involved, such as loyalty, boundaries, matters of insecurity, and the uncertainty of the future.

SUBSTANCE ABUSE

Family therapists undoubtedly encounter cases in which drug or alcohol abuse is a contributing factor to a dysfunction in family dynamics. Although the treatment of substance abuse is usually done on an individual basis for the identified patient, certain techniques and interventions used in couple and family therapy can be used while the identified substance abuser is in individual treatment. The focus of this section is on those particular cognitive-behavioral interventions that may be helpful in dealing with couples who have substance abuse problems.

Research has supported the hypothesis that the inclusion of a spouse and family members in the treatment of alcohol or substance abusers' leads to a slightly better treatment outcome (Steinglass, Bennet, Wolin, & Reiss,

1987; Noel & McCrady, 1993). Typically, the spouse and family members are not the focus of therapy; however, when they come for couple or family therapy, the issue of substance abuse has particular implications. Specific aspects of treatment may place emphasis on the alteration of the substance abusers' behavior, as well as the spouse's and family members' behaviors that may trigger or reinforce the substance use. It must be emphasized that spouses' and family members' behaviors do not cause alcohol or substance use, but may, without intention, reward or classically enable substance or alcohol use. Behaviors that involve protecting the abuser from negative consequences need to be highlighted, along with helping spouses and family members to understand their roles and the part they play in the enabling process. This is where the specific work outlined earlier in the text discussing schemas, particularly individual as well as relationship schemas, is extremely important.

It is also important to focus on the aspects in the couple or family relationship that may need enhancement in terms of avoiding relapse and the need for substance use (Paolino & McCrady, 1977). Increasing positive values and rewards in the relationship may take the place of substance use behaviors. Additional treatment interventions, such as assertiveness training and problem solving, which are discussed in this book, are extremely important in addressing issues in relationships that center on substance abuse.

There are also various questionnaires and inventories that address alcohol and substance abuse, one of which is the Drinking Patterns Questionnaire (DPQ; Zitter & McCrady, 1993). This is an inventory that both spouses complete to identify items that they believe may be associated with alcohol consumption, assigning a rank of importance to each set of items. Ten major areas are involved, including environment, work, financial factors, physiological states, interpersonal situations, marital problems, relationships with parents, problems with children, emotional factors, and recent major life stresses (Zitter & McCrady, 1993). This inventory also focuses on the major positive and negative consequences of alcohol consumption in order to pinpoint the reinforcing agents that can contribute to alcohol consumption and backslides.

There is also the Spouse Behavior Questionnaire (SBQ; Orford et al., 1975). This questionnaire lists various behaviors that individuals might use to control or cope with alcohol consumption by a spouse. There are separate forms given to spouses that relate to types and frequency of each nonabusing spouse's behavior in the last 12 months. These items, again, center on specific behaviors that nonabusing spouses may engage in that trigger or reinforce drinking, or contribute to relapse.

Further techniques that are very effective are stimulus control procedures, contingency rearrangements, cognitive restructuring, and the use of alternative behaviors, as outlined in O'Farrell and Fals-Stewart (2006) and Beck, Wright, Newman, and Leise (1993).

Other aspects of the relationship that need to be addressed are obviously the changes in the relationship dynamics due to the substance use. When there is one substance-misusing partner in a couple, the partners experience increased stress and decreased levels of enjoyment, both with one another and with life in general. Usually, the partner who does not use may feel abandoned or unappreciated as the substance use escalates, because more time is being given to the substance abuse than to the relationship. The probability of violence increases proportionately with the choice of substances, whether legal or illegal, and the length of time the substance is used, as well as the individual's comorbid personality structure. Lack of time, energy, and nurturance of the relationship often results in emotional distance, alienation, and resentments that are difficult to deescalate without external assistance.

The situation becomes even more difficult when both partners in a relationship are substance abusers and find that they need to be intoxicated or high to show signs of affection or talk about problems in the relationship. This, again, is an aspect that requires individual intervention for both spouses during the relationship treatment. Many of the protocols used with individuals can also be used with couples. See the excellent chapter by Morgillo-Freeman and Storie (2007), as well as the popular text by Beck et al. (1993).

DOMESTIC ABUSE

Domestic abuse and violence are on the rise in a number of countries, particularly in the United States. Data from a recent national Violence Against Women survey indicates that, in their lifetimes, 22.1% of women experience physical violence, 7.7% are raped by their intimate partners, and 4.8% are stalked (Tjaden & Thoennes, 2000). It should be noted that violence between spouses can go either way, although the majority of cases reported typically involve male violence against female partners.

Therapeutic intervention is vitally important in matters such as this because, without intervention, the cycle of violence typically continues over an extended period of time.

The effect of violence on the victim is often profound and may lead to psychological, as well as physical, health problems. Often, victims of domestic abuse develop "cognitive rules," derived from a variety of sources, including messages from society in general, formal and informal "helpers," and the batterers (Hamberger & Holtzworth-Monroe, 2007). This is often why couples who present for treatment don't always report abuse as a presenting problem. Epstein and Werlinich (2003), for instance, found that only 5% of persons calling a university clinic to request couple therapy cited abuse in response to an open-ended questionnaire on presenting problems. Therefore, to increase the likelihood of disclosure, assessment techniques should utilize structured and multimethod assessment procedures. Spouses should be directed to complete self-report measures separately and in private, without collaboration. They should also be administered well rated measures, such as the Conflict Tactics Scale—Revised (CTSR; Straus et al., 1996). A detailed list of measures can be found in La Taillade, Epstein, and Werlinich (2006, p. 398).

Consequently, addressing cognitions that pertain to attributions of responsibility for the violence or for keeping the relationship together are important, along with assumptions about the individual spouse's inability to survive outside a violent relationship. Issues of dependence and loyalty, often accompanied by cognitive distortions, are matters that need to be addressed. Hamberger and Holtzworth-Monroe (2007) discuss a number of areas that need to be addressed among victims of domestic violence. These aspects affect both victim and perpetrator and the essential dynamics of the relationship. It is vital to address the cognitions of violent spouses that can increase the risk of continued perpetrating behaviors, which also have a profound effect on a family's offspring.

It is strongly recommended that the first step in addressing abuse issues is always to ensure safety. Making sure that both spouses are safe from further abuse may involve contracting, as well as separation, and seeing them in treatment either with another party present or in another location other than an intimate office setting. Depending on the dynamics of the abuse, separation may be an initial step to take. Safety planning may also involve the use of shelters.

The second step is to develop a plan of intervention that all parties can agree to. This may also involve a danger assessment and a determination of the potential for violence in the future. Often, the individual who is the actual perpetrator of the physical abuse undergoes a danger assessment, but it is also important for the victim to understand his or her particular role in the enabling process and his or her contributions to escalation in the physical abuse process. After it has been determined that interventions are in place for ensuring safety and a cooperative plan of action has been established, the typical cognitive-behavioral techniques for addressing relationship dysfunction and triggers for abusive outbursts are adhered to. Recommending individual therapy for each spouse is also important. Cognitive restructuring of the escalation behavioral process, in terms of alternative behavioral interaction, is preferred. In addition, stress inoculation techniques may be used, as well as methods for devictimization of the battered spouse.

When therapy progresses to the point where both spouses can be seen in the same room the therapist may exercise caution by allowing the battered spouse to leave before the perpetrator, so that he or she can exit the premises safely.

Finally, it is essential for all therapists to make sure that safety precautions are in place for their own welfare, as well. Therapists need to be careful to respect their instincts and not allow themselves to be put in a position of danger.

Therapists who may be afraid for their own safety, in what could potentially become a heated exchange during the course of the therapeutic hour, need to treat this concern as real. If necessary, they can reduce the threat by insisting that the initial phase of therapy with violent batterers is conducted in separate locations, using speaker phones.

In addition, each spouse needs to assume complete responsibility for his or her own role in the violence cycle. The offender is ultimately responsible for his or her own violent behaviors. The victim is responsible for taking steps to ensure his or her own safety, either through prevention and avoidance strategies or by escaping from any potential abuse.

Empathic Joining

Some of the recent work of Andrew Christensen and associates highlights the aspects of *empathic joining, unified detachment,* and *tolerance building* in their work with couples (Christensen, Sevier, Simpson, & Gattis, 2004). In this approach, the authors suggest that the therapist elicit feelings associated with couple problems. In this case, these would involve the dynamics of the abuse exchange. The idea is to bring to the surface any unexpressed feelings that may be harbored and may later build up and contribute to explosive abusive outbursts. The aim is then to elicit, from the partners, more constructive and sympathetic responses to each other in advance of the dynamic display going awry. These authors suggest having partners discuss problems by verbalizing the "hard feelings" and "rigid thoughts" they experience and then try to look at the softer, more vulnerable thoughts and feelings that may coexist with the harsher ones. This exercise helps them to balance out their thoughts and emotions.

Unified Detachment

With *unified detachment,* the emphasis is on creating objective, intellectual distancing from the problem as opposed to the emotional focus of *emphatic joining.* In empathic joining, the therapist alters an ongoing battle between spouses by helping them to notice and attend to each other's wounds. This, in essence, enables the couple to move to a better vantage point so that they can observe their ongoing battle and develop a different perspective. In unified detachment, the therapist often has the couple engage in a descriptive analysis of the sequence of behavior that leads to a particular problematic interaction—in this case, abuse. Thus, specific actions are identified that can enable them to deescalate and heal.

The authors go on to state that promoting emotional acceptance through unified detachment and emphatic joining are conceptually distinct in that the former is focused on objective analysis of a problem, whereas the latter is focused on an emotional exploration of the problem (Christenen et al., 2004, p. 302). In using these two strategies together, the authors further illustrate that in debriefing an incident, the therapist may help the spouses not only to articulate the important behaviors that unfolded in the sequence of their interaction, and how these behaviors are similar to or different from their usual pattern (unified detachment), but also to explore the emotional reactions that each experienced at different points in the sequence (empathic joining). It is the use of these two strategies together that gives way to greater *relationship mindfulness* or a nonjudgmental awareness of negative relationship roles and interaction patterns with less emotional participation in the roles or patterns (p. 302).

Tolerance Building

An important aspect of Christensen's work has to do with *tolerance building*, or what others in CBT may refer to as "inoculation" (Meichenbaum, 1977). This concept centers on the assumption that problems will reappear and that therefore the need to focus on management, as opposed to unrealistic elimination, is important in preparing spouses for potential problems in the future. The authors also recommend that spouses enact negative behaviors within sessions so that the therapist can instruct them on how to deal with clearly defined negative behaviors that are part of their perceptual problem. The procedure is to enact an episode when either of the partners is feeling the requisite emotions so that they can discuss methods for control and management and look at alternative ways to respond and desensitize themselves in advance of the usual provocative behaviors that contribute to explosive exchanges. The goal here is for the therapist to follow an enactment of problematic behavior with instructions for appropriate problem management. In addition, the therapist may engage spouses in an analysis of the positive benefits that result from differences that partners normally experience as negative. In this respect, their strategy serves as a kind of balancing function, in which the view of one spouse may balance the opposite view of the other. The basic message to couples in using tolerance building is that they should prepare for the fact that their problem may reappear, but can be managed effectively.

These interventions also serve as a type of relapse prevention mechanism during the course of treatment. This is essential, particularly in situations of domestic abuse and violence, because this is such a serious matter.

In addition, Epstein and associates (Epstein et al., 2005) have designed a program known as the Couples Abuse Prevention Program (CAPP), which is a cognitive-behavioral model that focuses on risk for intimate partner violence. It includes components that focus on psychoeducation about abusive behavior and its negative consequences, increasing partners' use of effective anger management skills during conflict, improving a couple's communication and problem-solving skills, helping the couple recover from past trauma and broken trust, and increasing partners' mutual support and shared positive activities.

The following is a synopsis of the 10-week CAPP protocol and what is involved with the session content. Although the empirical research is only in its early stage, studies have thus far yielded positive results (LaTaillade et al., 2006).

- *Initial sessions.* During the initial two sessions, spouses are presented with an overview of the cognitive-behavioral treatment program and the structure of the sessions (e.g., review of homework that was set at the previous meeting). A history of the relationship is taken, including a focus on strengths as well as the presenting problems that will be the focal point of treatment. In addition, the spouses complete a no-violence contract (including a commitment to reduce verbal aggression).

In addition, the spouses are specifically taught cognitive and behavioral strategies for anger management, including, but not limited to, self-soothing procedures, time outs, and cognitive restructuring of anger-eliciting thoughts (Epstein & Baucom, 2002; Heyman & Neidig, 1997). Spouses are provided with additional education about the consequences of constructive versus destructive forms of communication and are taught strategies for effective conflict containment (e.g., making a conciliatory statement rather than reciprocating a negative message from one's partner). They are further instructed to practice anger management strategies between sessions as a homework assignment.

- *Sessions 3 and 4.* Expressive and receptive skills are taught (Baucom & Epstein, 1990; Epstein & Baucom, 2002; Dattilio & Padesky, 1990) and rehearsed during both sessions. Spouses begin practicing their newly acquired skills with relatively benign topics. As they progress, the significance of the topics increases so that they are able to practice the skills with topics involving moderate to severe conflict). During these sessions, the homework focuses on additional practice of communication skills as well as continued use of anger management techniques.

- *Sessions 5 through 7.* Beginning with the fifth session, spouses are taught problem-solving skills (Baucom & Epstein, 1990; Epstein & Baucom, 2002) for resolving conflict without abuse. Partners are coached in combining communication and problem-solving skills and in applying those skills to increasingly conflictual topics. An emphasis is placed on applying these skills to the spouses' areas of concern about their relationship.

There is a specific focus on the identification and modification of spouses' negative cognitions that interfere with problem solving. Each session concludes with plans for the spouses' homework assignment for the following week and a renewed commitment to use their anger management skills whenever needed.

• *Sessions 8 through 10.* In the final sessions of the protocol, the spouses continue with the application of communication and problem-solving skills. This is supplemented with relationship recovery and enhancement strategies. Clinicians emphasize recovery from traumatic events, including past domestic violence, and the need to exercise patience as the spouses work together for the common good of the relationship. Clinicians encourage the formerly abusive partner to be empathic and supportive when the recipient of prior abuse continues to exhibit trauma symptoms (e.g., startle and anxiety responses, defensive withdrawal) and to assist his or her partner appropriately in efforts to cope with the symptoms more effectively.

Readers are also referred to some of the other fine literature on stress inoculation and anger control outlined by Novaco (1975) and Meichenbaum (1977). The therapist may also refer to the work of Dutton (2007) on the abusive personality.

CONTRAINDICATIONS AND LIMITATIONS OF THE COGNITIVE-BEHAVIORAL APPROACH

Like any form of treatment, the cognitive-behavioral model has contraindications and limitations. As noted previously, cognitive-behavioral couple therapy has been subjected to more controlled outcome studies than any other therapeutic approach (Baucom, 1987). These studies present strategies that are particularly effective in reducing relationship distress, especially as additions to a program that includes communications training, problem-solving training, and behavioral contracts.

However, there are some caveats to be considered in the use of the cognitive-behavioral model. One of these is the importance of training and skill in applying the cognitive-behavioral principles. Cognitive-behavioral interventions necessitate extensive study, training, and practice and often require the therapist to be fully grounded in the theory and approach. However, these interventions are best used against the backdrop of a systems approach, inasmuch as members of a family simultaneously influence and are influenced by each other's thoughts, emotions, and behaviors, which is important for the effectiveness of CBT techniques (Dattilio, 2001a; Leslie, 1998).

When CBT is used in the strictest sense, it tends to be linear and may have less impact on couples and families because of the need to address circularity and the couple or family as a system, rather than as individuals. Some of the cognitive-behavior therapies that place emphasis away from exploring an individual's past may also be a hindrance, particularly in regard to issues of family of origin.

Another potential limitation is the misuse of the therapist's perceived power through his or her imposing ideas of what constitutes rational or balanced thinking. Sometimes clients may feel pressured to adopt the therapist's values and goals for therapy. Obviously, some spouses and family members may have trouble with confrontational styles, especially if a strong therapeutic alliance has not been established. The therapist should help clients to explore their own assumptions and not lecture them on what they should or should not do.

One of the areas drawing the highest criticism in the past concerns how emotions and affect are used in treatment. Often, the cognitive-behavioral approach may attract practitioners who are drawn to it because they are uncomfortable in working with feelings. Therefore, CBT should be enhanced by placing greater emphasis on the affective and emotional aspects, particularly when it is called for in a particular case. This issue is addressed in more depth in Chapter 2.

Cultural sensitivity may sometimes be overlooked in the cognitive-behavioral approach. One of the shortcomings of applying CBT to diverse cultural groups pertains to the hesitation of some clients to question their basic cultural values. For example, some Mediterranean and Middle Eastern cultures have strict rules in regard to religion, marriage, family, and child-rearing practices (Dattilio, 1995) that may be in conflict with the cognitive-behavioral suggestions of disputation (attacking thoughts based on erroneous thinking). For example, in one particular case that I worked with in Egypt, my suggestion to a wife that she question her husband's motives went over like a lead balloon. I was later informed that such behavior is forbidden in Egypt and in many of the Mideastern and Asian cultures. Although, this happened years ago and the tides may be changing to some degree, it is still an issue that may surface with various cultures.

Clinicians may also encounter difficulty with the cognitive end of the cognitive-behavioral approach in working with couples who are intellectually limited. Sometimes, the cognitive strategies may have to be modified or abandoned for the use of behavioral interventions, owing to clients' intellectual limitations or lack of insight.

The ability to maintain flexibility within the cognitive-behavioral domain is probably one of any therapist's greatest assets. Depending on the characteristics of the couples or families that are treated, they might find a didactic approach to be insulting or unduly educational, and this, of course, would need to be modified in order to address varying needs.

In general, the more flexible a cognitive-behavioral therapist can be in working with couples and families, the better. One of the beauties of this approach is that it lends itself to integration with other modalities, particularly in working with couples and families.

COUPLES AND FAMILIES IN CRISIS

Occasionally, therapists may be faced with families who come in during a crisis. If the crisis session is the first visit a therapist has with a family, then, obviously, the protocol will deviate significantly from the typical course. Because crisis situations do not usually afford the opportunity of conducting a detailed history or forming a case conceptualization of a couple's or family's general functioning, a modified approach must be used to address the crisis by targeting the current thoughts and behaviors that are contributing to the immediate concerns of the dysfunction and escalating it into a crisis.

Because the focus in such situations is on defusing the immediate crisis itself, a modified version of a step-by-step procedure is recommended, depending on the situation at hand. This may involve a host of cognitive or behavioral strategies up front, such as the use of deescalation techniques, instituting contracts, or teaching some emergency problem-solving skills so that the volatility of the situation can be reduced. This is analogous to clearing away the smoke in order to determine the extent of the flames, paving the way for the identification of individual or joint schemas, at which point the restructuring process may unfold.

Modified Step-by-Step Procedure

The strategies used in a crisis setting are similar to those typically suggested for inpatient units (Miller, Keitner, Epstein, Bishop, & Ryan, 1993), but have been adapted here for crisis situations in CBT.

1. Define the crisis at hand. Attempt to establish some level of agreement among family members about the nature of the problem and the family in general. This assessment may include evaluating the impact of the crisis on the family members and their style of processing it.

2. Maintain a definite, directive stance in entering the family unit and attempting to introduce any change or modification of the symptoms displayed or the family members' process of dealing with the situation.

3. Attempt to gather and understand some general dynamics of the couple or family members and their standards for dealing with crisis. This may involve delving into issues stemming from the family of origin or even past relationships, which may lead into the subsequent step.

4. Identify schemas derived from the spouses' or parents' families of origin, relative to the present crisis or similar situations, and how these impinge on the overall situation at hand.

5. Introduce the concept of automatic thoughts and schemas through psychoeducation and the various methods of identifying cognitive distortions. Introduce the Dysfunctional Thought Record and explain how it can be used to modify affect and behavior.

6. Introduce the use of behavioral contract agreements, couple and family support methods, and alternatives for additional consultation sessions (i.e., seeing a physician for medication, etc.).

7. Introduce the concept of agreeing to behavioral contracts in an attempt to defuse the current crisis. If the crisis is ongoing, this intervention must be conducted over the course of multiple visits.

8. Move toward permanent schema restructuring and behavioral change enactment.

9. Address conversation skills and improve problem-solving strategies.

10. Reinforce the implementation of the afore-mentioned strategies as a measure of inoculation against future crisis situations.

11. Determine if ongoing counseling or therapy is required, and make appropriate referrals.

It is essential to defuse the volatility of a marital or family crisis prior to focusing on permanent schemas and behavioral change. If the couple or family members learn to deal effectively with crisis, their therapy is less likely to be derailed by any other crises that may arise, and they can focus on permanent change. See Dattilio (2007) for a full-length case study of a family in crisis and more explicit details on techniques and interventions.

Sometimes a crisis serves as an impetus for change. That is, couples or families will sometimes address certain dynamics or conflicts only after a crisis brings the situation to a head. As a result, therapists need to focus on what this says about a particular couple or family situation. The tone of treatment differs slightly in such cases.

SAME-SEX COUPLES AND THEIR CHILDREN

Working with same-sex couples and their offspring is a topic that has appeared increasingly in the professional literature. Same-sex couples seek treatment for many of the same reasons that heterosexual couples do (Dattilio & Padesky, 1990). As a result, many of the same interventions apply, usually with some alterations, depending on the circumstances. The therapist needs to be aware that there are special issues and pressures that couples and families face with same-sex unions. It is important for the therapist to become familiar with some of the myths that often surround same-sex couples (American Psychological Association, 1985).

Probably one of the most salient issues that arise concerning same-sex relationships is the external pressure to which individuals are exposed. The added stress of isolation in times of relationship distress may be problematic, particularly isolation from family, friends, or coworkers. Other stressors include adopting children and relationships with extended family. It is important to help couples realize that many of the conflicts they experience are very similar to those that heterosexual couples experience. Helping them to feel more normalized about their relationship is typically an important aspect of treatment.

Not all therapists have the expertise to treat same-sex couples. Therefore, they should consider referring to another resource if necessary.

ATYPICAL COUPLE AND FAMILY CONSULTATIONS

The majority of therapists have centered on the more traditional modes of therapy with couples and families who apply for treatment. However, during the course of a therapist's professional career, atypical consultations arise that fall outside the normal realm of treatment. One of these addresses crisis situations, which are discussed in the preceding section. However, there are other types of consults that fall under the rubric of interventions. Some of these situations are discussed in the following sections.

Second-Opinion Consultations

Occasionally, mental health professionals are contracted by other treating therapists to provide a second opinion or a case consultation. This request may even come, at times, from a couple or members of a family themselves who want another opinion on the course of their treatment. In these cases, the consulting therapist is usually limited to a handful of visits in order to conduct an assessment and render an opinion on the course and direction of treatment. In such instances, the steps for assessment are recommended and an opinion given as to whether progress is being made, along with any recommendations for changes in interventions. Therapists providing a second opinion can still adhere to the basic principles of CBT without proceeding to the full extent of treatment. Within the general framework of an assessment, the therapist may wish to assess by using the guidelines offered in Chapter 4 and part of Chapter 5, always being respectful of the referring clinician, not overstepping boundaries, and not proceeding with treatment unless other arrangements are made with all parties.

It is suggested that the therapist providing a second opinion should talk by telephone or in person with the referring therapist and subsequently provide a written report on the assessment and recommendations.

Consultation to the Court System

Couples and, sometimes, families (in situations involving custody) may be referred by the court system in order to get a therapist's opinion on the direction taken regarding a marital or familial situation. For example, many states and provinces have mandatory counseling requirements for spouses or family members in certain situations, especially when one spouse is suing for divorce or custody and the other is contesting the action. In such cases, the therapist, again, may find him- or herself providing a quick assessment (typically three to five sessions) as to whether a particular relationship is salvageable and what should be recommended. Therapists also need to advise clients in such consults about their limits of confidentiality and their need to provide a written report directly to the court system.

Brief Inpatient Consultation

Psychiatric units in hospitals, drug and alcohol rehabilitation centers, and other institutionalized settings often use family therapists to address marital and family issues for patients admitted to the facility for treatment. Such involvement may consist of ongoing treatment consultations during the length of the inpatient stay or simply brief exit visits to address remaining issues in treatment. See the excellent chapters on inpatient family therapy in Wright, Thase, Beck, and Ludgate (1993) for a detailed discussion.

Once again, as in court consultations, clients must be made aware of the limits of confidentiality and the need for collaboration and consultation with other healthcare providers who may be involved.

Family-of-Origin Consultations

On occasion, therapists also receive requests for family-of-origin consultations. As stated earlier, such consultations have been more popular in other modalities of family therapy, such as that introduced by the late James Framo (1992). Family-of-origin visits may occur under two circumstances during the course of normal couple or family therapy. In some cases the therapist and one spouse/parent may elect to meet with his or her family of origin to address specific issues. In other cases, the entire intervention may involve one individual who wishes to meet with the specific family of origin for the sake of addressing any of a number of subjects, ranging from a particular incident to family dysfunction. For example, a certain case involved a man who came to individual therapy complaining of depression because he had had a falling-out with his parents and siblings some 20 years prior; he now wanted to reach out to them and reunite. This involved the therapist's contacting the man's parents and siblings directly and inviting them to a family-of-origin session. On occasion, such sessions may be more difficult to arrange and have to involve telephone conferencing. Sometimes, depending on the circumstances, marathon weekend sessions are held, especially if family members have to fly in from different areas. (This is the reason that holiday seasons are often great times to hold family-of-origin sessions.)

In cases such as that of the aforementioned client's, much of the same format is used as in the case of crisis consultation, in that a specific area of focus is pinpointed quickly because of the limited amount of time available. The focus is often restricted to a single issue, which may entail anything from incest, to estrangement, to death of a family member, and so forth. This focus is usually more of a problem-solving and reuniting interaction, which may later blossom into ongoing visits with one or all family members, depending on whatever is arranged.

In other circumstances, a parent may wish to have a special consultation for two—with only one of his or her offspring—instead of meeting with the entire family of origin. Although, in some cases, more may be accomplished by having the entire family of origin in for several sessions, sometimes limited consults may be beneficial. This must be left to the therapist's judgment.

There may also be occasions when only one spouse shows up for marital therapy with a specific request to not include his or her spouse. Although this is unusual, it often has to do with issues of power and control, unless, of course, the other spouse has refused to submit to treatment (see the section "Handling Roadblocks and Resistance to Change" in Chapter 6). Once again, therapists must make a clinical call and use their ethical judgment in such situations. Sometimes therapeutic gain can be accomplished, although limited. This may also be a prelude for drawing a spouse or other family members into treatment at a later date.

On occasion, therapists may be confronted by family members who are estranged. Often, the family members who struggle most with the estrangement may seek help in order to either cope with the estrangement or find ways of reconnecting with the estranged family member(s).

In cases such as this, the therapist might elect to contact the estranged member(s) and invite them in. Whether or not the therapist is successful in gathering all the family members together, many of the CBT techniques discussed earlier in this book can be applied to this situation as well, particularly the issue of schema and how it relates to the estrangement and the rigid beliefs that contribute to the ongoing separation of family members. Once the therapist is successful in assembling family members in treatment, a schema-focused approach can be very effective in addressing distorted beliefs and emotional wounds that exist with family members. This process strays from the traditional type of family therapy in that it involves more of a time-limited atmosphere and one in which a therapist only has a brief opportunity to make inroads before certain family members withdraw due to the volatile circumstance at hand.

COTHERAPY WITH COUPLES AND FAMILIES

Occasionally, therapists may elect to use a cotherapist in treatment. When treating couples, I often work along with my wife, Maryann, who is a wonderfully talented psychotherapist. This approach is more typical in couple therapy than in family therapy; however, it can be used with either. Couples often find it more constructive for a husband-and-wife therapy team to work with them during the course of treatment in order to balance out gender-related issues or simply to provide them with an expanded perspective.

Although financial and logistical considerations often prevent a therapist from working with a cotherapist, if this can be arranged, it is often very effective. Cotherapy can also be conducted with a same-sex cotherapist, particularly if the situation so dictates, such as with same-sex couples. Research has suggested that male–female cotherapy teams are the best therapeutic combination (Sonne & Lincoln, 1965).

In some cases, cotherapy might make a therapy situation more complex and create added difficulties if treatment is not orchestrated properly. However, when the members of a well-experienced cotherapy team work together and use the same modality of treatment, their shared experience and insight can enhance the therapeutic climate. For an expanded discussion on this topic, see the works of the late James L. Framo (1992).

Cognitive-behavioral therapists should keep in mind that cotherapy must always be coordinated in the best interest of the client. Typically, the agenda for each session should be planned in advance, and potential challenges and pitfalls should always be discussed. The same types of procedures outlined in this text that are used by solo therapists are also used in cotherapy.

MULTILEVEL TREATMENT

Some cases require therapists to work on multiple levels, which means that they may have to do some individual, as well as family work in more than one area.

The following is an example of therapy with a family that presented with an adolescent female who was suffering from a history of depression, suicidal behavior, and trichotillomania (chronic hair-pulling). This example illustrates how a combination of techniques was used to address cognitive, emotional, and behavioral issues, as well as to deal with the family's stress in regard to the adolescent's problems. The case also addresses issues of inpatient consultation regarding the child's psychopathology, as well as follow-up outpatient treatment.

"YOU MAKE ME PULL MY HAIR OUT": THE CASE OF LILLIAN[3]

Lillian was a 15-year-old girl referred by a local hospital's psychiatric unit subsequent to a voluntary admission because of suicidal ideation of disturbing frequency. On admission to the hospital, she was depressed and anxious, but friendly and cooperative with her doctors and the inpatient treatment team. There were also reports that she had begun pulling hair out of her head and eyebrows. She was placed on 20 mg of Fluovaxitine and 50 mg of trazodone at bedtime for sleep. After a few weeks she reported a cessation of suicidal ideation and was engaged in individual, group, and occupational therapy. Lillian remained in the hospital for only 1 week more and was subsequently discharged to her parents. She was followed by a psychiatrist and a therapist for counseling on an outpatient basis. Unfortunately, Lillian and her parents did not think that the therapy was very effective, particularly with the problems of tension between her and her parents and her compulsive hair pulling. Consequently, the family physician referred the family to me for consultation.

In my first session with Lillian and her parents, the parents told me that Lillian was pulling out her hair and eyebrows and was also cutting herself superficially with a razor blade on her forearms. She had apparently broken up with her boyfriend and was very distressed over the loss of what she described as her "true love."

Lillian told me that she had made an earlier suicide attempt at age 14 because of "family problems." She was diagnosed with major depressive disorder which subsequently reconstituted to a dysthymic disorder. She was also diagnosed with obsessive–compulsive disorder. Lillian's mother claimed that she was particularly unhappy with her daughter's previous treatment, because she did not feel that she was included enough in the process of therapy. I was informed that Lillian had received a full medical workup, including a blood profile, CT scan, and additional diagnostic tests, all of which yielded negative results.

---

[3]Portions of this case first appeared in Dattilio (2005d). Adapted with permission from Elsevier, Ltd.

At the initial family session, Lillian informed me that she had started pulling her hair out in an attempt to express her anger, as well as to alleviate guilt. Although it is unusual for teenagers to speak so openly in the presence of their parents, Lillian was so angry that, at this point, she didn't care. Lillian felt that everything that had happened in her life with her parents and her relationship with her boyfriend was her fault. (She also experienced anxiety in dealing with her relationship with her boyfriend.)

Background information indicated that Lillian was an only child and was always very independent. She first began pulling out individual hairs from her head at age 14, owing to feelings of frustration and anger. She tried to stop her hair pulling, but her anxiety and depression would increase each time she attempted to refrain from such behavior. She felt tormented by her obsessive thoughts and hence felt compelled to revert to pulling out what she deemed to be "unwanted hairs." She also experienced thoughts such as "I'm a loser" and "I'm stupid." In addition, there was a perfectionistic aspect to her thinking. Lillian pulled only the dark hair out of her head. When I mentioned that it was ironic that her mother had very dark hair (unlike her own, which was strawberry blonde), she became quiet and made no comment.

The family therapy session involved mother, father, and Lillian. We began to explore some of Lillian's family dynamics. Lillian explained to me that she experienced a considerable amount of guilt and that the hair pulling was really more of an expression of her anger and resentment for her mother, who she always felt was intrusive in her life. She was also somewhat angry with her father, who she felt was too passive and subservient to his wife's demands. Lillian felt that her father should have stood up more for her against her mother. Lillian considered his inaction to be abandonment.

The initial phase of treatment focused on the tension in the family and moved away from Lillian's self-abuse. Lillian's symptoms were dealt with separately in individual sessions, with the use of a cognitive-behavioral approach involving exposure and response prevention techniques.

Lillian's mother came across as overbearing and intrusive, but it seemed she had evolved into this posture because her husband had assumed such a passive role since the beginning of their relationship. She always pushed Lillian very hard to succeed in life, which is why, Lillian believed, she developed a perfectionistic belief system. In some sense, Lillian wanted to comply with her mother's requests; at the same time, she resented her mother's intrusiveness and did not feel as though she could live up to her mother's expectations. This feeling of being stuck drove her to literally pulling her hair out.

Lillian's father, unfortunately, maintained the homeostasis in the family by simply going along and trying to keep peace with his wife and daughter. At the same time, he tried to avoid any confrontation with either of them. It would have been easy to allow this situation to evolve into therapy between Lillian and her mother because her father maintained such a passive stance. I repeatedly encouraged the father to join the conversation and gradually called him on his passiveness, slowly integrating him more into the therapy process. This met with quite a bit of resistance from the mother who, at times, strove for power and control over her husband, until she was informed repeatedly that one of the problems in the family was that there was an insufficient balance of power between her and her husband. Interestingly, during this phase of treatment, Lillian reported that her hair pulling increased, almost as a way of trying to symbolically distract herself from intervening in her parents' dispute.

Surprisingly, despite their initial resistance, Lillian's parents proved to be open to my suggestions. I suggested that they enter into marital therapy to address some of their conflicts over power and control in their own relationship. They also focused on their methods for dealing with anger and resentment and their respective unfulfilled needs.

Much of my individual work with Lillian involved using *in vivo* exposure and response prevention, which is the technique of choice in CBT with trichotillomania (compulsive hair pulling). Lillian was repeatedly exposed to hair on her *head* that she felt tempted to pull out and was asked to refrain from pulling, forcing her to feel her anxiety. She was then instructed to wait it out until her anxiety level decreased on its own. Any kind of motivations toward self-mutilating behaviors, such as cutting or scratching herself, were addressed in the same fashion, based on a graded hierarchy. When Lillian became agitated and depressed, cognitive restructuring techniques were utilized to help her process her thoughts and emotions and challenge them. For example, she was educated in the use of the Dysfunctional Thought Record in an attempt to weigh the evidence supporting the statements she made to herself and to weigh them against the cognitive distortions discussed in the section "Testing and Reinterpreting Automatic Thoughts" in Chapter 5.

Lillian's father was also requested to assist her as a coach. I asked that her mother not become directly involved, but that she support her husband's work with Lillian. This served to balance out the power and control in the family and allowed Lillian to bond with her father. Lillian also dealt with the symbolic notion that her pulling only the dark hairs from her head was a way of pulling her mother out of her life. It seemed that she learned from her father to be afraid to stand up to her mother. Therefore, she rebelled in self-destructive ways.

My objective was to teach Lillian how to exchange her self-destructive behavior for a way to assert herself more openly. Consequently, part of our work involved Lillian's becoming more assertive with her mother and confronting her. I spent several individual sessions with Lillian, using the technique of assertiveness training mentioned in the section "Behavioral Techniques" in Chapter 6. We utilized systematic role play, which I modeled for her first by pretending that I was Lillian and she was her mother. We then reversed roles, and I played her mother while she expressed herself to me. Treatment also highlighted the notion that Lillian needed to accept the fact that she was not perfect and would never meet all of her mother's expectations. This objective was achieved through both individual and conjoint sessions. Conjoint sessions also served as a conduit for Lillian's father to eventually become more assertive, thus allowing Lillian's mother to redirect her own behaviors and to be less overbearing. At first, there was, obviously, tremendous resistance to making these changes, inasmuch as my interventions were disrupting the family's homeostasis. Lillian's mother also felt that she often became the "bad guy" in the relationship and that I was intimating that everything was her fault. I suggested that, because she was the more demonstrative parent, it appeared that she was the majority of the blame. But I explained this as a result of the family dynamics and her husband's decision to assume a more subservient role in the parenting process. As I began to redirect the members of this family to develop a new way of interacting and achieving a different balance of power and control, they began to accept my lead and to make some meaningful changes.

This is an interesting case of a family that experienced difficulty on a number of levels. For one, there were clearly cognitive distortions that fueled a negative behavioral exchange. However, the issue of attachment between Lillian and her mother was another important issue to address, as well as the manner in which the family members expressed emotion and dealt with crisis. A significant portion of therapy was directed to helping Lillian bond with her mother, as well as with her father, attempting to restore the balance in their relationships.

8

Enhancements to Cognitive-Behavioral Therapy

A number of ancillary treatments have been developed that often work well in concert with CBT. Although some authors promote them in their own right as wholly existing interventions, these are best suited, in my opinion, as enhancements to the CBT approach (Hofmann, 2008; Hofmann & Asmundson, 2008; Dattilio, 2009).

ACCEPTANCE-BASED TECHNIQUES

Some emergent therapeutic techniques promote a conscious posture of openness and acceptance of psychological events, even if they are "formally negative," irrational, or even psychotic (Hayes, 2004). The term *acceptance* has been employed to describe a variety of psychological processes and interactional behaviors.

According to Hayes the principle goal of acceptance and commitment therapy (ACT) is to treat emotional avoidance, excessive literal response to cognitive content, and the inability to make and keep commitments to behavior change (Hayes, 2004).

In working with couples and families, acceptance is not only viewed as a psychological phenomenon within a person, but also a transactional process between spouses, family members, or interpersonal contacts. Acceptance involves something a person does in response to his or her own private experience that is either accepted or not by others. This may be a thought, sensation, emotion, experience of arousal, desire or want, or other internal stimulus (Fruzetti & Iverson, 2004).

One form of acceptance may involve tolerating distress in a relationship. There may be a focus on transforming the initial stimulus for distress into a different stimulus with different responses. In this respect, the stimulus is transformed from discomfort to contentment. Acceptance of stress means living in a way that is consistent with one's own values or more likely to achieve one's goals. A minimal aspect of acceptance may also involve awareness that a problem exists and how it is relevant to the relationship situation. Fruzetti and Iverson (2004) define acceptance as having several components: (1) the phenomenon in question is within the person's awareness, (2) the person, regardless of the valence of the experience (pleasant or unpleasant, initially desired or not), is not currently focused exclusively on organizing his or her resources to change the experience or the stimulus (or stimuli) that elicits the experience, and (3) the person has an understanding (regardless of its accuracy or veracity) of the relationship between the present private experience and some stimulus (or stimuli) that preceded it. Fruzetti and Iverson (2004) go on to state that there are two levels of acceptance: (1) acceptance in the balance with change and (2) pure acceptance. Pure acceptance may involve simple tolerance or genuine or radical acceptance, in which the experience is transformed from one that is negative to one that is neutral or even positive.

These principles have been recommended as useful in treating couples who are in conflict. Christensen et al. (2004) suggest that acceptance work with couples may involve trying to create conditions in which partners naturally increase in their emotional acceptance of each other. They suggest that there are various strategies that may be used, which include empathic joining.

MINDFULNESS

Mindfulness has been studied extensively by Western researchers and practitioners, but it derived originally from Buddhism and other Eastern spiritual systems. Mindfulness is a component of most, if not all, successful therapies because it emphasizes contemplation and the cultivation of conscious attention. Mindfulness has essentially been defined as the direction of attention toward one's ongoing present experience in a manner characterized by curiosity, openness, and acceptance (Bishop et al., 2004).

Mindfulness has recently been applied to work with intimate relationships. One way to understand the development of relationship distress is as an outcome of maladaptive emotional repertoires in the context of challenging and vulnerable emotions. The concept of mindfulness is an open and receptive attention to the present moment in which one can promote a more accepting and less avoidant orientation to challenging emotions. In this way, a more responsive and relationally healthy mode of responding becomes possible (Wachs & Cordova, 2007). A recent study conducted by Wachs and Cordova (2007) explores the theoretical relationship between mindfulness emotion repertoires and marital adjustment. In a study using a sample of married couples, the investigators examined the association between self-reported mindfulness and relationship satisfaction, as well as emotional skills, which involve recognition and identification of emotions, empathy, and thoughtful responding in the context of anger. They also looked at both mindfulness and relationship satisfaction.

The findings suggested that emotional skills and mindfulness were both related to marital adjustment and that skilled emotional repertoires, specifically those associated with identifying and communicating emotions, as well the regulation of anger expression, fully mediated the association between mindfulness and marital quality. The upshot of the study supports the rationale for an increase in emotional tolerance, which suggests that paying sustained attention to ongoing experience places an individual in close proximity to his or her own thoughts and feelings, allowing the individual to grow more comfortable with his or her own emotional experience. The concept of mindfulness underscores the quality of one's conscious attention and how this may create conditions in which more adaptive emotional responding is possible. This type of metalevel awareness of the contents of consciousness has previously been referred to as "metacognitive awareness" (Teasdale et al., 2002).

Mindfulness is particularly appropriate in working with couples and their empathy levels. Preliminary work exploring empathy levels in association with mindfulness, furthermore, leads to the speculation that attunement to and concern for another's feelings is a skill set that may be associated with attention to the present moment. The construct of empathy captures the ability of an individual to remain sensitive to another person's emotional state and to reflect that emotion back to the other individual, indicating that he or she vicariously feels the same emotion (Johnson, Cheek, & Smither, 1983).

Several other authors have suggested that mindfulness may have considerable value for enhancing the quality of romantic relationships. Kabat-Zinn (1993) and Welwood (1996) have suggested that mindfulness promotes attunement, connection, and closeness in relationships. A further study examined the role of mindfulness in romantic relationship satisfaction and response to relationship stress. In the results, mindfulness was again shown to relate to relationship satisfaction, indicating that mindfulness may play an influential role in romantic relationship well-being (Barnes, Brown, Krusemark, Campbell, & Rogge, 2007).

Mindfulness may also help heighten attention and awareness, both of which are important in interpersonal relationships. There has also been an emphasis on the importance of attentive active listening for successful communication between members of a couple as well (Bavelas, Coates, & Johnson, 2000, 2002). The notion of mindfulness in the promotion of healthy romantic relationship functioning has also been supported by recent studies examining the efficacy of interventions designed to enhance mindfulness skills in a randomized wait-list control study of an 8-week mindfulness-based relationship enhancement program with nondistressed couples. Carson, Carson, Gil, and Baucom (2004) found that the intervention favorably influenced couples' relationship satisfaction, closeness, acceptance of the partner, relationship distress, and other relationship outcomes. The intervention also positively affected individual well-being.

Another study, conducted by Shapiro, Schwartz, and Bonner (1998), found that during an 8-week longitudinal study, mindfulness-based stress reduction and increased levels of mindfulness were associated with an increase in self-reported empathy, a characteristic that is particularly likely to influence the maintenance of relationships, predict positive adaptive behaviors, and ultimately lead to relationship satisfaction (Davis & Oathout, 1987, 1992; Hansson, Jones, & Carpenter, 1984).

Another way that mindfulness may play a role in relational adjustment is that mindful spouses have a tendency to engage in relationships that are lower in emotional and behavioral negativity. A positive relationship between mindfulness and positive affectivity, and an inverse relation with negative affectivity, suggests that mindful individuals in a romantic partnership may be less likely to experience the disproportionate dominance of negative affectivity that is predictive of relationship discord and disillusionment (Carrere & Gottman, 1999).

9

Case Examples

THE RETIREMENT TRAP

Warden and Viola (or Vie, as she preferred to be called) were a couple in their late 60s who had been married for 44 years. They had two children, a son and a daughter in their late 30s, who were both married. They also had several grandchildren. Both Warden and Vie were raised Pennsylvania German, otherwise known as Pennsylvania Dutch, which is a hard-working culture of the northeast section of Pennsylvania—descendants of early German settlers who arrived in the United States in the early part of the 19th century.

Vie and Warden reported that they had had a fairly good marriage through the years and never really experienced any significant difficulties aside from the usual stressors of raising a family. They recall experiencing very few arguments—that is, until they both retired.

Couples often function quite well when they are immersed in their careers and raising a family. However, in later years, once the children are grown and both spouses reach retirement age, many find themselves spending more time together than previously, are thrust into a more intense relationship, and sometimes experience trouble in adjusting. This was not the first time I had heard partners tell me that they were getting on each other's nerves and often wished the other would go back to work or spend more time away from home. I recall one woman in treatment referring to the situation as "the retirement trap." This was certainly the case with Warden and Vie, who presented as a very friendly, congenial couple who were enjoying their golden years. Unfortunately, during the first session, Warden and

Vie informed me that they were ready to kill each other and didn't know whether they could remain married.

Warden had been a cost estimator with a large accounting firm during his working years, and Vie had worked as a custom drapery manufacturer and designer. Both loved their work, as well as their family life, and always seemed to get along fairly well.

Warden retired first when he was in his late 50s. This is when some of the problems in the marriage started, or so they contended. Vie found Warden to be more agitated than normal once he was at home on a daily basis. At first she thought this had to do with the fact that he was taking high doses of corticosteroids for his asthmatic condition, which she felt might have been contributing to his "flipping out" at times over minor issues. Vie cited an incident when she brought home the wrong type of salad dressing from the market and Warden launched into a tirade. Vie stated that Warden was a little bit like this during their earlier years, although his behaviors were very mild. Since retiring, however, she reported that Warden had become worse and his outbursts more frequent.

Vie worked a few years longer than Warden. When she eventually retired, the "shit hit the fan." Vie and Warden referred to themselves as "snow birds," because they spend summers in the Northeast and winters in South Carolina. Despite the change of scenery and climate, they continued to experience arguments, both agreeing that their arguments had become worse in the past several years.

Warden was the first to own up, stating, "I know I have a problem, but it's not all me! A lot of it is her as well." It was Vie's impression that Warden was also struggling with depression. The spouses went on to inform me that they missed their working years, when they had gotten along fairly well and were absorbed with their jobs and the children. They admitted that they had had rough spots at times, but that they had usually occurred only when Warden consumed alcohol a little too much. He drank for the first 7 to 10 years of their marriage and then discontinued because he felt that he was becoming too dependent on alcohol. Both assured me that there had never been any physical or verbal abuse—just arguments.

Warden often worried too much about things that Vie felt were trivial. For example, Warden was a neat freak and nitpicky about everything being just right. "We used to balance each other out nicely in the past; now we can't seem to do that anymore." Both admitted that they had never sought marital counseling previously because they felt it would be giving in to failure and that they should be able to work out their problems on their own. "We're Pennsylvania Dutch," Warden said. "We wash our own laundry." Vie felt that Warden was always very controlling, but she simply absorbed it. Sometimes she would write letters, which she never gave to Warden, or talked to her girlfriends in order to express her feelings. She felt that she could never do this with Warden because it would just agitate him. Both admitted to me that their respective jobs served as a refuge for them and diverted many of their arguments.

But after Warden retired, Vie felt he became even more controlling and tried to tell her what to do with her business, as well as her friends. Vie said, "There is nowhere to run and sometimes I feel trapped." Warden spoke up, stating that he felt the same way. "She expects me to do what she wants to do all the time, and I don't care for some of the things she wants to do." He said that he becomes bored and depressed and feels like going off on his own. Warden also complained that, while in South Carolina, "Vie likes to go out with the 'old people,' whom I find boring. She is content with that, but I need to do something else."

After listening to this couple for approximately 40 minutes, it struck me that what Vie and Warden were complaining about appeared to be superficial issues. I wondered if their problems represented an underlying power struggle that had been going on for years. I decided to explore a little more with them and refrained from raising the issue of power and control. I asked, "How was it that two accomplished individuals in the prime of their lives can't seem to iron out what appears to be such a superficial matter?" Vie stated, "I don't know. This is what is bothering both of us. I have always been so tolerant of Warden, and I think now I have reached a point where I've had it, and I am not tolerating it any more and he doesn't know what to do with it. As a result, he blows up and I can't stand his behavior, so I leave." Vie believed that Warden did not have enough activities to keep himself busy in his retirement and that as a result, he sat around and worried and then became preoccupied with trivial matters, and this made him miserable.

Warden retorted, "I like sitting around and being by myself. I have projects to do around the house, which I enjoy, and I like the warm climate in South Carolina, but I prefer the Northeast. The problem is that there is a lot to do in South Carolina, but not the type of things that I like to do, and we're torn." Vie spoke up at that point: "It's more than that. Warden is sarcastic and makes a lot of caustic remarks, which I can't stand. I can never disagree with him because he flies off the handle. It's like walking on eggshells and I can't be my own person." At this point, Vie began to cry, saying that she felt as though she was losing a part of herself and sometimes felt the need to get away from Warden in order to be a "whole person" again. I observed Warden at the moment his wife began to cry. He seemed to sink into his chair like a little child who had just been scolded.

I asked Warden what his automatic thoughts were about his wife's statement, at which point he became a little loud and said, "Well, she shoots her mouth off without thinking and it just pisses me off! We were visiting our grandchildren not too long ago and apparently they were close to the neighbor's dog that had just died. So the first thing Vie says to the kids is, 'Oh, I'm so sorry to hear about the neighbor's dog,' and of course the kids got upset and started crying. And I thought to myself, 'What the hell did you have to go and say that for'?" It was Warden's impression that the timing was bad and that Vie didn't need to bring up the subject because they already knew the dog had died—it didn't make any sense. It was at this point that Vie chimed in, stating, "I just say what I feel, Warden. What's so bad about that?" She pointed to Warden and said, "You have to weigh every word you say, and I am not like that. I am constantly being told by you that I'm saying the wrong thing. I can't be myself when I am with Warden. I can't say what I feel. He wants to control everything that I say because it is the way he believes it should be."

It was at this point that I stopped both of them in their tracks and said to them, "You simply can't tolerate each other and your differences, can you?" The spouses hung their heads, saying very little. I said, "I think what happened here is that you were able to tolerate each other all these years because you had distracters, and now the spotlight is on the two of you because you have more time together. It has highlighted your differences, and your ability to tolerate each other's differences is just not there. But again, what troubles me is why you have so much difficulty coming up with strategies for dealing with these differences? You seem to be such capable individuals, yet you can't overcome this hurdle."

Both of them looked at me with a blank stare, almost as if to say that they both knew the answer but did not want to admit it to me, or to themselves. I looked at both of them and said, "I think you need to begin to tell me what's on your mind. Your faces are telling me a lot, but you're not stepping up to the plate." Warden rolled his eyes and said, "I guess it's a pissing contest. We don't want to give in to each other and I don't know why. It's crazy! This is the prime of our life and here we are fighting like cats and dogs. It's really stupid!"

It was at this point that I decided to shift gears a little because we were obviously at a standstill and I wanted them to think about this and allow it to resonate in their heads. I asked them a question that I often ask after I listen to a barrage of complaints about what isn't right with a relationship: "Can you tell me what works in your relationship?"

Vie answered first. "You know, sometimes when we're doing something that we both enjoy we really get along, and if it's nothing heavy and kind of lighthearted, we have a really good time. It seems to be when things get a little bit more complicated that the sparks fly." I asked them to provide me with an example of a couple of things they do well together and enjoy. They were able to tell me that they enjoyed visiting certain friends and playing cards, bridge mostly. They also enjoyed seeing their grandchildren, as well as going to the movies together.

They were not able to stay on these positive topics very long before Vie reverted to her complaints. "Warden just sugarcoats everything. He tells people what they want to hear, and I just tell it like it is. But that is when Warden shoots me looks that say 'shut up' and I just resent it." I looked at Warden for some confirmation, at which point he stated that he was just annoyed by some of things that his wife says because he thinks that Vie should be more reserved in what she says to people.

I asked Warden what harm is caused by Vie's saying what she feels. Warden admitted that she has never said anything that has been hurtful intentionally or usually created any problems. I began to introduce the idea that perhaps they tended to draw arbitrary inferences about each other's behavior, which has contributed significantly to the conflict they have experienced. Vie also went on to state, "Often, when we are going somewhere, Warden sometimes preps me beforehand not to say certain things or bring up certain issues, which really causes me to go into orbit. He'll say, 'Now don't bring this up, or don't say anything about that.' I just feel more relaxed when I'm by myself and I can't imagine this changing."

As we progressed through the first session, I tried to expand my conceptualization of exactly what was going on with this couple, because it seemed to me that many of the complaints were not as serious as others. It also seemed, however, that there was a deeper level of thinking with these spouses, which may have come from their respective families of origin. I decided to probe into this a little and ask them to each tell me something about their backgrounds.

Vie was an only child. Her parents had a very stormy marriage and always got on each other's nerves. She stated, "My mother was like Warden and my father was a lot like me. I favored my father and came to resent my mother through most of my upbringing." Vie went on to say, "It's interesting that I went and married my mother—what do you know about that?" I reminded her that this was actually not uncommon and that we often seek out attributes in our spouses, positive and negative, that hail from our families of origin. I asked Vie to think about whether Warden's behavior might sometimes trigger reactions in her that are reminiscent of her interaction with her mother. Vie felt that this was very likely. "Maybe I'm still battling with my mother when I argue with Warden." I suggested that Vie think about that and that we would address it later during the course of therapy.

Vie went on to inform me that Warden often compares her to her father. She recalled that her father would go out drinking with the guys, which bothered her quite a bit, but he was never abusive or disrespectful. It reminded her that this was another area in which she had problems regarding Warden's drinking. Vie informed me that identifying with her father contributed to her developing the belief that "you say what is on your mind and get it off your chest, and this is what contributes to one being a genuine person." Vie went on to elaborate: "My mother was often like Warden—she didn't say what she felt and minced words, but kept her true feelings to herself." Vie believed that this holding back was why her mother would later act out in a vicious fashion, much like Warden does. When I asked her what it was that attracted her to Warden, she stated that when she first met him, she found him to be a very steady, hardworking, and kind individual. She also thought that he would make a good family man and he always knew the right things to say to her. "I guess I just felt comfortable with him, in that he reminded me a little bit of both of my parents. And my parents liked Warden and that seemed to be a green light for me."

Warden's parents were the exact opposite of Vie's. His parents got along well. He was the third child of four. He recalls that his parents were strict, but they always kept things on an even keel. "My parents also never told me anything that they didn't want me to hear. Feelings were kept inside." Warden's family schema was, "Don't rock the boat and make other people feel bad, even though you may be burning inside. This was the motto we lived by." Warden was able to clearly relay the fact that this is why he holds things inside and doesn't always say what he feels. He also was able to link this to the fact that he later blows up when his emotions become overwhelming.

Much of this information was derived not only from my interview with Warden and Vie, but also from answers to selected questions from the Family of Origin Scale (Hovestadt et al., 1985). Interestingly, both reported little intimacy in their families of origin. There was also a low sensitivity for empathy or any emotion, which was an area that would later be addressed in treatment.

During the first session, I was able to help Warden and Vie understand a little about how the beliefs of their families of origin had been handed down and contributed to their own belief systems. I also informed them, however, that sometimes family-of-origin schemas work at the time during our upbringing, but don't necessarily work later in our own marriages. We began to explore the potential for modifying some of these beliefs and changing their behavior in ways that might have a positive impact on the relationship.

I decided to ask Warden and Vie to complete a homework assignment after the intake interview and write down their goals for therapy. I also asked them to make a list of the aspects that they felt they needed to change in their relationship and then construct a separate list of what each felt his or her spouse needed to change. I asked them not to collaborate on this assignment and told them that upon meeting for the second conjoint visit, we would discuss the assignment in detail. I also informed them that I would be meeting each of them separately for one visit in the interim in order to gather some additional information about their own conceptualizations of the problem in the relationship. I also asked each of them to complete the Marital Attitude Survey—Revised (Pretzer et al., 1991), along with the Relationship Belief Inventory (Eidelson & Epstein, 1982). It was my hope to obtain some additional information regarding their patterns of belief about the perceived ability to change, in regard to each partner him- or herself and to his or her spouse, as well as some of the underlying rigid beliefs they may have been harboring, keeping them gridlocked in their ongoing state of conflict.

Individual Sessions

I had a chance to meet with Vie for an individual visit, at which point she provided me with her responses to the two inventories I had asked her to complete. We also reviewed her goals for therapy. Vie informed me that she would really like to get along better with Warden and learn more of what that they had in common. She believed that she needed to try to be more tolerant of what he was saying, but felt that she could do this only if he were not so sarcastic. We discussed why she seemed to be so agitated all the time, at which point she told me that she suffered from fibromyalgia, which caused her a lot of pain on a daily basis. Vie went on to inform me that, in fact, she and Warden weren't able to have sexual relations because vaginal intercourse was too painful for her. Consequently, her libido was low and their sexual relations had been very bad for the past 2 years. She felt that this may also have been contributing to Warden's agitation. It was Vie's perception that this clearly made the problems in the relationship worse.

I informed Vie that I felt that one of the first lines of intervention was to at least reduce the tension in the relationship. I asked her what she felt she could do herself to ease the tension. "I guess maybe just let some of these things go and not react to them—I don't know." I asked her to give me some examples, at which point she informed that she sometimes allows Warden's comments to get on her nerves. I suggested that perhaps she consider just taking a different approach and begin to monitor the automatic thoughts she had about what his comments meant to her. It was at this point that I introduced to her the Dysfunctional Thought Record, and we did an example together. I oriented Vie to the CBT model and explained to her how her automatic thoughts tended to affect her emotions and behaviors. We then walked through an example in which she described for me a situation in which she and Warden were painting the living room and she became annoyed because Warden was so meticulous about using masking tape on the woodwork. She recalls that she became agitated with his obsessiveness and the amount of time that it consumed. When I asked her to close her eyes and imagine the situation and think back to what thoughts went through her mind, she stated, "Everything always has to be so controlled. Why can't he just let things go sometimes—like normal people." I worked with Vie as we put all of this on paper. Figure 9.1 is the result of our efforts.

I spent a little time helping Vie think about what she was telling herself and what it may have reminded her of. It was this door that I opened that allowed us to discuss the images of her own mother, who used to agitate her with the same type of finickiness, and how Vie perceived this as her mother's means of controlling her. It was at this point that we talked about the fact that Vie may be superimposing some of the anger she had about her mother's need to control, onto Warden's behaviors and interpreting them as being controlling when, in fact, this was just his way of doing a good job and feeling good about his work. I then suggested to Vie that she consider running this same scenario through the Dysfunctional Thought Record in which she addressed the issues of her automatic thoughts—separating the fact that Warden was not her mother and that it was not fair to assign the same emotions to his behaviors. We took this opportunity to talk a bit about her mother and father and how she tended to superimpose the emotions she had for her parents' actions on some of the same behaviors that her husband displayed.

Part of the individual session also addressed the issue of helping Vie to begin to separate these emotions and consciously remind herself that Warden is not her mother or father, but a different person and that the same behaviors cannot be associated with the negative emotions she experienced with her parents. We also spent some time talking about how she might resolve some of her issues from her family of origin, particularly her hostility toward her parents and some of the leftover resentment she still maintains, despite the fact that her parents have passed away.

Another issue that surfaced during the course of our individual therapy was Vie's feeling that now that they were retired, she and Warden needed to spend all their time together. We talked about how this was an unrealistic expectation and, maybe, because she was pushing this in the beginning, it had backfired and caused some tension in the relationship. Vie went on to inform me, "I always believed that once you were retired, you spent days and nights together, and I guess maybe that's unrealistic." We talked about the idea that, ironically, her attempt to do that has caused her to now desire to spend less time with Warden. I proposed the idea that perhaps some space between them might help them get along a little better and appreciate their time with each other.

Finally, the issue of her fibromyalgia was addressed and how her own

Directions: When you notice your mood getting worse, ask yourself, "What's going through my mind right now?" and as soon as possible jot down the thought or mental image in the automatic thoughts column.

Date Time	Situation	Automatic Thoughts	Emotions(s)	Distortion	Alternative Response	Outcome
	Describe: 1. Actual event leading to unpleasant emotion, or 2. Stream of thoughts, daydreams, or recollection, leading to an unpleasant emotion, or 3. Distressing physical sensations.	1. Write automatic thought(s) that preceded emotions(s). 2. Rate belief in automatic thought(s) 0–100%.	Describe: 1. Specify sad, anxious/ angry, etc. 2. Rate degree of emotion 0–100%.	1. All-or-nothing thinking 2. Overgeneralization 3. Mental filter 4. Disqualifying the positive 5. Jumping to conclusions 6. Magnification or minimization 7. Emotional reasoning 8. Should statements 9. Labeling and mislabeling 10. Personalization	1. Write a rational response to automatic thought(s). 2. Rate belief in alternative response 0–100%.	1. Rerate belief in automatic thought(s) 0–100%. 2. Specify and rate subsequent emotions 0–100%.
	Warden and I were painting the living room, and I became annoyed because Warden was so meticulous about the masking tape	*Why does he have to be so meticulous? Why can't he let some things go?*	*Irate, agitated*	*Magnification* *Disqualifying the positive*	*Maybe this is just Warden's way of making our house look nicer. Maybe it just makes him feel good and in control. That's not such a bad thing. I need to relax with it. Why do I get so upset over something so trivial?*	*Anxiety and agitation reduced*

Questions to help formulate the ALTERNATIVE RESPONSE: (1) What is the evidence that the automatic thought is true? Not true? (2) Is there an alternative explanation? (3) What's the *worst* that could happen? Could I live through it? What's the *best* that could happen? What's the *most realistic* outcome? (4) What should I do about it? (5) What's the effect of my believing the automatic thought? What could be the effect of changing my thinking? (6) If _____ (person's name) _____ was in this situation and had this thought, what would I tell him/her?

FIGURE 9.1. Vic's Dysfunctional Thought Record.

feelings of being out of control with her physical illness contributed to her frustration and agitation.

During the rest of this session, I also tried to assess Vie's amenability to going forward in the relationship and using some of the interventions I proposed. She convinced me that she was a willing participant and was open to my lead in treatment. She also reassured me that she truly did love Warden and wanted to work out—it was just that she also felt a little discouraged that things had been so tense lately in the relationship and wondered whether she was jumping to conclusions. We talked about the role of cognitive distortions and how powerful they are. I also suggested that she begin to use the Dysfunctional Thought Record and work through some of her distortions as they arose on an individual basis.

Individual Session with Warden

I had time to meet with Warden for a separate session. I followed some of the same course of questioning that I used with Vie in her individual session and oriented him to the cognitive-behavioral model. I also reviewed the Dysfunctional Thought Record and had Warden begin to address some of his own issues. Warden admitted that he had been "itchy" since he hadn't been working and told me that he often wonders whether he made a mistake by completely retiring. "Sometimes, I wish I was working part-time since I'm a 'doer' and I just need to keep busy. I know I drive my wife nuts sometimes with things I do around the house, and maybe that's just because I should be elsewhere, working part-time." During the course of our meeting, Warden would often offer up self-deprecating maxims such as "Well you know Doc, I'm not always the sharpest knife in the drawer," which was his indirect way of indicating that he knew that he was at fault a lot in the marital relationship. Such self-condescending statements may also have been Warden's way of soliciting empathy from me that he "wasn't such a bad guy." We discussed the idea that maybe getting a part-time job wouldn't be a terrible thing for him, or that he could at least find a hobby where he could rechannel some of his energies.

I also addressed the issue of what I perceived to be his perfectionism. Warden admitted that this was the "accountant" in him and had always been part of his fabric. I suggested to him that it wasn't a bad quality to have, but that, sometimes, in regard to his relationship with his wife, maybe it wasn't always the best thing. I had him begin to think a bit about changing his perspective on things and addressing the issue of why it was so important that everything always be perfect. I began to have him challenge some of his distorted beliefs through the use of the Dysfunctional Thought Record and also suggested that he try relaxing some of this behavior and see what types of reactions surface.

Part of what Warden had recorded on his surveys, particularly the Marital Attitude Questionnaire, was that he felt he needed to remain very structured in his life or things in the relationship would become too unstructured because of his wife's attitude. Warden did admit that this was a control feature in the relationship, and he gave some thought to my suggestion that perhaps he consider an alternative behavior that might relax the tension in his marriage.

Second Conjoint Session

I met with Warden and Vie for a second visit, during which we tied in some of the content that we discussed in the individual visits and targeted some goals for initially reducing the tension in the relationship and making some agreements. Both wholeheartedly agreed that the first order of business was to reduce the tension in the relationship so that we could focus on some of the positive aspects of their interchange. We also agreed that they would consider spending some separate times enjoying their own activities so that they could minimize the intensity in the time they spent together. This involved Warden's exploring the possibility of a part-time job, even if it was without remuneration, just to stay busy and focused. This would be offset by Vie's spending time with some of her friends whom Warden didn't find necessarily enjoyable. I also suggested that each of them share with the other their Dysfunctional Thought Records and how they began to address some of the restructuring of their respective thinking and a number of distortions. It was interesting that both of them sort of got a laugh out of what the other was processing and seemed to be very supportive of each other's efforts toward change.

We also discussed the issue of Vie's fibromyalgia and how this caused her a great deal of pain. Surprisingly, Warden was very sensitive to this issue and seemed quite concerned. It happened to be an area in which he was able to express his emotions and be supportive. We discussed what he should do when he became agitated, particularly regarding issues involving sexual relations, as well as Vie's need to say what was on her mind. Part of the mutual exchange was for both to make some exceptions to their expectations in the relationship and engage in "give and take." For example, I suggested to Warden that he build some tolerance to the fact that his wife was prone to express her thoughts, regardless of whether they were appropriate. This discussion was also helping Warden realize that he didn't have to take responsibility for things that Vie said and that he should let her take responsibility if there were negative repercussions. At the same time, I asked Vie to consider consulting with Warden, at her discretion, to get his opinion before she said certain things, rather than necessarily being chided or scolded by him. It was interesting to see how they actually served as consultants to each other in a harmonious way instead of getting under each other's skin about what was said.

I thought that this was a rather successful session. I suggested that they consider some of the homework that we had discussed and that we meet in approximately 10 days. Much to my surprise and, somewhat, chagrin, I received a telephone message from Warden saying that he and Vie were canceling the next visit with me and would call me in the future if they wanted to return. I found this rather intriguing and called them back, requesting that they both get on the phone. At that point, I asked them why they decided not to return, and Warden spoke up, stating that things were going pretty well and they didn't think that they needed to return for additional sessions. I told them that I thought that it was good that things were going well, but I still felt uncomfortable about leaving the situation hanging; therefore, I asked both of them if they would come in for a visit so that we could at least talk about this change in more in detail. Both agreed to maintain their previously scheduled appointment.

When I saw Warden and Vie together, they said that things had miraculously gotten better and they were no longer fighting. I warned them that this is what we sometimes call the "honeymoon period" and that things might automatically get better just because the anxiety about their situation had dropped, but that they still needed to come in and work on their conflicts. It was interesting that, at this session, some very important aspects of the relationship came to the surface.

I started the session by asking them to tell me what they had done in the interim that contributed to things going better in the relationship. Both Warden and Vie informed me that they had been working hard to monitor their automatic thoughts and think before they reacted. They had also taken some steps to communicate with each other, which they hadn't done before. However, it struck me that they were still quite guarded and avoidant of each other, at which point I decided to go out on a limb and raise the question that had been lurking in the back of my mind since I first started working with them.

"Do you think that maybe the two of you avoid being intimate with each other and this is really what all of this arguing and friction has been about?" Warden and Vie got very quiet and, at first, looked at me as though unsure of what I was asking. I then got blunter and said, "It just strikes me sometimes, based on your upbringing, that the two of you have avoided becoming more intimate, and the way you do this is to simply manufacture reasons for avoiding the intimacy by focusing on superficial, nitpicky issues and getting into arguments."

Vie said, "I think you're right. I've been thinking recently that what's been missing in our relationship is more of the intense type of closeness that I see between other couples. This is something we never had, but I've always desired."

Warden, on the other hand, didn't think that this was important to him and he felt that there was enough intimacy in the marriage for him.

At this point, we began to discuss what intimacy meant for each of them and how they had developed these ideas in their respective families. It became quite clear that Vie had a greater need for the traditional type of intimacy, which she just did not feel that Warden was capable of providing. In essence, this is what she was doing when she went out with her friends in South Carolina, drawing a healthy intimacy from others in her relationships. With time, we were able to determine that this was something that was foreign to Warden and that he misinterpreted many of Vie's overtures for intimacy as being "demanding." Consequently, he responded to her by being overtly controlling and chastising, which halted her in her tracks and had obviously led to the present dilemma.

My goal with the spouses at this point was, in large part, to develop their awareness about this issue and get them on the same page with being able to fulfill each other's needs. In many ways, Warden and Vie portrayed what is referred to in systems theory as the "pursuer–distancer dynamic" (Fogarty, 1976). This dynamic suggests that the more one presses for communication and togetherness, the more the other distances—goes for a walk, stays late at the office, and so forth. It was my impression that Warden, unfortunately, was not really very capable of addressing these issues because of his emotional limitations, and this was something that Vie had to accept and learn to tolerate. Consequently, the tolerance building that Christensen and associates (2004) recommended was used with her on this issue, along with helping Vie explore her own inner emptiness. It was my hope that this recommendation would open the space for Warden to move closer on his own terms.

Warden also went on to inform me, "I sort of know what she wants because she's often indicated it when we've watched movies about the kind of closeness that she would like from me. However, this just isn't my way and I've told her many times that I can't be like that." We did discuss ways in which Warden felt that he could engage in closeness that were comfortable for him. Much of the focus was on helping Vie accept Warden's best effort and encouraging Warden to remain aware of his need to try harder.

What also became important to Vie was the mere fact that Warden was willing at least to address and talk about the issue of their intimacy needs. We went on to discuss some of the cognitive distortions that centered on their misperceptions of each other's behaviors, as well as some of the content that had been addressed earlier in treatment.

I also had to accept the fact that I was limited in terms of where I could go in treatment with this couple and that the best I could hope for in terms of a goal was for the partners to maintain some sense of stabilization and reduce the friction between them. Often, major cognitive restructuring in older clients is not always realistic, and, depending on what people have been through in their lives and how set in their ways they have become, a therapist may risk losing them for the sake of attempting to change long ingrained habits of thinking and acting. I also had to realize that I had no control over how frequently this couple would decide to return for therapy. The notion of remaining in treatment on an ongoing basis was antithetical to this couple, although I always felt that Vie was more amenable than Warden was to coming in on a regular basis. I did see them two or three times subsequently, and they seemed to accept many of the traditional cognitive-behavioral strategies I suggested, such as monitoring their distorted automatic thoughts and adjusting their levels of expectations of each other, as well as simply learning to relax in the relationship and have more discussions about issues of intimacy and what each needed of the other.

This is a good case example of how a therapist sometimes needs to be willing to modify his or her approach in order to accommodate the various cases that come through the door. Although it was my intention to do a lot more with this couple, that simply was not going to happen, given the partners' resistance. Therefore, I made my best attempt to modify the approach in order to address at least some of their immediate needs. It was also my feeling that, had I pushed any harder with these spouses, they probably would have just bailed out and not returned to therapy at all.

FAMILY OF GLUTTONS[1]

Over the course of 30 years of my doing couple and family therapy, cases have been referred to me in many different ways. Usually they come through direct referral, but occasionally they may be referred circuitously, which is what happened with the Steigerwalts.

One day, in the late afternoon, I received a joint telephone call from two teenage children, who had picked my name out of the telephone book at random. They were each calling from an extension phone at their home, and they asked whether I did family therapy. When I said I did, they asked about my fees and subsequently proceeded to schedule an appointment. Because they sounded so young, I inquired about their ages. They told me that they were 14 and 16, respectively. I said that they would have to get their parents' consent for me to treat them. They thanked me and hung up.

---

[1]Portions of this case first appeared in Dattilio (1997). Adapted with permission from Rowman & Littlefield.

I didn't hear from these two teenagers again. But about a week later, I received a telephone call from their father, who said he wanted to schedule an appointment for the family. Mr. Steigerwalt quickly made the connection for me that his two kids had contacted me the week before. An appointment was made, and I promptly saw this family a week later. The Steigerwalts were an attractive, well-dressed middle-class family. At first glance, they would not arouse suspicion that there was anything wrong and, in many ways, they appeared to be quite a charming family.

During the initial session, I asked them how it was that they came to therapy and how I could help them. The two teenagers—Rollie, the 16-year-old son, and Janice, the 14-year-old daughter—piped up immediately, voicing their discontent. Rollie and Janice seemed well poised. They were both neat and appropriately groomed and made an impressive appearance. However, what came out of their mouths shocked me. "We're sick of our parents telling us what to do and we'd just as soon live somewhere else—divorced from them." This took me aback; I had never heard such a statement come out of a child's mouth in 30 years of doing therapy. The parents sat silently through this declamation, which gave me the distinct impression that this was not the first time this song had been sung in the Steigerwalt household.

Bob, a 48-year-old draftsman, worked for a large national automation firm, a job that had moved the family around the United States quite a bit during the course of his 19-year marriage. Carole, his wife, was a 43-year-old who worked full-time as an administrator at a nursing home. Carole would later tell me how she resented the moves they made over the years, particularly in light of Bob's failure to be promoted or given a significant salary increase. The Steigerwalts reported having had a tense, distant marriage up until 3 years ago, when they sought marital therapy. All of this was coming at me too fast and I realized that I had to slow things down.

I asked the family members what it had been like for them, living in their household during the last year or so, causing the children to make such a profound move as to contact a family therapist and then ask for a divorce from their parents. "They both act like a couple of 'dicks,'" said Rollie, motioning toward his parents in almost a cavalier fashion. "They're stupid, they fight all of the time, they drag us into the middle of their dumb fights and I can't stand it." "It is not fair," piped up Janice, who began to tear up when talking about the dissension in the home.

I looked at the parents, at which point Carole shocked me by saying, "They're right. We are miserable! There's been a constant tension in the house for more than a year." I noticed, out of the corner of my eye, that Bob was rolling his eyes and shaking his head as he looked down. "Bob, what's going through your mind?" I inquired. "It's not that bad," he said. "They're blowing this all out of proportion. I go through this crap all the time with them." Carole shot him a look, "Bob, you're always minimizing things. It's never that bad, nobody's feelings matter. When are you going to wake up?" "Yeah, Dad—you're like the biggest dick in this whole family," said Rollie. I couldn't believe that these kids were talking to their parents like this and, even more, that these parents tolerated it. I asked Rollie, "Do you always speak to your parents like this?" "Sometimes," Rollie smirked, "but it's because we're usually upset. Everybody gets like that in our family when we are upset, but we don't really mean it. It's .... it's just like we're so sick of everything."

I was trying to catch my breath to understand what exactly was going on with them. Thus far, my initial impression was that there was a lot of animosity and a great deal of blurring of boundaries; sometimes it seemed to me as if I were dealing with four adults rather than a family of two parents and two children.

One of the best techniques I learned in my early years of family therapy training was that, at times, it is best to just remain silent and let things unfold—absorb as much as I could and let it sink in. I did just that, at which point the mother emerged as the spokesperson. "We've actually had these problems for years. This is nothing new." I asked the family to tell me a little about what life had been like in the home before Mom and Dad went to couple therapy. I directed my question to Bob and Carole. "Was there as much dissension in the home, or was it mainly between the two of you?" In reply, Carole offered the following scenario:

"Actually, things weren't so bad at one time. Because Bob traveled so much with his work, I naturally spent more time with the kids. When Bob would come home, he was tired and usually didn't want to interact too much with the family, so he would sort of go off and stay to himself. When I would try to get him to become part of the family unit, he would get nasty and start to become verbally abusive to me." Carole continued, "Things kind of went down hill from there. I found myself getting increasingly angry and isolated from him. That is when we weren't getting along at all. It got real bad at one point, which is when we sought marital therapy and were in treatment for about 8 months."

I asked her if the therapy was successful. "Kind of," she said, looking at Bob. I waited for Bob to respond, but all he said while looking at his wife was, "Go ahead, you have the floor." "Well," said Carole, "things have gotten better, but the problem that still exists is with Bob's occasional verbal attacks on me—and now the children. Still, I don't understand why they're so unhappy. I mean, we have our tensions, but it's not that bad. This is crazy—asking for a divorce from us."

I noticed Bob shaking his head and kind of snickering. He said, "It's weird. Things got better between Carole and me, and now the kids seem to be unhappy. It doesn't make a lot of sense, does it?"

"Well, in some ways it does," I said. "Maybe because things shifted in the family dynamics, it's had an impact on everyone, and this new expression of emotion and behavior is the result."

It dawned on me that the children's dissatisfaction with their parents had seemed to surface around the time that Bob and Carole had started working on their marriage and becoming more unified. Rollie and Janice explained that, although they were good kids, their parents treated them unfairly. For example, their parents kept changing their minds, giving them permission to go away with their friends on the weekends, then later rescinding their permission and making it conditional by saying, "Well, you can go only if you do this or do that first." Both kids complained that this and other examples of inconsistency were terribly unfair, and they felt "jerked around" by their parents. They also didn't want to hear what either of their parents had to say any more.

One of the basic tenets of family therapy is that when there is a major shift in the parents' relationship, the entire family system, or homeostatic balance, changes. I suspect that this was at the root of the children's rebellion. What I found interesting, however, were the spontaneous automatic thoughts that these children had, particularly about what they seemed to assume were their rights. There was a major issue in regard to boundaries that formed as part of the family constitution, and I started to wonder what schemas were handed down early in this family unit that gave the message to these children that it was OK for them to challenge their parents on basic rules, regulations, and freedoms, and, most of all, to speak out against them so disrespectfully. I was intrigued and appalled at how these parents just sat there and let it go.

It was at that point that Bob chimed in and stated that, prior to marital therapy, they had been quite lax with discipline and setting boundaries. Carole agreed and said, "If anything, we are guilty of that behavior, and I think now we are trying to mop up after the mess, and the kids are getting older and are challenging us." Rollie and Janice spoke up to tell me that their parents had never agreed on anything in the past, and now, all of a sudden, they had become extremely strict, even though they maintain no set of rules in the household and simply make things up as they go along. Carole acknowledged that she and Bob often shoot from the hip and deal with situations as they come up. I thought that this inconsistency had probably had a major impact on the children's current rebellion.

Carole went on to inform me that when she and Bob were experiencing marital difficulties, they were more divided about parenting. She was the one in the children's camp, and Bob was in his own camp. Most clients eventually act out their family dynamics, often right in my office, and I soon had a chance to see the Steigerwalts in their battle mode.

As Carole talked about what used to happen, she and the two children began denouncing Bob for being verbally abusive. Bob shot back, "Talk about verbally abusive. What about the things that the kids say to me? They call me a 'bull-fucker' and choice statements like that."

"Who called you that?" I asked. "I did," said Janice, "Because he called me his fat little tomato."

Janice began to cry as Bob and Rollie started snickering in unison, and Carole threw up her hands and said, "See, this is the way it goes all the time. Bob always picks on Janice's weight, and that only makes things worse. It's really disgusting."

This continued nastiness among family members really shocked me. "Do you two permit this kind of language?" I asked, looking at both Carole and Bob. Embarrassed, Carole said, "Well, I think Bob set the precedent with his swearing in the house over the years. It's really terrible, but we all do it."

Rollie said, "Yeah, we talk like that to them because they talk like that to us."

It was at that point that I wondered whether these kids were following in their parents footsteps by forming an alliance, much in the way that Bob and Carole had done after their marital therapy. Their marital therapy had achieved some success. Bob and Carole were a bit more cohesive and seemed to work together, and this may have had a profound effect on Janice and Rollie's teaming up together. I suggested that the children's idea of how the family should operate may have come out of the chaotic atmosphere they had been exposed to until recently, and now they were both confused by the shift in their parents' behavior. They were unhappy about the loss of autonomy and power they once enjoyed.

Rollie went on to say that he used to regard his parents as friends rather than parents and that he missed having that type of relationship with them. Janice, however, still viewed her mother as somewhat of a friend, but saw her father as a "big pain" and a "jerk." And now, "Mom is starting to be the same way and I feel like we are losing her."

I certainly got a whiff of this family after 45 minutes and began to understand a little about how things had gone awry. I decided to ask how everyone felt about being in family therapy. The children had informed me in the beginning that they had never been in family therapy, that only Bob and Carole had sought marital therapy. "We're just here because we want to know how we can get out of this situation," said Rollie. "Well, you can't," I said, "unless you run away, and that's not acceptable."

I decided to take a risk by assuming an authoritative stance, just to see how everyone would react to it. Surprisingly, it wasn't rebuked. "Why do you need to get out if maybe we can work things out here?" "I don't know," said Rollie, "It just seems impossible and we're getting older and I just don't want to be here anymore." "Well, I understand that," I said, "but why don't we give this process a little bit of a chance? If I could help things improve a little for everyone in the relationship, would you decide to stick around?" Rollie was quiet, but shook his head affirmatively. I looked at Janice and she said, as she was tearing up, "I don't want to go anywhere, I want to be a family again, but not like this."

At that point, I looked at both Bob and Carole and said, "Well, look. You spent some time in marital therapy; you know it can be helpful. How do you feel about meeting as a family together for another visit?" Bob shrugged and said, "Sure, I mean it's not good the way it is." Carole said, "Hey, I'm all for it. I am very much supportive of therapies and I read a lot." I suggested that we meet a number of times to see if we could make some changes. I also assured the kids, "Certainly, file for divorce if things don't work out." They snickered as if they realized how ridiculous their initial request had been.

At that point, Bob asked, "So, who needs the help here?" I said, "Well, that's a good question, Bob, because actually the entire family needs help. There is no one individual person whom we target as the patient. We look at the family as a system, and the system is sort of broken right now, although I am sure it has a lot of good attributes. Right now, everyone seems to be unhappy with the way things are working, and we need to address the situation from a familial standpoint. So, we will all be meeting together every time, if that is OK with you." "I'm fine with that, I guess," Bob said, "as long we work it through our schedules."

I noticed out of the corner of my eye that the kids seemed to beam a little, which told me that maybe they were truly more motivated to work things out than they initially projected at the beginning of the session.

I also decided to give the family a homework assignment in this initial session for several reasons. First, I wanted to gather some additional information about the family dynamics and, second, I needed to see if they did their homework, which would also be a sign to me that they were truly motivated to move forward. I talked with them a little about the importance of family of origin and how it is essential that we look at our belief systems and some of the customs that we hand down transgenerationally. I also said that I was very much interested in learning about the types of households Mom and Dad were exposed to during their own upbringing.

With that, I asked the parents to complete the Family of Origin Scale (Hovestadt et al., 1985). The purpose of completing this scale was to measure some of the attributes that they each brought to the family from their respective families of origin. Part of the focus of this inventory centers on autonomy and intimacy as two key concepts in life, and how these form the perception of intimacy and family relationships. I was particularly interested in the aspect of autonomy and boundaries—how these two concepts were perceived in their own families of origin and how this translated into the mix that I witnessed before me in this initial session.

I also asked all family members to complete the Family Beliefs Inventory (FBI; Roehling & Robin, 1986). This inventory consists of two parallel forms, for parents and adolescents, and is designed to measure historic beliefs regarding relationship. The FBI for Parents (FBI-P) assesses six distorted beliefs, which include ruination, perfectionism, approval, obedience, self-blame, and malicious intent. The *FBI for Adolescents* (FBI-A) measures four beliefs, which include ruination, unfairness, autonomy, and approval.

Unfortunately, it was a couple of weeks before I got to see the family again because of father's travel schedule. In the meantime, I had everyone mail his or her completed inventory to me, which I had a chance to review. The responses that the mother and father had completed with the Family of Origin Scale on the issues of autonomy and intimacy were quite telling. Both Bob and Carole had experienced low levels of intimacy with their families of origin and portrayed their family members as keeping to themselves. There were also rather rigid boundaries in both families of origin, suggesting that there was little interaction. Both reported difficulties with conflict and very few signs of affection. They specifically portrayed family dynamics in which the father called the shots and everybody listened and did whatever he said. Carole, however, reported her father's being relatively absent from the home and her mother's being the inconsistent matriarch. Rules and regulations were often loose, although boundaries were tight so that no one really knew what was allowed or off-limits. It was easy to see how all of this had a trickle-down effect on their immediate family.

On the Family Beliefs Inventory, all family members had responded in a manner that suggested that perfectionism, approval, and obedience were rated very low. There was a clear indication of a loose family structure with poor cohesiveness, yet, interestingly, a desire for more cohesiveness did exist. It seemed that the family members were simply unclear on what constituted a salubrious and cohesive family dynamic.

The family was also administered the Family Awareness Scale (FAS; Green, Kolevzon, & Vosler, 1985). This scale is a 14-item instrument to measure family competence in areas of family structure, mythology (how the family views itself), goal-directed negotiation, autonomy of its members, and the nature of the family expression. All members viewed the family as being poor at problem solving and very unclear in regard to telling each other about their respective thoughts and feelings. There was also an indication that family members would not readily admit they were at fault and take responsibility for their own past or present behaviors and that there was an overall disengagement, with which everyone was uncomfortable.

What I would go on to piece together was that Bob and Carole maintained similar schemas about parenting and family life, which subsequently affected how they parented together. Basically, they failed to provide the appropriate balance between permissiveness and discipline. Earlier in the treatment, I had Bob and Carole complete the Family of Origin Scale (Hovestadt, Anderson, Piercy, Cochran, & Fine, 1985), which provided me with additional information about their upbringing. Figure 9.2 is an example of one of their joint schemas.

I had also gotten a signed Consent Form to Release Information from the parents and obtained their permission to contact their former marital therapist. Once I received permission, I had an opportunity to speak with the marital therapist, who informed me that she had experienced quite a bit of difficulty with Bob and Carole as a couple because of their problems with intimacy. It was her impression that they were both very insulated and protective of themselves. She also underscored for me the fact that Bob had significant problems with emotional regulation and often hid his emotions for fear of his own vulnerability.

Session 2

Although I originally had a specific agenda for the second session with this family, it was, unfortunately, thwarted by an incident that came up in the interim. I thought that it would be prudent to address this issue immediately inasmuch as it seemed to be at the heart of the matter with this family.

DATTILIO: Well, I'm glad to see that all of you agreed to return. Before we get started, I'm wondering what's happened in the past 2 weeks. Everyone seemed kind of tense when you came in this evening.

CAROLE: We had a terrible week. I think the tension in the family is at an all-time high. It's so depressing.

DATTILIO: Oh, really. What happened?

CAROLE: Well, it started with Bob being verbally abusive to all of us last Friday night and ...

BOB: (*interrupting abruptly*) Now wait a goddamn minute! Right off the fucking bat you're all over my case. I am responsible for the lousy week—it's *my* fault!

JANICE: Well, you started, Dad, with the stupid pizza.

DATTILIO: Hold it! What does "stupid pizza" have to do with it? Help me, I'm lost here. (*Kids begin to snicker.*)

BOB: Friday night I brought home pizza, like I usually do on weekends. I

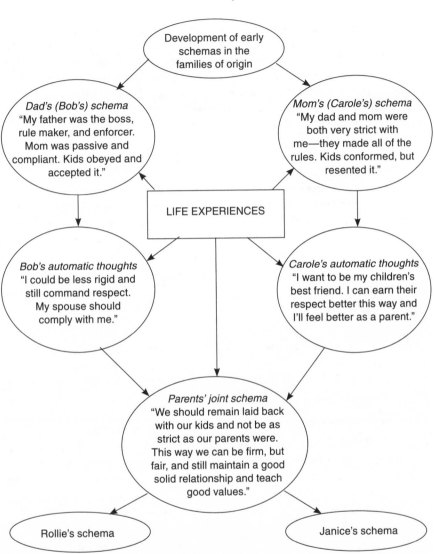

FIGURE 9.2. Family-of-origin schemas for Bob and Carole.

called Carole from the office and we agreed that neither of us felt like cooking, so I picked up a pizza.

DATTILIO: OK, sounds good to me.

BOB: Yeah, well, I come in the door, laid the pizza on the kitchen table, and went into the hallway to hang up my coat in the closet. Well, the three of them swoop down like vultures, each grabbing two pieces of pizza and scurry off to wherever. They leave two thin little pieces for me with hardly any cheese on them. So this really ticked me off. I lost my temper and called them all "a family of gluttons." I said that they were ingrates. And I guess a few other choice words ... I don't know. I don't remember.

CAROLE: Well, I remember! You called Rollie an asshole and Janice and I pigs. (*Rollie and Bob start snickering.*)

DATTILIO: OK. I get the picture. So let's get right into it and pick up where we left off last time. Dad, let's go back to Friday night when you brought the pizza home. Do you remember what you were feeling?

BOB: Uh, I don't know, I guess I was tired, hungry, just like everybody else.

DATTILIO: Anything else?

BOB: What do you mean?

DATTILIO: Well, "tired, hungry"—they're sort of vague terms. I'd like to know more about your mood and, more important, your thoughts surrounding your mood.

BOB: I don't know. I really can't say.

I really didn't want to push Bob too much, this early in the game, about his emotions because I suspected that he wasn't in touch with them. I decided to address things on a cognitive level and lead into the affective component later, particularly because of his guardedness.

DATTILIO: So you brought this pizza home and set it down on the kitchen table to share with everyone. First let me ask you, what did you anticipate would happen? What were your expectations?

BOB: Ah ... I don't know, I didn't think about it. I guess that everyone would just sort of sit down and we'd eat the pizza normally. You know, like you're supposed to. Like human beings do! (*Glares at Rollie and Janice.*)

DATTILIO: So, when everyone kind of just dove in, this had a major impact on you.

CAROLE: Well, wait a minute! Bob set the pizza down and yelled, "Pizza's here," and then went in to hang up his coat. He must have done something else because he didn't come right back to the kitchen immediately. The kids were watching a TV program and they ran in and grabbed their pizza—which they normally do—and took it and sat in front of the television to eat it.

DATTILIO: So, Bob, this violated your expectation of what you thought should be?

BOB: Yeah, I guess so.

DATTILIO: All right, and that no doubt aggravated you to some degree?

BOB: Yes. Then when I came in and saw the two slices of pizza with hardly any cheese left on them, I flipped.

DATTILIO: All right, stop right there! What thoughts went through your mind at that moment?

BOB: (*Stops and thinks for a minute.*) Ah, I don't know. I don't remember.

DATTILIO: Let's try this—close your eyes for a minute and try to visually recall yourself back in that situation.

ROLLIE: No, don't tell him to do that, he'll fall asleep. (*Everyone laughs.*)

DATTILIO: Bob, close your eyes and try to imagine this scene. Let me know when you have an image in your head.

BOB: OK—I'm there (*grinning with his eyes closed*).

DATTILIO: Good. Now think about what you were wearing, where you were standing, and the surrounding atmosphere—the smells, and so forth.

BOB: Yes—OK.

DATTILIO: Can you remember what your thoughts were upon seeing those two measly, pathetic pieces of pizza lying in the box—just staring at you?

BOB: Yeah. I thought, "What gluttons—this is just typical."

DATTILIO: What's typical?

BOB: You know, this selfishness, this disregard for me. I bring the damn pizza home and no one sits with me. They aren't even considerate enough to see that I get a decent piece of pizza. They just don't care.

DATTILIO: So what is the schema attached to this?

BOB: I'm not sure what you mean.

DATTILIO: Well, your automatic thought is, "They aren't considerate of me." That means what?

BOB: Well, that means that they don't care. They're just using me. I'm just a meal ticket.

CAROLE: Aw, come on, Bob!

DATTILIO: No, wait, Carole. Let him finish!

BOB: That's all I am. They don't give a shit about me.

DATTILIO: So your schema, or core belief, is that no one in the family really cares about you, and your worth to them is symbolized by the lean pieces of pizza that they left for you, after you went through all the trouble to pick it up, pay for it, and so forth—correct?

BOB: Yep, that's it in a nutshell.

DATTILIO: All right now, here's the important question, What evidence, other than the pizza incident, do you have that truly substantiates the blanket statement "They don't give a shit about me. I am just a meal ticket"?

BOB: Uh, well, lots of evidence. I mean, this is just one day in the life of Robert Steigerwalt. My family's been treating me like this for years. I get kicked around at work, almost in the same fashion. Sometimes, I just feel like a piece of shit.

DATTILIO: Tell me about the family's behavior in the past. What other events have occurred like this?

BOB: I don't know, there have been times.

DATTILIO: A lot? Enough to substantiate such a strong statement?

BOB: Uh, well, no, not a lot, but it's happened.

DATTILIO: So, you don't have a lot of evidence, just a few incidences.

BOB: Yeah, maybe one other time.

DATTILIO: So, could there possibly be some cognitive distortions at work here?

BOB: Well, yeah, maybe, but still, I don't think that it was unreasonable to be irritated by this. It was very selfish of them.

DATTILIO: No, I am not disputing that issue with you. I am sure that you were looking forward to cheese on your pizza too; so, to end up with two slices of "sauce-covered bread" is a big letdown, I'm sure—especially when you're hungry (*kids begin to snicker*). But to say that this equates to their not caring at all—I just don't see where this is an accurate assumption.

BOB: Well, I guess not, but it's frustrating.

DATTILIO: Sure, but the emotion attached to what you tell yourself about your value and worth makes a significant difference in how you react emotionally and behaviorally. You can see this clearly if we plot it out on the Dysfunction Thought Record. Let's map it out.

I began to write this out on a chalkboard so that the entire family could see an example of it:

SITUATION	AUTOMATIC THOUGHTS	EMOTION(S)	COGNITIVE DISTORTION
Everyone helps him- or herself to the best pieces of pizza, leaving the lean pieces for Dad.	They just don't give a shit about me! I am just a meal ticket.	Agitated/angry, devalued	1. Arbitrary inference 2. Maximization 3. Dichotomous thinking

DATTILIO: All right. So, when we break it down like this, it is easy to see the distortions that are occurring and how the statements that you are making to yourself are erroneously based.

BOB: Yeah. I guess I can see that.

DATTILIO: So the emotions and behavior that follow are what set the stage for your reactions and what this evokes in the other members of the family.

BOB: So I am the one who is wrong.

DATTILIO: No, not entirely. I've just taken the opportunity to highlight this situation to use as an example for the family because it has come up today. Let's look at the thoughts that occurred with everyone else. Carole, what happened when Bob reacted the way he did?

CAROLE: Well, I thought that he clearly jumped the gun. I mean, I would have been angry also, but he could have said to the rest of us, "Come on, guys, how about leaving me some pieces with more cheese on them?" I mean, they were still left. The kids hadn't eaten them all yet. They could have put some of them back. We also could have just ordered another pizza. The place is only about 5 minutes away from our house.

DATTILIO: But how did this affect the rest of you?

ROLLIE: Well, I wasn't even sure what happened, and the next thing you know, Dad's yelling and he's calling me an ungrateful asshole. So I got mad.

DATTILIO: Janice? What about you?

JANICE: I don't know. I just kept eating my pizza. (*Everyone laughs.*)

DATTILIO: But something must have gone through your mind.

JANICE: Well, I thought, "Here he goes again. He's always making everyone miserable."

DATTILIO: So it caused a lot of disruption. If Dad had come to you with a little less fury and said that he wanted his share of the decent slices of pizza, how would you have responded?

ROLLIE: No problem—I would have given him the other piece. I don't want to be unfair.

DATTILIO: So it wasn't your deliberate intention to cheat your father or leave him with the scraps—you're not really gluttons, are you?

ROLLIE and JANICE: (*laughing*) No, it's just that he's slower than we are and we were starving.

DATTILIO: So that's it, "every man for himself"?

ROLLIE: No, we don't share most of the time.

DATTILIO: All right, but can you understand how your father felt?

ROLLIE and JANICE: Yeah, I guess. I mean, we all sort of "dis" each other in our family a lot. It's not good.

DATTILIO: And Dad, you are aware now that the conclusion you arrived at was a bit exaggerated?

BOB: Yeah, I exaggerated, I guess.

DATTILIO: Mom, what are you thinking—you're awfully quiet.

CAROLE: Well, I am just thinking about how typical this is of our family. I mean this stuff just goes on all the time and I think that you have made a very good point here tonight. We jump the gun a lot with our thinking—sometimes to the point that it really gets us all in serious trouble.

DATTILIO: Well, yes. I can see that. But I also think that there's something else going on here with your emotions. You really don't seem to express emotions evenly until there is some sort of a crisis or upheaval and then they come out in a highly charged way.

As can be seen in this scenario, I encouraged all members of the family to begin to think about the dynamics that were occurring with their thought processes and how easily they can distort things. More important, I opened the door for them to begin to make a connection between their thoughts and how they were linked to their emotions—and how this specifically led to conflicts in their relationships with one another.

This family also had problems with emotional expression, particularly intimacy. Much of this difficulty stemmed from the parents and their families of origin and had no doubt trickled down to influence how this family functioned on an emotional, cognitive, and behavioral level.

I deliberately chose the father to use as a role model because I believed that, in many ways, he set the main tone for the family. This strategy was certainly not meant to pick on him, but it presented itself as an available inroad to start addressing an important problem with this family. The mother, who had a special strength and control of her own, watched quietly as I made these maneuvers with her husband. My thought was that the restructuring process might have had less of an impact had I chosen her as a role model. Moreover, I wanted to silently disarm her power by shifting the focus away from her and onto the father. This would be less threatening to this family at this point in treatment than to do the reverse, because it was still early in the therapy process.

DATTILIO: So, what about the rest of the family? Do you all recognize how you may have had similar experiences—when your own automatic thoughts affected how you responded emotionally to situations that came up with your family?

ROLLIE: Well, yeah, I do—but sometimes I just get so upset about things, I can't stop and think straight. I mean, for me to slow things down is real hard. Also, I don't see why I have to do this if no one else does.

DATTILIO: Well, that's sort of the point, Rollie. You see, everyone will need to begin to examine the way he or she thinks things through and learn to challenge thoughts and distortions that cause conflict. One of the ways we can begin to do this is by asking ourselves the following questions when we catch ourselves engaging in distorted thinking. We call this "questioning your interpretations."

It was at this juncture in treatment that I began to orient the family to the model of therapy. This was the educational component that set the tone for how we would proceed in future sessions. I listed the questions I wanted them to use in understanding their thought content:

1. "What is the evidence in favor of my interpretation?"
2. "What evidence is there contrary to my interpretation?"
3. "Does it logically follow from my family member's actions that he [or she] has the motive that I assign to him [or her]?"
4. "Is there an alternative explanation for his [or her] behavior?"

I told them to take an example in which one of the members of the family spoke harshly or in some other way that upset or annoyed them and to ask themselves these questions:

1. "Does it follow that because he [or she] spoke sharply that he or she was angry at me?"
2. "Are there alternative explanations for his [or her] tone of voice? For example, he [or she] could have a cold or be strained or bothered by something else."
3. "Even if he [or she] is angry, does it follow that:
   • He [or she] doesn't care about me or is devaluing me in some way?
   • Or that he [or she] is always this way?
   • Does it necessarily mean that he [or she] will make life miserable for me?
   • That I have done something wrong?"

DATTILIO: (*to the entire family*) Do you see how this might be helpful?

CAROLE: Yes, I do, now we just need to learn how to slow things down in our family and remember to do this without being so emotional.

DATTILIO: Well, yes. That's the tough part. But I also don't want to downplay emotions, because they are a vital part of therapy. We certainly need to learn how to regulate them better. I think we can do that by first examining some of our thought content and better understanding how it affects our emotion and behavior. Families are interesting but complicated systems that operate on principles or assumptions. These assumptions can significantly affect our emotions and behaviors.

I then went on to explain to the Steigerwalts in a simplified fashion some of the assumptions that were posited by Schwebel and Fine (1994).

• *Assumption 1*: All members of a family seek to maintain their environment in order to fulfill their needs and wants. They attempt to understand their environment and how they can function most effectively in it, even if it sometimes means testing the boundaries (e.g., Rollie may exceed his curfew by a half hour). As family members gather data about how the family operates, they use this information to guide their behaviors and to aid in building and refining family-related cognitions. This leads to the development of an individual's construct of family life and family relationships. So, in Rollie's case, he may begin to develop the concept that he can stretch the limits and not be chastised, thus inferring that rules may be broken with little consequence.

• *Assumption 2*: Individual members' cognitions affect virtually every aspect of family life. Five categories are identified as cognitive variables that determine these cognitions: (1) selective attention (Bob and Carole's focus on the children's negative behaviors), (2) attributions (Bob's explanations for why the children act up), (3) expectations (Bob's expectation that Carole and the children will do as he asks without question), (4) assumptions (Janice's view that life is not fair), and (5) standards (Rollie's thoughts about how the world should be).

• *Assumption 3*: Certain "obstacles" to satisfaction lie within individual family members' cognitions (for example, Carole's belief that she needs to be her children's best friend).

• *Assumption 4*: Unless family members become more aware of their family-related cognitions and how these cognitions affect them in certain situations, they will not be able to identify areas that cause distress and replace them with healthy interaction.

These assumptions are usually unspoken within a family structure and simply exist and are maintained on an unconscious level. In a sense, they occur automatically and often form the rules by which a family operates.

ROLLIE: But it seems as though our rules or assumptions are all screwed up. I mean, that's what gets us crazy about the family, that half the time we don't know what's what. The rules are always changing.

DATTILIO: I am not clear on what you are saying, Rollie—could you be more specific?

JANICE: (*interrupting*) I think that what he is trying to say is that my parents shift things around a lot. They confuse us. They do what they think is right at the time.

DATTILIO: OK, but, Janice, let Rollie speak for himself. I think it's important that he say it himself.

CAROLE: All right, I'll buy that, I think that's fair to say. But you guys (*pointing to Rollie and Janice*) then take it and run with it and manipulate the hell out of your father and me.

JANICE: Well, yeah, we're kids, what do you expect?

DATTILIO: You know, it just struck me that perhaps Rollie and Janice are waiting for you and Bob to come down on them more firmly, but until you do, they act out or give you a hard time.

CAROLE: But that's what they are complaining about, that we're too hard on them or, in Rollie's words, "give them crap." It's like we are damned if we do and damned if we don't.

DATTILIO: No, that's not what I'm hearing. You (*to Rollie and Janice*) can correct me if I'm wrong, but what I am hearing is that it's the inconsistency that you are reacting to. In fact, I believe that this has been the issue all along.

BOB: You mean the inconsistency?

DATTILIO: Sure. My guess is that they feel as though they are in somewhat of a double bind, and it's confusing and disruptive to them.

CAROLE: Well—again, I think that I am the one who is guilty of that, because I would flip-flop so much. I usually struggle with playing the role of the tough guy and also trying to be their best friend at the same time.

DATTILIO: And it's my impression that Bob would react to that by assuming a more rigid posture, thus polarizing the two of you. When this occurs, it gives the kids a lot of room to do what they want, causing conflict in the family.

CAROLE: God, what a mess. Do you think that you can help us straighten all of this out?

DATTILIO: I am sure going to try—as long as everybody gives me his or her best effort.

At this point I reaffirmed the family's commitment to working with me in treatment. This was very important, because the volatility and vying for power among these family members was such that the cohesion could quickly deteriorate, depending on what I did.

In the subsequent five visits, the most of my focus centered on addressing family schemas about rules and regulations and, more important, how family members truly felt about one another. I also made connections for the parents in regard to how their own experiences from their families of origin had affected how they thought and emoted and handled situations, such as boundaries, consistency, and so forth.

The following is an excerpt from the sixth session:

DATTILIO: Janice, a moment ago you mentioned something about your parents' not really being concerned about what you are going through right now. I'd like to hear more about your thoughts.

JANICE: Well, I am sick of my parents getting on me about my weight. I know I am overweight and I can't help it. And they talk to me like it's so easy to just stop eating and lose weight.

DATTILIO: This sounds like a really emotional issue for you.

JANICE: (*Begins crying.*) It is. I feel so rejected.

DATTILIO: What are the specific thoughts that go through your mind when you hear another family member make a remark about your weight?

JANICE: I feel hurt and frustrated.

DATTILIO: OK, that's what you feel, but what about the thought that precedes your feelings?

JANICE: (*Takes a moment to think.*) Well, that they don't care about how it might hurt me. That they are not thinking that I can't help it.

DATTILIO: Good! Now how do you think that this affects how you react to them, how you behave?

JANICE: Well, for one, it makes me want to eat more.

CAROLE: Ah, that's interesting, I never knew that.

DATTILIO: You mean you actually experience anger and engage in overeating?

JANICE: Yes. All the time.

DATTILIO: It also sounds retaliatory. As though you then try to get back at them for being insensitive to you.

JANICE: Right.

DATTILIO: It's sort of like insulation, your eating.

BOB: Yeah, literally! (*Rollie and Bob snicker. Janice begins to cry.*)

CAROLE: Ah, you see, Bob? That's what I mean. It's wisecracks like that, that are really destructive.

BOB: All right, I'm sorry (*still snickering*). I just couldn't help myself.

DATTILIO: I can't help but notice that laughing seems to serve a very special purpose in this family.

CAROLE: How is that?

DATTILIO: Well, every time someone expresses his or her feelings or really shows any vulnerability, family members either lash out or laugh and make fun of it. What do you think that means?

ROLLIE: We're screwed up?

DATTILIO: Well, but something more than that. It's almost as though you have trouble handling intimacy. You, as a family, almost avoid it, either by arguing or making fun of each other.

CAROLE: Oh, I couldn't agree more.

DATTILIO: What could we say about the family schema regarding intimacy and expressing our emotions? What form does intimacy take in your family?

BOB: Well, it kind of is expressed in jest. Like when I call Janice my fat little tomato queen. I really mean it affectionately.

DATTILIO: Yes, but the word "fat" is hardly a term of endearment. How is that affectionate?

BOB: Well, that word isn't.

DATTILIO: So, what does it mean that you throw that word in there?

BOB: Anger, I guess.

DATTILIO: Anger about what?

BOB: That she's overweight at this young stage of her life. It shouldn't be.

DATTILIO: So why can't this just be said to each other as opposed to being disguised in a joke or negative statement?

BOB: I don't know. That's a really good question. I guess it's just a really sensitive issue.

DATTILIO: Well, I think it's a sensitive issue and also one that I think you have difficulty talking about. That is, if what Janice really needed is for you to comfort her, I think you have difficulty doing that.

BOB: Well, it's true, I don't do that well. That's part of my wife's complaint, although we've gotten better at that and maybe—I guess—we just have to work on that with therapy. This is just something I feel awkward expressing and—you know—I've never been comfortable with expressing my feelings. The way I grew up, we didn't show affection, and it's just kind of awkward for me.

DATTILIO: Well, I think part of what we can focus on in therapy is how to express this nurturance to each other in a way that will help each of you grow. That is, you can grow by learning how to express yourself in a more productive fashion, and certainly Janice and the rest of the family members will grow and benefit from your expressing your love in a different way.

BOB: I never intended for them to misunderstand my love for them. They are the apples of my eye.

For the first time, I saw Bob start to tear up, which then unleashed a cascade of crying by both children and a welling up in Carole's eyes. It was really amazing to see this trigger point and how it really unleashed a lot of emotions that I suspected were harbored beneath all of this anger, jest, and ridicule.

I decided that this was enough for this session, and I told the family members that I would look forward to meeting them again.

The subsequent session, interestingly, yielded a lot more calm and respectful interaction between family members in the 10 days since I had last seen them. Most of my work with this family went on to focus on the restructuring of its members' individual and family schemas about mutual respect, boundaries, display of affect, and emotional regulation, as well as learning new methods for exchange of intimacy. This, obviously, took some time and a lot of hard work. I went on to meet this family for another 15–20 sessions over the course of a year. I was surprised that its members really hung in there and made some great strides. One of the consistent distortions among these family members was the idea that expressing emotions related to their fear of exposing their individual vulnerabilities to each another. Once this issue was successfully addressed, they all appeared to be able to make headway in displaying more productive expression between each other.

Therapy eventually ended on a positive note, with family members reporting improvement in their relationships and a major reduction in arguing and bickering. The greatest delight of all was, of course, that Rollie and Janice decided not to file for divorce.

10

Epilogue

The scientific and clinical literature in CBT has burgeoned, and it is too broad to capture within the confines of this text. I have made a real attempt to include what I feel is the most salient information, as well as some direction to obtain additional resources on specific topics. Likewise, the field of family therapy is constantly expanding, and readers should continue to update their knowledge by reading whatever they can in order to strengthen their skills.

Keep in mind that CBT is an integrative modality that can be used with other approaches to couple and family therapy. Therefore, practitioners of various modalities may find the techniques and strategies in this book helpful, even as adjuncts to their existing approaches.[1]

I tried to convey throughout this text that therapists need to remain flexible in their work with couples and families, yet, at the same time, to add as many techniques to their therapeutic toolbox as they can. Continuing to be knowledgeable about a range of interventions is a key ingredient in doing good work.

Finally, I want to make clear that there are many ways to employ CBT techniques with couples and families. Practitioners need to blend their own unique styles of treatment with the techniques and strategies that are evidence based in order to achieve the most effective results with their clients.

---

[1]This is illustrated very clearly in *Case Studies in Couple and Family Therapy: Systemic and Cognitive Perspectives* (Dattilio, 1998a), in which CBT is nicely integrated with a number of therapeutic modalities.

In my opinion, this is the heart and soul of doing good therapy and is what affords clinicians the freedom to do what they do best in order to help couples and families in need.

Given CBT's fine track record in the past half-century, I am hopeful that it will continue to remain an efficacious approach to the future needs of couples and families throughout the world.

Appendix A

Questionnaires and Inventories for Couples and Families

Questionnaires and Inventories for Couples

- Communication Patterns Questionnaire (CPQ; Christensen, 1988)
- Dyadic Adjustment Scale (DAS; Spanier, 1976)
- Marital Attitude Questionnaire—Revised (Pretzer, Epstein, & Fleming, 1991)
- Marital Communication Inventory (Bienvenu, 1970)
- Marital Happiness Scale (MHS; Azrin, Master, & Jones, 1973)
- Marital Satisfaction Inventory (MSI; Snyder, 1981)
- Primary Communication Inventory (Navaran, 1967)

Questionnaires and Inventories for Families

- Adolescent–Family Inventory of Life Events and Change (McCubbin & Thompson, 1991)
- The Revised Conflict Tactics Scales (CTS-2; Straus, Hamby, Bonley-McCoy, & Sugarman, 1996)
- Family Adaptability and Cohesion Evaluation Scale (FACES-III; Olson, Portner, & Lavee, 1985)
- Family Assessment Device (FAD; Epstein, Baldwin, & Bishop, 1983)
- Family Awareness Scale (FAS; Green, Kolevzon, & Vosler, 1985)
- Family Beliefs Inventory (FBI [forms P & A]; Roehling & Robin, 1986)
- Family Coping Inventory (FCI; McCubbin & Thompson, 1991)
- Family Functioning Scale (FFS; Tavitian, Lubiner, Green, Grebstein, & Velicer, 1987)
- Family of Origin Scale (FOS; Hovestadt, Anderson, Piercy, Cochran, & Fine, 1985)

- Family Sense of Coherence (FSOC) and Family Adaptation Scales (FAS; Antonovsky & Sourani, 1988)
- Kansas Family Life Satisfaction Scale (KFLS; Schumm, Jurich, & Bollman, 1986)
- Parent–Child Relationship Survey (PCRS; Fine & Schewebel, 1983)
- Self-Report Family Instrument (SFI; Beavers, Hampson, & Hulgus, 1985)

Appendix B

Dysfunctional Thought Record

Directions: When you notice your mood getting worse, ask yourself, "What's going through my mind right now?" and as soon as possible jot down the thought or mental image in the automatic thoughts column.

Date Time	Situation	Automatic Thoughts	Emotions(s)	Distortion	Alternative Response	Outcome
	Describe: 1. Actual event leading to unpleasant emotion, or 2. Stream of thoughts, daydreams, or recollection, leading to an unpleasant emotion, or 3. Distressing physical sensations.	1. Write automatic thought(s) that preceded emotions(s). 2. Rate belief in automatic thought(s) 0–100%.	Describe: 1. Specify sad, anxious/ angry, etc. 2. Rate degree of emotion 0–100%.	1. All-or-nothing thinking 2. Overgeneralization 3. Mental filter 4. Disqualifying the positive 5. Jumping to conclusions 6. Magnification or minimization 7. Emotional reasoning 8. Should statements 9. Labeling and mislabeling 10. Personalization	1. Write a rational response to automatic thought(s). 2. Rate belief in alternative response 0–100%.	1. Rerate belief in automatic thought(s) 0–100%. 2. Specify and rate subsequent emotions 0–100%.

Questions to help formulate the ALTERNATIVE RESPONSE: (1) What is the evidence that the automatic thought is true? Not true? (2) Is there an alternative explanation? (3) What's the *worst* that could happen? Could I live through it? What's the *best* that could happen? What's the *most realistic* outcome? (4) What should I do about it? (5) What's the effect of my believing the automatic thought? What could be the effect of changing my thinking? (6) If _____ (person's name) _____ was in this situation and had this thought, what would I tell him/her?

References

Abrahms, J., & Spring, M. (1989). The flip flop factor. *International Cognitive Therapy Newsletter, 5*(1), 7–8.

Abrams, S., & Spring, J. (1996). *After the affair: Healing the pain and rebuilding trust when a partner has been unfaithful.* New York: Harper Collins.

Abrams, S., & Spring, J. (2004). *How can I forgive you?* New York: Harper Collins.

Ainsworth, M. D. S. (1967). *Infancy in Uganda: Infant care and the growth of attachment.* Baltimore: Johns Hopkins University Press.

Ainsworth, M. D. S., Blehar, M. C., Waters, E., & Wall, S. (1978). *Patterns of attachment: A psychological study of the strange situation.* Hillsdale, NJ: Erlbaum.

Alberti, R. & Emmons, M. (2001). *Your perfect right.* Atascadero, CA: Impact.

Albrecht, S. L., Bahr, H. M., & Goodman, K. L. (1983). *Divorce and remarriage: Problems, adaptations and adjustments.* Westport, CT: Greenwood Press.

Alexander, J. F., & Parsons, B. V. (1982). *Functional family therapy.* Monterey, CA: Brooks/Cole.

Alexander, P. C. (1988). The therapeutic implications of family cognitions and constructs. *Journal of Cognitive Psychotherapy 2,* 219–236.

Alford, B. A., & Beck, A. T. (1997). *The integrative power of cognitive therapy.* New York: Guilford Press.

American Psychological Association. (1985). *A selected bibliography of lesbian and gay concerns in psychology: An affirmative perspective.* Washington, DC: Author.

Antonovsky, A., & Sourani, T. (1988). Family sense of coherence and family adaptation. *Journal of Marriage and Family, 50,* 79–92.

Aron, A., Fisher, H., Mashek, D. J., Strong, G., Li, H., & Brown, L. L. (2005). Reward, motivation, and emotion systems associated with early-stage intense romantic love. *Journal of Neurophysiology, 94,* 327–337.

Ascher, L. M. (1980). Paradoxical intention. In A. Goldstein & E. B. Foa (Eds.),

Handbook of behavioral interventions: A clinical guide (pp. 129–148). New York: Wiley.

Ascher, L. M. (Ed.). (1984). *Therapeutic paradox*. New York: Guilford Press.

Atkinson, B. J. (2005). *Emotional intelligence in couples therapy: Advances from neurobiology and the science of intimate relationships*. New York: Norton.

Azerin, N. H., Naster, B. J., & Jones, R. (1973). A rapid learning-based procedure for marital counseling. *Behavior Research and Therapy, 11*, 365–382.

Baldwin, M. W. (1992). Relational schemas and the processing of social information. *Psychological Bulletin, 112*, 461–484.

Barnes, S., Brown, K. W., Krusemark, E., Campbell, W. K., & Rogge, R. D. (2007). The role of mindfulness in romantic relationship satisfaction and responses to relationship stress. *Journal of Marital and Family Therapy, 33*(4), 482–500.

Bartholomew, K., & Horowitz, L. M. (1991). Attachment styles among young adults: A test of the four category model. *Journal of Personality and Social Psychology, 61*, 276–244.

Barton, C., & Alexander, J. F. (1981). Functional family therapy. In A. S. Gurman & D. P. Kniskern (Eds.), *Handbook of family therapy* (pp. 403–443). New York: Brunner/Mazel.

Bateson, G., Daveson, D. D., Haley, J., & Weakland. J. (1956). Toward a theory of schizophrenia. *Behavior Sciences, 2*, 251–264.

Baucom, D. H. (1987). Attributions in distressed relations: How can we explain them? In S. Duck & D. Perlman (Eds.), *Heterosexual relations, marriage and divorce* (pp. 177–206). London: Sage.

Baucom, D. H., & Epstein. N. (1990). *Cognitive-behavior marital therapy*. New York: Brunner/Mazel.

Baucom, D. H., Epstein, B. B., Daiuto, A. D., Carels, R. A., Rankin, L., & Burnett, K. (1996). Cognitions in marriage: The relationship between standards and attributions. *Journal of Family Psychology, 10*, 209–222.

Baucom, D. H.. Epstein, N., Rankin, L.A., & Burnett, C. K. (1996b). Assessing relationship standards: The Inventory of Specific Relationship Standards. *Journal of Family Psychology, 10*, 72–88.

Baucom, D. H., Epstein, N., Sayers, S., & Sher, T. G. (1989). The role of cognitions in marital relationships: Definitional, methodological, and conceptual issues. *Journal of Consulting and Clinical Psychology, 57*, 3–38.

Baucom, D. H., Shoham, V., Mueser, K. T., Daiuto, A. D., & Stickle, T. R. (1998). Empirically supported couples and family therapies for adult problems. *Journal of Consulting and Clinical Psychology, 66*, 53–88.

Bavelas, J. B., Coates, L., & Johnson, T. (2000). Listeners as co-narrators. *Journal of Personality and Social Psychology, 79*, 941–952.

Bavelas, J. B., Coates, L., & Johnson, T. (2002). Listener responses as a collaborative process: The role of gaze. *Journal of Communication, 52*, 566–580.

Beach, S. R. H. (2001). *Marital and family process in depression: A scientific process for clinical practice*. Washington, DC: American Psychological Association.

Beavers, W. R., Hampson, R. B., & Hulgus, Y. F. (1985). The Beavers systems approach to family assessment. *Family Process, 24*, 398–405.

Beck, A. T. (1967). *Depression: Clinical, experimental and theoretical aspects*. New York: Hoeber.

Beck, A. T. (1976). *Cognitive therapy and the emotional disorders*. New York: International Universities Press.

Beck, A. T. (1988). *Love is never enough*. New York: Harper & Row.

Beck, A. T. (2002). Cognitive models of depression. In R. L. Leahy & T. E. Dowd (Eds.), *Clinical advances in cognitive psychotherapy: Theory and application* (pp. 29–61). New York: Springer.

Beck, A. T., Rush, A. J., Shaw, B. F., & Emery, G. (1979). *Cognitive therapy of depression*. New York: Guilford Press.

Beck, A., Wright, F., Newman, C., & Leise, B. (1993). *Cognitive therapy of substance abuse*. New York: Guilford Press.

Beck, J. S. (1995). *Cognitive therapy: Basics and beyond*. New York: Guilford Press.

Becvar, D. S., & Becvar, R. J. (2009). *Family therapy: A systemic integration* (7th ed.). Boston: Allyn & Bacon.

Bedrosian, R. C. (1983). Cognitive therapy in the family system. In A. Freeman (Ed.), *Cognitive therapy with couples and groups* (pp. 95–106). New York: Plenum Press.

Bennun, I. (1985). Prediction and responsiveness in behavioral marital therapy. *Behavioral Psychotherapy, 13*, 186–201.

Bevilacqua, L. J., & Dattilio, F. M. (2001). *Brief family therapy homework planner*. New York: John Wiley.

Bienvenu, M. J. (1970). Measurements of marital communication. *The Family Coordinator, 19*, 26–31.

Birchler, G. R. (1983). Behavioral-systems marital therapy. In J. P. Vincent (Ed.), *Advances in family intervention, assessment and theory* (Vol. 3, pp. 1–40). Greenwich, CT: JAI Press.

Birchler, G. R., & Spinks, S. H. (1980). Behavioral-systems marital and family therapy: Integration and clinical application. *American Journal of Family Therapy, 8*, 6–28.

Bishop, S. R., Lau, M., Shapiro, S., Carlson, L., Anderson, N., & Carmody, J. (2004). Mindfulness: A proposed operational definition. *Clinical Psychology: Science and Practice, 11*, 230–242.

Bitter, J. M. (2009). *Theory and practice of family therapy and counseling*. Belmont, CA: Brooks/Cole.

Bless, H., Hamilton, D. L., & Mackie, D. M. (1992). Mood on the organization of personal information. *European Journal of Social Psychology, 22*, 497–509.

Bless, H., Mackie, D. M., & Schwartz, Z. (1992). Mood effects on attitude judgments: Interdependent effects of mood before and after message elaboration. *Journal of Personality and Social Psychology, 63*, 585–595.

Bornstein, P. H., Krueger, H. K., & Cogswell, K. (1989). Principles and techniques of couple paradoxical therapy. In L. M. Ascher (Ed.), *Therapeutic paradox* (pp. 289–309). New York: Guilford Press.

Bowen, M. (1978). *Family therapy in clinical practice*. New York: Jason Aronson.

Bowlby, J. (1969). *Attachment and loss: Vol. 1. Attachment*. New York: Basic Books.

Bowlby, J. (1973). *Attachment and loss: Vol. 2. Separation, anxiety, and anger*. New York: Basic Books.

Bowlby, J. (1979). *The making and breaking of affectional bonds.* London: Tavistock.

Bowlby, J. (1982). *Attachment and loss: Vol. 1. Attachment* (2nd ed.). New York: Basic Books. (Original work published 1969)

Bradbury, T. N., & Fincham, F. D. (1990). Attributions in marriage: Review and critique. *Psychological Bulletin, 107,* 3–33.

Bramlett, M. D., & Mosher, W. D. (2002). Cohabitation, marriage, divorce and remarriage in the United States. *Vital Health Statistics, 23*(22). Hyattsville, MD: National Center for Health Statistics.

Brizendine, L. (2006). *The female brain.* New York: Broadway Books.

Brown, G. W., & Harris, T. (1978). *Social origins of depression: A psychiatric disorder in women.* London: Tavistock.

Bryant, M. J., Simons, A. D., & Thase, M. E. (1999). Therapist skill and patient variables in homework compliance: Controlling the uncontrolled variable in cognitive therapy outcome research. *Cognitive Therapy and Research, 23,* 381–399.

Cahill, L. (2003). Sex-related influences on the neurobiology of the emotionally influenced memory. *Annals of the New York Academy of Sciences, 985,* 168–173.

Carrere, S., & Gottman, J. M. (1999). Predicting divorce among newly weds from the first three minutes of marital conflict discussion. *Family Process, 38,* 293–301.

Carson, J. W., Carson, K. M., Gil, K. M., & Baucom, D. H. (2004). Mindfulness-based relationship enhancement. *Behavior Therapy, 35,* 471–494.

Cassidy, J., & Shaver, P. S. (Eds.). (1999). *Handbook of attachment: Theory, research and clinical applications.* New York: Guilford Press.

Chae, P. K., & Kwon, J. H. (2006). *The psychology of happy marriage.* Seoul: Jibmoon-Dang.

Choi, S. C. (1998). The third-person psychology and the first-person psychology: The perspectives on human relations. *Korean Social Science Journal, 25,* 239–264.

Christensen, A. (1988). Dysfunctional interaction patterns in couples. In P. Noller & M. A. Fitzpatrick (Eds.), *Perspectives on marital interaction* (pp. 31–52). Clevedon, UK: Multilingual Matters.

Christensen, A., & Heavey, C. L. (1999). Interventions for couples. *Annual Review of Psychology, 50*(1), 165–190.

Christensen, A., Sevier, M., Simpson, L. E., & Gattis, K. S. (2004). Acceptance, mindfulness and change in couple therapy. In S. C. Hayes, V. M. Follette, & M. M. Linehan (Eds.), *Mindfulness and acceptance: Expanding the cognitive-behavioral tradition.* New York: Guilford Press.

Cierpka, M. (2005). Introduction to family assessment. In M. Cierpka, V. Thomas, & D. H. Sprenkle (Eds.), *Family assessment: Integrating multiple clinical perspectives.* Cambridge, MA: Hogrefe.

Clayton, D. C., & Baucom, D. H. (1998, November). *Relationship standards as mediators of marital equality.* Paper presented at the Annual Meeting of the Association for the Advancement of Behavior Therapy, Washington, DC.

Cook, J., Tyson, R., White, J., Rushe, R., Gottman, J. M., & Murray, J. (1995). The mathematics of marital conflict: Qualitative dynamic mathematical modeling of marital attraction. *Journal of Family Psychology, 9,* 110–130.

Coontz, S. (2005). *Marriage: A history from obedience to intimacy or how love conquered marriage.* New York: Viking Press.

Coyne, J. C., & Benazon, N. R. (2001). Not agent blue: Effects of marital functioning on depression and implications for treatment. In S. R. H. Beach (Ed.), *Marital and family processes in depression: A scientific foundation for clinical practice* (pp. 25–43). Washington, DC: American Psychological Association.

Crespi, T. D., & Howe, E. A. (2001). Facing the family treatment crisis: Changing parameters in marriage and family and marriage therapy education. *Family Therapy, 28*(1), 31–38.

Damasio, A. R. (1999). *The feeling of what happens: Body and emotion in the making of consciousness.* New York: Harcourt, Brace.

Damasio, A. R. (2001). Emotion and the human brain. *Annals of the New York Academy of Sciences, 935*(1), 101–106.

Dattilio, F. M. (1983, Winter). The use of operant techniques and parental control in the treatment of pediatric headache complaints: Case report. *Pennsylvania Journal of Counseling, 1*(2), 55–58.

Dattilio, F. M. (1987). The use of paradoxical intention in the treatment of panic disorder. *Journal of Counseling and Development, 66*(2), 66–67.

Dattilio, F. M. (1989). A guide to cognitive marital therapy. In P. A. Keller & S. F. Heyman (Eds.), *Innovations in clinical practice: A source book* (Vol. 8. pp. 27–42). Sarasota, FL: Professional Resource Exchange.

Dattilio, F. M. (1993). Cognitive techniques with couples and families. *Family Journal, 1,* 51–56.

Dattilio, F. M. (1994). Families in crisis. In F. M. Dattilio & A. Freeman (Eds.), *Cognitive-behavioral strategies in crisis intervention* (pp. 278–301). New York: Guilford Press.

Dattilio, F. M. (1995). Cognitive therapy in Egypt. *Journal of Cognitive Psychotherapy, 9*(4), 285–286.

Dattilio, F. M. (1997). Family therapy. In R. L. Leahy (Ed.), *Practicing cognitive therapy: A guide to interventions* (pp. 409–450). Northvale, NJ: Jason Aronson.

Dattilio, F. M. (Ed.). (1998a). *Case studies in couple and family therapy: Systemic and cognitive perspectives.* New York: Guilford Press.

Dattilio, F. M. (1998b). Cognitive-behavior family therapy. In F. M. Dattilio (Ed.), *Case studies in couple and family therapy: Systemic and cognitive perspectives* (pp. 62–84). New York: Guilford Press.

Dattilio, F. M. (1998c). Finding the fit between cognitive-behavioral and family therapy. *Family Therapy Networker, 22*(4), 63–73.

Dattilio, F. M. (2000). Families in crisis. In F. M. Dattilio & A. Freeman (Eds.), *Cognitive-behavioral strategies in crisis intervention* (2nd ed., pp. 316–338). New York: Guilford Press.

Dattilio, F. M. (2001a). Cognitive-behavior family therapy: Contemporary myths and misconceptions. *Contemporary Family Therapy, 23,* 3–18.

Dattilio, F. M. (2001b). The ripple effects of depressive schemas on psychiatric patients [Letter to the editor]. *Archives of Psychiatry and Psychotherapy, 3*(2), 90–91.

Dattilio, F. M. (2001c). The pad and pencil technique. In R. E. Watts (Ed.), *Favorite counseling techniques with couples and families* (Vol. 2, pp. 45–47). Alexandria, VA: American Counseling Association.

Dattilio, F. M. (2002). Homework assignments in couple and family therapy. *Journal of Clinical Psychology, 58*(5), 570–583.

Dattilio, F. M. (2003). Family therapy. In R. E. Leahy (Ed.), *Overcoming roadblocks in cognitive therapy* (pp. 236–252). New York: Guilford Press.

Dattilio, F. M. (2004a). Cognitive-behavioral family therapy: A coming-of-age story. In R. L. Leahy (Ed.), *Contemporary cognitive therapy: Theory, research and practice* (pp. 389–405). New York: Guilford Press.

Dattilio, F. M. (2004b, Summer). Extramarital affairs: The much-overlooked PTSD. *The Behavior Therapist, 27*(4), 76–78.

Dattilio, F. M. (2005a). Homework for couples. In N. Kazantzis, F. P. Deane, K. R. Ronan, & L. L'Abate (Eds.), *Using homework assignments in cognitive-behavior therapy* (pp. 153–170). New York: Brunner-Routledge.

Dattilio, F. M. (2005b). Restructuring family schemas: A cognitive-behavioral perspective. *Journal of Marital and Family Therapy, 31*(1), 15–30.

Dattilio, F. M. (2005c). Cognitive-behavioral therapy with an East Indian family. *Contemporary Family Therapy, 27*(3), 367–382.

Dattilio, F. M. (2005d). Clinical perspectives on involving the family in treatment. In J. L. Hudson & R. M. Rapee (Eds.), *Psychopathology and the family* (pp. 301–321). London: Elsevier.

Dattilio, F. M. (2005e). Rejoinder to Webster. *Australian and New Zealand Journal of Family Therapy, 26*(2), 81.

Dattilio, F. M. (2006a). Case-based research in family therapy. *Australian and New Zealand Journal of Family Therapy, 27*(4), 208–213.

Dattilio, F. M. (2006b). Cognitive behavior therapy in the wake of divorce. In C. A. Everett & R. E. Lee (Eds.), *When marriages fail: Systemic family therapy interventions and issues* (pp. 217–228). New York: Haworth Press.

Dattilio, F. M. (2006c). Restructuring schemata from family-of-origin in couple therapy. *Journal of Cognitive Psychotherapy, 20*(4), 359–373.

Dattilio, F. M. (2007). Breaking the pattern of interruption in family therapy. *Family Journal, 15*(2), 163–165.

Dattilio, F. M. (2009). Foreword. In N. Kazantzis, M. Reinecke, & A. Freeman (Eds.), *Cognitive and behavioral theories in clinical practice* (pp. xi–xiii). New York: Guilford Press.

Dattilio, F. M., & Epstein, N. B. (2003). Cognitive-behavior couple and family therapy. In I. L. Sexton, O. R. Weeks, & M. S. Robbins (Eds.), *The family therapy handbook* (pp. 147–175). New York: Routledge.

Dattilio, F. M., & Epstein, N. B. (2005). Introduction to the special section: The role of cognitive-behavioral interventions in couple and family therapy. *Journal of Marital and Family Therapy, 31*, 7–13.

Dattilio, F. M., Epstein, N. B., & Baucom, U. H. (1998). An introduction to cognitive-behavioral therapy with couples and families. In F. M. Dattilio (Ed.), *Case studies in couple and family therapy: Systemic and cognitive perspectives* (pp. 1–36). New York: Guilford Press.

Dattilio, F. M., Freeman, A., & Blue, J. (1998). The therapeutic relationship. In A.

S. Bellack & M. Hersen (Eds.), *Comprehensive clinical psychology* (pp. 224–229). Oxford, UK: Elsevier Science.

Dattilio, F. M., & Jongsma, A. E. (2000). *The Family Therapy Treatment Planner.* New York: Wiley.

Dattilio, F. M., Kazantzis, N., Shinkfield, G., & Carr, A. G. (in press). A survey of homework use, experiences of barriers to homework, and attitudes about the barriers to homework among couples and family therapists. *Journal of Marital and Family Therapy.*

Dattilio, F. M., L'Abate, L., & Deane, F. (2005). Homework for families. In N. Kazantzis, F. P. Deane, K. R. Ronan, & L. L'Abate (Eds.), *Using homework assignments in cognitive-behavior therapy* (pp. 171–190). New York: Brunner-Routledge.

Dattilio, F. M., & Padesky, C. A. (1990). *Cognitive therapy with couples.* Sarasota, FL: Professional Resource Exchange.

Dattilio, F. M., Tresco, K. E., & Siegel, A. (2007). An empirical survey of psychological testing and the use of the term "psychological": Turf battles or clinical necessity. *Professional Psychology: Research and Practice, 38*(6), 682–689.

Dattilio, F. M., & Van Hout, G. C. M. (2006). The problem solving component in cognitive-behavioral couples therapy. *Journal of Family Psychotherapy, 17*(1), 1–19.

Daveson, D. D. (1965). Family rules. *Archives of General Psychiatry, 12,* 589–594.

Davis, M. H., & Oathout, H. A. (1987). Maintenance of satisfaction in romantic relationships: Empathy and relational competence. *Journal of Personality and Social Psychology, 53,* 397–410.

Davis, M. H., & Oathout, H. A. (1992). The effect of dispositional empathy on romantic relationship behaviors: Heterosocial anxiety as a moderating influence. *Personality and Social Psychology Bulletin, 18,* 76–83.

Davis, S. D., & Piercy, F. P. (2007). What clients of couple therapy model developers and their former students say about change: Part 1. Model dependent common factors across three models. *Journal of Marital and Family Therapy, 33*(3), 318–343.

Dawson, G. (1994). Frontal electroencephalographic correlates of individual differences in emotional expression of infants: A brain systems perspective on emotion. In N. A. Fox (Ed.), The development of emotional regulation: Biological and behavioral considerations. *Monographs of the Society of Research in Child Development, 59*(2–3, Serial No. 240), 135–151.

DeRubeis, R. J., & Beck, A. T. (1988). Cognitive therapy. In K. S. Dobson (Ed.), *Handbook of cognitive behavioral therapies* (pp. 273–306). New York: Guilford Press.

DeShazer, G. (1978). Brief therapy with couples. *International Journal of Family Counseling, 6,* 17–30.

Diamond, G. M., Diamond, G. S., & Hogue, A. (2007). Attachment-based family therapy: Adherence and differentiation. *Journal of Marital and Family Therapy, 33*(2), 177–191.

Doss, B. D., Simpson, L. E., & Christensen, A. (2004). Why do couples seek marital therapy? *Professional Psychology: Research and Practice, 35*(6), 608–614.

Dowd, E. T., & Swoboda, J. S. (1984). Paradoxical interventions in behavior therapy. *Journal of Behavior Therapy and Experimental Psychiatry, 15*(3), 229–234.

Dudek, D., Zieba, A., Jawor, M., Szymaczek, M., Opila, J., & Dattilio, F. M. (2001). The impact of depressive illness on spouses of depressed patients. *Journal of Cognitive Psychotherapy, 15*(1), 49–57.

Duncan, B. L. (1989). Paradoxical procedures in family therapy. In L. M. Ascher (Ed.), *Therapeutic paradox* (311–348). New York: Guilford.

Dunlap, K. (1932). *Habits, their making and unmaking.* New York: Liverright.

Dutton, D. G. (2007). *The abusive personality: Violence and control in intimate relationships* (2nd ed.). New York: Guilford Press.

Eidelson, F. I., & Epstein, N. (1982). Cognition and relationship maladjustment: Development of a measure of dysfunctional relationship beliefs. *Journal of Consulting and Clinical Psychology, 50*, 715–720.

Ellis, A. (1977). The nature of disturbed marital interactions. In A. Ellis & F. Grieger (Eds.), *Handbook of rational-emotive therapy* (pp. 170–176). New York: Springer.

Ellis, A. (1982). Rational-emotive family therapy. In A. M. Home & M. M. Ohlsen (Eds.), *Family counseling and therapy* (pp. 302–328). Itasca, IL: Peacock.

Ellis, A., & Harper, F. A. (1961). *A guide to rational living.* Englewood Cliffs, NJ: Prentice-Hall.

Ellis, A., Sichel, J. L., Yeager, R. J., DiMattia, D. J., & DiGiuseppe, R. (1989). *Rational-emotive couples therapy.* New York: Pergamon Press.

Epstein, N. B. (1982). Cognitive therapy with couples. *American Journal of Family Therapy, 30*, 5–16.

Epstein, N. B., Baldwin, L. M., & Bishop, D. S. (1983). The MacMaster Family Assessment Device. *Journal of Marital and Family Therapy, 9*, 171–180.

Epstein, N. B., & Baucom, D. H. (1993). Cognitive factors in marital disturbance. In K. S. Dobson & P. C. Kendall (Eds.), *Psychopathology and cognition* (pp. 351–385). San Diego, CA: Academic Press.

Epstein, N. B., & Baucom, D. H. (2002). *Enhanced cognitive-behavior therapy for couples: A contextual approach.* Washington, DC: American Psychological Association.

Epstein, N. B., & Baucom, D. H. (2003). Couple therapy. In R. L. Leahy (Ed.), *Roadblocks in cognitive-behavior therapy: Transforming challenges into opportunities for change* (pp. 217–235). New York: Guilford Press.

Epstein, N. B., & Baucom, D. H., & Rankin, L. A. (1993). Treatment of marital conflict: A cognitive-behavioral approach. *Clinical Psychology Review, 13*, 45–57.

Epstein, N. B., & Eidelson, R. J. (1981). Unrealistic beliefs of clinical couples: Their relationship to expectations, goals and satisfaction. *American Journal of Family Therapy, 9*, 13–22.

Epstein, N. B., & Schlesinger, S. E. (1996). Treatment of family problems. In M. A. Reinecke, F. M. Dattilio, & A. Freeman (Eds.), *Cognitive therapy with children and adolescents: A casebook for clinical practice* (pp. 299–326). New York: Guilford Press.

Epstein, N. B., Schlesinger, S. E., & Dryden, W. (1988). Concepts and methods of cognitive-behavior family treatment. In N. Epstein, S. E. Schlesinger, & W. Dryden (Eds.), *Cognitive-behavior therapy with families* (pp. 5–48). New York: Brunner/Mazel.

Epstein, N. B., & Werlinich, C. A. (2003, November). *Assessment of physical and psychological abuse in an outpatient marital and family therapy clinic: How much abuse is revealed under what conditions and with what relation to relationship distress?* Paper presented as part of the symposium, "Assessment of psychological and physical abuse in couples: What can we learn through different methods?" at the annual meeting of the Association for Advancement of Behavior Therapy, Boston.

Epstein, N. B., Werlinich, C. A., LaTaillade, J. J., Hoskins, L. H., Dezfulian, T., Kursch, M. K., et al. (2005, October). *Couple therapy for domestic abuse: A cognitive-behavioral approach.* Paper presented at the annual convention of the American Association for Marriage and Family Therapy, Kansas City, MO.

Fadden, G., Bebbington, P., & Kuipers, L. (1987). The burden of care: The impact of functional psychiatric illness on the patient's family. *British Journal of Psychiatry, 150,* 285–292.

Falloon, I. R. H. (Ed.). (1988). *Handbook of behavioral family therapy.* New York: Guilford Press.

Falloon, I. R. H., Boyd, B. L., & McGill, C. W. (1984). *Family care of schizophrenia.* New York: Guilford Press.

Falloon, I. R. H., & Lillie, F. (1988). Behavioral family therapy: An overview. In I. R. H. Falloon (Ed.), *Handbook of behavioral family therapy* (pp. 3–26). New York: Guilford Press.

Fincham, F. D., Beach, S. R. H., & Nelson, O. (1987). Attribution processes in distressed and nondistressed couples: Causal and responsibility attributions for spouse behavior. *Cognitive Therapy and Research, 11,* 71–86.

Fine, M. A., & Schwebel, A. I. (1983). Long-term effect of divorce on parent–child relationships. *Developmental Psychology, 19,* 703–713.

Finn, S. E., & Tonsager, M. E. (1997). Information-gathering and therapeutic models of assessment: Complementary paradigms. *Psychological Assessment, 9*(4), 374–385.

Firth, C., & Johnstone, E. (2003). *Schizophrenia: A very short introduction.* Oxford, UK: Oxford University Press.

Fogarty, T. F. (1976). Marital crisis. In P. J. Guerin (Ed.), *In family therapy: Theory and practice* (pp. 55–65). New York: Gardner Press.

Forgatch, M., & Patterson, G. R. (1998). Behavioral family therapy. In F. M. Dattilio (Ed.), *Case studies in couple and family therapy: Systemic and cognitive perspectives* (pp. 85–107). New York: Guilford Press.

Framo, J. (1992). *Family of origin therapy: An intergenerational approach.* New York: Brunner/Mazel.

Frankl, V. E. (1960). Paradoxical intention: A logo-therapeutic technique. *American Journal of Psychotherapy, 14,* 520–535.

Fredman, N., & Sherman, R. (1987). *Handbook of measurements of marriage and family therapy.* New York: Brunner/Mazel.

Freud, S. (1952). Inhibitions, symptoms and anxiety (A. Strachey, Trans.). In R. M. Hutchins (Ed.), *Great books of the Western world* (pp. 718–734). Chicago: Encyclopedia Britannica. (Original work published 1926)

Friedberg, R. D. (2006). A cognitive-behavioral approach to family therapy. *Journal of Contemporary Psychotherapy, 36,* 159–165.

Fruzetti, A. E., & Iverson, K. M. (2004). Mindfulness, acceptance, validation, and "individual" psychopathology in couples. In S. C. Hayes, V. M. Follette, &

M. M. Linehan (Eds.), *Mindfulness and acceptance: Expanding the cognitive-behavioral tradition* (pp. 168–191). New York: Guilford Press.

Gardner, H. (1985). *The mind's new science.* New York: Basic Books.

Geiss, S. K., & O'Leary, K. D. (1991). Therapists' ratings of frequency and severity of marital problems: Implications for research. *Journal of Marital and Family Therapy, 7,* 515–520.

Ginsberg, B. G. (1997). *Relationship enhancement family therapy.* New York: Wiley.

Ginsberg, B. G. (2000). Relationship enhancement couples therapy. In F. M. Dattilio & L. J. Bevilacqua (Eds.), *Comparative treatments for relationship dysfunction* (pp. 273–298). New York: Springer.

Glass, S. P. (2000). The harder you fall, the farther you fall. In J. R. Levine & H. J. Markman (Eds.), *Why do fools fall in love?* New York: Jossey-Bass.

Glass, S. P. (2002). Couple therapy after the trauma of infidelity. In A. S. Gurman & N. S. Jacobson (Eds.), *Clinical handbook of couple therapy* (3rd ed.). New York: Guilford Press.

Glass, S. P. (2003). *Not "just friends": Protect your relationship from infidelity and heal the trauma of betrayal.* New York: Free Press.

Gleick, J. (1987). *Chaos: Making a new science.* New York: Viking.

Goldenberg, I., & Goldenberg, H. (2000). *Family therapy: An overview* (5th ed.). Belmont, CA: Brooks/Cole.

Goldenberg, I., & Goldenberg, H. (2008). *Family therapy: An overview* (8th ed.). Belmont, CA: Brooks/Cole.

Goldstein, S., & Thau, S. (2004). Integrating attachment theory and neruoscience in couple therapy. *International Journal of Applied Psychoanalytic Studies, 1*(3), 214–223.

Goleman, D. (1995). *Emotional intelligence.* New York: Bantam Books.

Gordon, K. C., & Baucom, D. H. (1998). Understanding betrayals in marriage: A synthesized model of forgiveness. *Family Process, 37,* 425–450.

Gordon, K. C., & Baucom, D. H. (1999). A multitheoretical intervention for promoting recovery from extramarital affairs. *Clinical Psychology: Science and Practice, 6,* 382–399.

Gottman, J. M. (1994). *What predicts divorce?* Hillsdale, NJ: Erlbaum.

Gottman J. M. (1999). *The marriage clinic: A scientifically based marital therapy.* New York: Norton.

Gottman, J. M., & Gottman, J. S. (1999). Marital survival kit: A research based marital therapy. In R. Berger & M. T. Hannah (Eds.), *Preventive approaches in couples therapy* (pp. 304–330). New York: Brunner/Mazel.

Gottman, J. M., & Levenson, R. W. (1986). Assessing the role of emotion in marriage. *Behavioral Assessment, 8,* 31–48.

Gottman, J. M., Notarius, C., Gonso, J., & Markman, H. J. (1976). *A couples guide to communication.* Champaign, IL: Research Press.

Granvold, D. K. (2000). Divorce. In F. M. Dattilio & A. Freeman (Eds.), *Cognitive-behavioral strategies in crisis intervention* (2nd ed., pp. 362–384). New York: Guilford Press.

Green, R. G., Kolevzon, M. S., & Vosler, N. R. (1985). The Beavers–Timberlawn Model of Family Competence and the Circumplex Model of Family Adaptability and Cohesion: Separate, but equal? *Family Process, 24,* 385–398.

Guerin, P. J. (2002). Bowenian family therapy. In J. Carlson & D. Kjos (Eds.), *Theories and strategies of family therapy* (pp. 126–157). Boston: Allyn & Bacon.

Guerney, B. G. (1977). *Relationship enhancement*. San Francisco: Jossey-Bass.

Haley, J. (1976). *Problem solving therapy: New strategies for effective family therapy*. San Francisco: Jossey-Bass.

Hamberger, L. K., & Holtzworth-Monroe, A. (2007). Spousal abuse. In F. M. Dattilio & A. Freeman (Eds.), *Cognitive-behavioral strategies in crisis intervention* (3rd. ed., pp. 277–299). New York: Guilford Press.

Hansson, R. O., Jones, W. H., & Carpenter, B. N. (1984). Relationship competence and social support. In N. P. Shaver (Ed.), *Review of personality and social psychology* (Vol. 5, pp. 265–284). Beverly Hills, CA: Sage.

Harvard Health Publications. (2007). *Couples therapy: Methods couples therapists use during couples therapy*. Retrieved from *https://www.health.harvard.edu/press_releases/couples*.

Hayes, S. C. (2004). Acceptance and commitment therapy and the new behavior therapies: Mindfulness, acceptance and relationship. In S. C. Hayes, V. M. Follette, & M. M. Linehan (Eds.), *Mindfulness and acceptance: Expanding the cognitive-behavioral tradition*. New York: Guilford Press.

Hazan, C., & Shaver, P. (1987). Romantic love conceptualized as an attachment process. *Journal of Personality and Social Psychology, 52*, 511–524.

Heitler, S. (1995). *The angry couple: Conflict-focused treatment* (videotape, 73 min.). New York: Newbridge Professional Programs.

Heyman, R. E., Eddy, J. M., Weiss, R. L., & Vivian, D. (1995). Factor analysis of the Marital Interaction Coding System (MICS). *Journal of Family Psychology, 9*, 209–215.

Heyman, R. E., & Neidig, P. H. (1997). Physical aggression in couples treatment. In W. K. Halford & H. J. Markman (Eds.), *Clinical handbook of marriage and couples intervention* (pp. 589–617). Chichester, UK: Wiley.

Hofmann, S. G. (2008). Acceptance and commitment therapy: New wave or morita therapy? *Clinical Psychology: Science and Practice, 15*(4), 280–285.

Hofmann, S. G., & Asmundson, G. J. (2008). Acceptance and mindfulness based therapy: New wave or old hat? *Clinical Psychology Review, 28*, 1–16.

Holtzworth-Munroe, A., & Jacobson, N. S. (1985). Casual attributions of married couples: When do they search for causes? What do they conclude when they do? *Journal of Personality and Social Psychology, 48*, 1398–1412.

Homans, G. C. (1961). *Social behavior: Its elementary forms*. New York: Harcourt, Brace Jananovich.

Hovestadt, A. J., Anderson, W. T., Piercy, F. P., Cochran, S. W., & Fine, M. (1985). Family of origin scale. *Journal of Marital and Family Therapy, 11*(3), 287–297.

Jacob, T., & Tennenbaum, D. L. (1988). *Family assessment: Rationale, methods and future directions*. New York: Plenum.

Jacobson, N. S. (1992). Behavioral couple therapy: A new beginning. *Behavior Therapy, 23*, 493–506.

Jacobson, N. S., & Margolin, G. (1979). *Marital therapy: Strategies based on social learning and behavior exchange principles*. New York: Brunner/Mazel.

James, I. A., Reichelt, F. K., Freeston, M. H., & Barton, S. B. (2007). Schemas as memories: Implications for treatment. *Journal of Cognitive Psychotherapy,* 21(1), 51–57.

Johnson, J. A., Cheek, J. M., & Smither, R. (1983). The structure of empathy. *Journal of Personality and Social Psychology,* 45(6), 1299–1312.

Johnson, P. L., & O'Leary, K. D. (1996). Behavioral components of marital satisfaction: An individualized assessment approach. *Journal of Consulting and Clinical Psychology,* 64, 417–423.

Johnson, S. M. (1996). *The practice of emotionally focused marital therapy: Creating connection.* New York: Brunner/Mazel.

Johnson, S. M. (1998). Emotionally focused couple therapy. In F. M. Dattilio (Ed.), *Case studies in couple and family therapy: Systematic and cognitive perspectives* (450–472). New York: Guilford Press.

Johnson, S. M., & Denton, W. (2002). Emotionally focused couple therapy: Creating secure connections. In A. S. Gurman & N. S. Jacobson (Eds.), *Clinical handbook of couple therapy* (3rd ed., pp. 221–250). New York: Guilford Press.

Johnson, S. M., & Greenberg, L. S. (1988). Relating process to outcome in marital therapy. *Journal of Marital and Family Therapy,* 14, 175–183.

Johnson, S. M., Hunsley, J., Greenberg, L., & Schindler, D. (1999). Emotionally focused couples: Status and challenges. *Clinical Psychology: Science and Practice,* 6, 67–79.

Johnson, S. M., & Talitman. E. (1997). Predictors of success in emotionally focused marital therapy. *Journal of Marital and Funnily Therapy 23,* 135–152.

Johnson, S. M., & Whiffen, V. E. (Eds.). (2003). *Attachment processes in couple and family therapy.* New York: Guilford Press.

Kabat-Zinn, J. (1993). Mindfulness meditation: Health benefits of an ancient Buddhist practice. In D. Goleman & J. Garin (Eds.), *Mind/body medicine* (pp. 259–276). Yonkers: Consumer Reports.

Kaslow, F. (1995). *Projective genogramming.* Sarasota, FL: Professional Resource Press.

Katz, E., & Bertelson, A. D. (1993). Effects of gender and response style on depressed mood. *Sex Roles, 29,* 509–514.

Kazantzis, N., & Dattilio, F. M. (in press). A survey of psychologists who use homework in clinical practice: Definitions, types, and perceived importance. *Journal of Clinical Psychology.*

Kazantzis, N., Deane, F. P., & Ronan, K. P. (2000). Homework assignments in cognitive-behavioral therapy: A meta-analysis. *Clinical Psychology: Science and Practice, 7,* 189–202.

Kazantzis, N., Whittington, C. J., & Dattilio, F. M. (in press). Meta-analysis of homework effects in cognitive and behavior therapy: A replication and extension. *Clinical Psychology: Science and Practice.*

Kelly, G. A. (1955). *The psychology of personal constructs.* New York: Norton.

Kelly, H. H. (1979). *Personal relationships: Their structures and processes.* Hilldale, NJ: Erlbaum.

Kerr, M., & Bowen, M. (1988). *Family evaluation.* New York: Norton.

Kidman, A. D. (2007). *Schizophrenia: A guide for families.* St. Leonards, NSW: Biochemical and General Sciences.

Kirby, J. S., & Baucom, D. H. (2007). Integrating dialectical behavior therapy and cognitive-behavioral couples therapy: A couples skills group for emotion dys-regulation. *Cognitive and Behavioral Practice, 14,* 394–405.

L'Abate, L. (1985). A training program for family psychology: Evaluation, prevention and therapy. *American Journal of Family Therapy, 13,* 7–16.

L'Abate, L. (1998). *Family psychopathology: The relational roots of dysfunctional behavior.* New York: Guilford Press.

LaTaillade, J., Epstein, N. B., & Werlinich, C. A. (2006). Conjoint treatment of intimate partner violence: A cognitive-behavioral approach. *Journal of Cognitive Psychotherapy, 20*(4), 393–410.

Laumann, E. O., Gagnon, J. H., Michael, R. T., & Michaels, S. (1994). *The social organization of sexuality.* Chicago: University of Chicago Press.

Lazarus, A. A. (1976). *Multimodal behavior therapy.* New York: Springer.

Leahy, R. L. (1996). *Cognitive therapy: Basic principles and applications.* Northvale, NJ: Jason Aronson.

Leahy, R. L. (2001). *Overcoming resistance in cognitive therapy.* New York: Guilford Press.

LeBow, M. D. (1976). Behavior modification for the family. In G. D. Erickson & T. P. Hogan (Eds.), *Family therapy: An introduction to theory and technique* (pp. 347–376). New York: Jason Aronson.

LeDoux, J. (1994). Emotion, memory and the brain. *Scientific American, 270*(6), 50–57.

LeDoux, J. (1996). *The emotional brain.* New York: Simon & Schuster.

LeDoux, J. (2000). Emotional circuits in the brain. *Annual Review of Neuroscience, 23,* 155–184.

Leon, K., & Jacobvitz, D. B. (2003). Relationships between adult attachment representations and family ritual quality: A prospective longitudinal study. *Family Process, 42,* 419–432.

Leslie, L. A. (1988). Cognitive-behavioral and systems models of family therapy: How compatible are they? In N. B. Epstein, S. E. Schlesinger, & W. Dryden (Eds.), *Cognitive-behavior therapy with families* (pp. 49–83). New York: Brunner/Mazel.

Lewis, T., Amini, F., & Lannon, R. (2002). *A general theory of love.* New York: Vintage Press.

Liberman, R. P. (1970). Behavior approaches to couple and family therapy. *American Journal of Orthopsychiatry, 40,* 106–118.

Linehan, M. M. (1993). *Cognitive-behavioral treatment of borderline personality disorder.* New York: Guilford Press.

Margolin, G., & Weiss, R. L. (1978). Comparative evaluation of therapeutic components associated with behavior marital treatments. *Journal of Consulting and Clinical Psychology, 46,* 1476–1486.

Markman, H. J. (1984). The longitudinal study of couples' interaction: Implications for understanding and predicting the development of marital distress. In K. Halweg & N. S. Jacobson (Eds.), *Marital interaction: Analysis and modification* (pp. 253–281). New York: Guilford Press.

Markman, H. J., Stanley, S., & Blumberg, S. L. (1994). *Fighting for your marriage.* San Francisco: Jossey-Bass.

McCubbin, H. I., Larsen, A., & Olsen, D. (1996). Family coping coherence index (FCCI). In H. I. McCubbin, A. I. Thompson, & M. A. McCubbin (Eds.), *Fam-*

ily assessment resiliency coping and adaptation inventories for research and practice (pp. 703–712). Madison: University of Wisconsin.

McCubbin, H. I., & Thompson, A. I. (Eds.). (1991). *Family assessment: Inventories for research and practice.* Madison: University of Wisconsin.

McCubbin, M. A., & McCubbin, H. L (1989). Theoretical orientation to family stress and coping. In C. R. Figley (Ed.), *Treating stress in families* (pp. 3–43) New York: Brunner/Mazel.

McGoldrick, M., Gerson, R., & Petry, S. (2008). *Genograms: Assessment and intervention* (3rd ed.). New York: Norton.

McGoldrick, M., Giordano, J., & Garcia-Preto, N. (Eds.). (2005). *Ethnicity and family therapy* (3rd ed.). New York: Guilford Press.

McGoldrick, M., Giordano, J., & Pearce, J. K. (Eds.). (1996). *Ethnicity and family therapy* (2nd ed.). New York: Guilford Press.

McKay, M., Fanning, P., & Paleg, K. (2006). *Couple skills: Making your relationship work.* Oakland, CA: New Harbinger.

Meichenbaum, D. (1977). *Cognitive-behavior modification: An integrative approach.* New York: Plenum Press.

Miklowitz, D. J. (1995). The evolution of family-based psychopathology. In R. H. Mikesell, D. D. Lusterman, & S. H. McDaniel (Eds.), *Integrating family therapy: Handbook of family psychology and systems theory* (pp. 183–197). Washington, DC: American Psychological Association.

Mikulincer, M., Florian, V., Cowan, P. A., & Cowan, C. P. (2002). Attachment security in couple relationships: A systemic model and its implications for family dynamics. *Family Process, 41,* 405–434.

Mikulincer, M., & Shaver, P. R. (2007). *Attachment in adulthood: Structure, dynamics and change.* New York: Guilford Press.

Miller, G. E., & Bradberry, T. N. (1995). Refining the association between attributions and behavior in marital interaction. *Journal of Family Psychology, 9,* 196–208.

Miller, I. W., Keitner, G. I., Epstein, N. B., Bishop, D. S., & Ryan, C. E. (1993). Inpatient family therapy: Part A. In J. H. Wright, M. E. Thase, A. T. Beck, & J. W. Ludgate (Eds.), *Cognitive therapy with inpatients: Developing a cognitive milieu* (pp. 154–190). New York: Guilford Press.

Milner, B., Squire, L. R., & Kandel, E. R. (1998). Cognitive neuroscience and the study of memory. *Neuron, 20,* 445–468.

Minuchin, S. (1974). *Families and family therapy.* Cambridge. MA: Harvard University Press.

Minuchin, S., & Nichols, M. P. (1998). Structural family therapy. In F. M. Dattilio (Ed.), *Case studies in couple and family therapy: Systemic and cognitive perspectives* (pp. 108–131). New York: Guilford Press.

Moos, R. H., & Moos, B. H. (1986). *Family environment scale manual* (2nd ed.). Palo Alto, CA: Consulting Psychologists Press.

Morgillo-Freeman, S., & Storie, M. (2007). Substance misuse and dependency: Crisis as a process or outcome. In F. M. Dattilio & A. Freeman (Eds.), *Cognitive-behavioral strategies in crisis intervention* (3rd ed., pp. 175–198). New York: Guilford Press.

Mueser, K. T., & Glynn, S. M. (1999). *Behavior family therapy for psychiatric disorders* (2nd ed.). Oakland, CA: New Harbinger.

Navaran, L. (1967). Communication and adjustment in marriage. *Family Process,* 6, 173–184.

Nelson, T. S., & Trepper, T. S. (1993). (Eds.). *101 Interventions in family therapy.* New York: The Haworth Press.

Nelson, T. S., & Trepper, T. S. (1998). *101 More interventions in family therapy.* New York: The Haworth Press.

Nichols, M. P. (1995). *The lost art of listening: How learning to listen can improve your relationships.* New York: Guilford Press.

Nichols, M. P., & Schwartz, R. C. (2001). *Family therapy: Concepts and methods* (5th ed). Boston: Allyn & Bacon.

Nichols, M. P., & Schwartz, R. C. (2008). *Family therapy: Concepts and methods* (8th ed.). Boston: Allyn & Bacon.

Noel, N. E., & McCrady, B. S. (1993). Alcohol-focused spouse involvement with behavioral marital therapy. In T. J. O'Farrell (Ed.), *Treating alcohol problems: Marital and family interventions* (pp. 210–235). New York: Guilford Press.

Nolen-Hoeksema, S. (1987). Sex difference in unipolar depression: Evidence and theory. *Psychological Bulletin, 101,* 259–282.

Northey, W. F. (2002). Characteristics and clinical practices of marriage and family therapists: A national survey. *Journal of Marital and Family Therapy, 28,* 487–494.

Novaco, R. (1975). *Anger control: The development and evaluation of an experimental treatment.* Lexington, MA: Heath.

O'Leary, K. D., Heyman, R. E., & Jongsma, A. E. (1998). *The couples psychotherapy treatment planner.* Hoboken, NJ: Wiley.

O'Farrell, T. (1993). Couples relapse prevention sessions after a behavioral marital therapy couples group program. In T. J. O'Farrell (Ed.), *Treating alcohol problems: Marital and family interventions* (pp. 305–326). New York: Guilford Press.

O'Farrell, T., & Fals-Stewart, W. (2006). *Behavioral couples therapy for alcoholism and drug abuse.* New York: Guilford Press.

Ohman, A. (2002). Automaticity and the amygdala: Nonconscious responses to emotional faces. *Current Directions in Psychological Services, 11,* 62–66.

Olson, D. H., Portner, J., & Lavee, Y. (1985). *FACES-III, Family social sciences.* St. Paul: University of Minnesota.

Olson, M. M., Russell, C. S., Higgins-Kessler, M., & Miller, R. B. (2002). Emotional processes following disclosures of an extramarital affair. *Journal of Marital and Family Therapy, 28,* 423–434.

Orford, J., Guthrie, S., Nicholls, P., Oppenheimer, E., Egert, S., & Hensman, C. (1975). Self-reportive coping behavior of wives of alcoholics and its association with drinking outcome. *Journal of Studies on Alcohol, 36,* 1254–1267.

Paley, B., Cox, M. J., Kanoy, K. W., Harter, K. S. M., Burchinal, M., & Margand, N. A. (2005). Adult attachment and marital interactions as predictors of whole family interactions during the transition to parenthood. *Journal of Family Psychology, 19,* 420–429.

Palmer, C. A., & Baucom, D. H. (1998, November). *How our marriages lasted: Couples' reflections on staying together.* Paper presented at the Annual Meeting of the Association for the Advancement of Behavior Therapy, Washington, DC.

Paolino, T., & McCrady, B. (1977). *The alcoholic marriage: Alternative perspectives*. New York: Grune & Stratton.

Patterson, G. R. (1974). Interventions for boys with conduct problems: Multiple settings treatment criteria. *Journal of Consulting and Clinical Psychology, 42*(1), 471–481.

Patterson, G. R., & Forgatch, M. S. (1985). Therapist behavior as a determinant for client resistance: A paradox for the behavior modified. *Journal of Consulting and Clinical Psychology, 5*, 237–262.

Patterson, G. R., & Hops, H. (1972). Coercion, a game for two: Intervention techniques for marital conflict. In R. E. Ulrich & P. Mountjoy (Eds.), *The experimental analysis of social behavior*. New York: Appleton-Century-Crofts.

Patterson, G. R., McNeal, S., Hawkins, N., & Phelps, R. (1967). Reprogramming the social environment. *Journal of Child Psychology and Psychiatry, 8*, 181–195.

Pessoa, L. (2005). To what extent are emotional visual stimuli processed without attention and awareness? *Current Opinion in Neurobiology, 15*, 188–196.

Pessoa, L. (2008). On the relationship between emotion and cognition. *Nature Reviews/Neuroscience, 9*, 148–158.

Piaget, J. (1950). [Psychology of Intelligence] (M. Piercy & D, E. Berlyne, Trans.). New York: Harcourt, Brace. (Original work published 1947)

Pretzer, J., Epstein, N., & Fleming, B. (1991). Marital Attitude Survey: A measure of dysfunctional attributions and expectancies. *Journal of Cognitive Psychotherapy: An International Quarterly, 5*, 131–148.

Prochaska, J. O., DiClemente, C. C., & Norcross, J. C. (1992). In search of how people change: Applications for addictive behaviors. *American Psychologist, 47*, 1102–1114.

Psychotherapy Networker. (2007). The top 10: The most influential therapists of the past quarter-century. *Psychotherapy Networker, 31*(2), 24–68.

Regency Films (2002). *Unfaithful*. www.unfaithful.com.

Roehling, R. V., & Robin, A. L. (1986). Development and validation of the Family Beliefs Inventory: A measure of unrealistic beliefs among parents and adolescents. *Journal of Consulting and Clinical Psychology, 54*, 693–697.

Satir, V. M., & Baldwin, M. (1983). *Satir step by step: A guide to creating change in families*. Palo Alto, CA: Science and Behavior Books.

Schore, A. M. (2003). *Affect regulation and the repair of the self*. New York: Norton.

Schore, A. N. (1994). *Affect regulation and the origin of self: The neurobiology of emotional development*. Mahwah, NJ: Erlbaum.

Schore, A. N. (2001). The effects of secure attachment relationships on right brain development, affect regulation and infant mental health. *Infant Mental Health Journal, 22*, 7–66.

Schuerger, J. M., Zarrella, K. L., & Hotz, A. S. (1989). Factors that influence the temporal stability of personality by questionnaire. *Journal of Personality and Social Psychology, 56*, 777–783.

Schumm, W. R., Jurich, A. P., & Bollman, S. R. (1986). Characteristics of the Kansas Family Life Satisfaction Scale in a regional sample. *Psychological Reports, 58*, 975–980.

Schwebel, A. I., & Fine, M. A. (1992). Cognitive-behavior family therapy. *Journal of Family Psychotherapy, 3*, 73–91.

Schwebel, A. I., & Fine, M. A. (1994). *Understanding and helping families: A cognitive-behavior approach*. Hillsdale, NJ: Erlbaum.

Segal, Z. V. (1988). Appraisal of the self-schema construct in cognitive models of depression. *Psychological Bulletin, 103*, 147–162.

Seligman, M. E. P. (1995). The effectiveness of psychotherapy: The Consumer Reports Study. *American Psychologist, 50*, 965–974.

Senchak, M., & Leonard, K. E. (1992). Attachment styles and marital adjustment among newlywed couples. *Journal of Social and Personal Relationships, 9*, 51–64.

Sexton, T. L., Weeks, G. R., & Robbins, M. S. (Eds.). (2003). *Handbook of family therapy*. New York: Brunner-Routledge.

Shapiro, S. L., Schwartz, G. E., & Bonner, G. (1998). Effects of mindfulness-based stress reduction on medical and paramedical students. *Journal of Behavioral Medicine, 21*, 581–599.

Shaver, P. R., Hazan, C., & Bradshaw, D. (1988). Love as attachment: The integration of three behavioral systems. In R. J. Sternberg & M. Barnes (Eds.), *The psychology of love* (pp. 68–99). New Haven, CT: Yale University Press.

Siegel, D. (1999). *The developing mind*. New York: Guilford Press.

Smith, T. W. (1994). *The demography of sexual behavior*. Menlo Park, CA: Henry J. Kaiser Family Foundation.

Snyder, D. K. (1981). *Marital Satisfaction Inventory (MSI) Manual*. Los Angeles: Western Psychological Services.

Snyder, D. K., & Aikman, G. G. (1999). The Marital Satisfaction Inventory—Revised. In M. E. Maruish (Ed.), *Use of psychological testing for treatment planning outcome assessment* (pp. 1173–1210). Mahwah, NJ: Erlbaum.

Snyder, D. K., Baucom, D. H., & Gordon, K. C. (2009). *Getting past the affair: A program to help you cope, heal and move on—together or apart*. New York: Guilford Press.

Snyder, D. K., Cavell, T. A., Heffer, R. W., & Mangrum, L. F. (1995). Marital and family assessment: A multifaceted, multilevel approach. In R. H. Mikesell, D. D. Lusterman, & S. H. McDaniel (Eds.), *Integrating family therapy: Handbook of family psychology and systems theory* (pp. 163–182). Washington, DC: American Psychological Association.

Snyder, D. K., Wills, R. M., & Grady-Fletcher, A. (1991). Long-term effectiveness of behavior versus insight-oriented marital therapy: A 4-year follow-up study. *Journal of Consulting and Clinical Psychology, 59*, 138–141.

Sonne, J. C., & Lincoln, G. (1965). Heterosexual co-therapy team experiences during family therapy. *Family Process, 4*, 177–197.

Spainer, G. B. (1976). Measuring dyadic adjustment: New scales for assessing the quality of marriage and similar dyads. *Journal of Marriage and the Family, 38*, 15–28.

Spitzer, R. L., Williams, J. B. W., Gibbon, M., & First, M. B. (1994). *Structured clinical interview for DSM-IV (SCID-IV)*. New York: Biometric Research Department, New York State Psychiatric Institute.

Sprenkle, D. H. (2003). Effectiveness research in marriage and family therapy: Introduction. *Journal of Marital and Family Therapy, 29*, 85–96.

Steinglass, P., Bennet, L., Wolin, S. J., & Reiss, D. (1987). *The alcoholic family*. New York: Basic Books.

Straus, M. A., Hamby, S. L., Boney-McCoy, S., & Sugarman, D. B. (1996). The Revised Conflict Tactics Scales (CTS2): Development and preliminary psychometric data. *Journal of Family Issues, 17,* 283–316.

Stuart, R. B. (1969). Operant-interpersonal treatment for marital discord. *Journal of Consulting and Clinical Psychology, 33,* 675–682.

Stuart, R. B. (1980). *Helping couples change: A social learning approach to marital therapy*. New York: Guilford Press.

Stuart, R. B. (1995). *Family of origin inventory*. New York: Guilford Press.

Sue, D., & Sue, D. M. (2008). *Foundations of counseling and psychotherapy: Evidence-based practices for a diverse society*. Hoboken, NJ: Wiley.

Swebel, A. (1992). The family constitution. *Topics in family psychology and counseling, 1*(1), 27–38.

Tavitian, M. L., Lubinar, J. L., Green, L., Grebstein, L. C., & Velicer, W. F. (1987). Dimensions of family functioning. *Journal of Social Behavior and Personality, 2,* 191–204.

Teasdale, J. D., Moore, R. G., Hayhurst, H., Pope, M., Williams, S., & Segal, Z. (2002). Meta-cognitive awareness and prevention of relapse and depression: Empirical evidence. *Journal of Consulting and Clinical Psychology, 70*(2), 275–287.

Teichman, Y. (1981). Family therapy with adolescents. *Journal of Adolescence, 4,* 87–92.

Teichman, Y. (1992). Family treatment with an acting-out adolescent. In A. Freeman & F. M. Dattilio (Eds.), *Comprehensive casebook of cognitive therapy* (pp. 331–346). New York: Plenum Press.

Terman, L. M. (1938). *Psychological factors in mental happiness*. New York: McGraw-Hill.

Thibaut, J., & Kelley, H. H. (1959). *The social psychology of groups*. New York: Wiley.

Tilden, T. & Dattilio, F. M. (2005). Vulnerability schemas of individuals in couples relationships: A cognitive perspective. *Contemporary Family Therapy, 27*(2) 137–160.

Tjaden, P., & Thoennes, N. (2000). Prevalence and consequences of male-to-female and female-to-male intimate partner violence as measured by the National Violence Against Women Survey. *Violence Against Women, 6,* 142–161.

Touliatus, J., Perlmutter, B. F., & Straus, M. A. (Eds.). (1990). *Handbook of family measurement techniques*. Newbury Park, CA: Sage.

Wachs, K., & Cordova, J. V. (2007). Mindful relating: Exploring mindfulness and emotion repertoires in intimate relationships. *Journal of Marital and Family Therapy, 33*(4), 464–481.

Wagner, T. D., & Phan, K. L. (2003). Valance, gender, and lateralization of functional brain anatomy in emotion: A meta-analysis of findings from neuroimaging. *Neuroimage, 19*(3), 513–531.

Wahler, R. G., Winkel, G. H., Peterson, R. F., & Morrison, D. C. (1971). Mothers as behavior therapists for their own children. In A. M. Graziano (Ed.), *Behavior therapy with children* (pp. 388–403). Chicago: Aldine.

Wallin, D. J. (2007). *Attachment in psychotherapy.* New York: Guilford Press.

Walsh, F. (1998). *Strengthening family resilience.* New York: Guilford Press.

Watson, D., & Tellegen, A. (1985). Toward the structure of affect. *Psychological Bulletin, 98,* 219–235.

Watzalawick, P., Beavin, J. H., & Daveson, D. D. (1967). *Pragmatics of human communication.* New York: Norton.

Watzlawick, P., Weakland, J., & Fisch, R. (1974). *Change: Principles of problem formation and problem resolution.* New York: Norton.

Webster, M. (2005). Speaking from the pained place: Engaging with Frank Dattilio. *Australian and New Zealand Journal of Family Therapy, 26*(2), 79–80.

Webster's New World College Dictionary (4th ed.). (2005). Cleveland, OH: Wiley.

Weeks, G. R., & L'Abate, L. (1979). A compilation of paradoxical methods. *American Journal of Family Therapy, 7,* 61–76.

Weeks, G. R., & L'Abate, L. (1982). *Paradoxical psychotherapy: Theory and practice with individuals, couples and families.* New York: Brunner/Mazel.

Weiss, R. L. (1980). Strategic behavioral marital therapy: Toward a model for assessment and intervention. In J. P. Vincent (Ed.), *Advances in family intervention, assessment and theory* (Vol. 1, pp. 229–271). Greenwich, CT: JAI Press.

Weiss, R. L. (1984). Cognitive and strategic interventions in behavior marital therapy. In K. Hahlweg & N. S. Jacobson (Eds.), *Marital interaction: Analysis and modification* (pp. 309–324). New York: Guilford Press.

Weiss, R. L., & Heyman, R. F. (1997). A clinical- research overview of couples interactions. In W. K. Halford & N. J. Markman (Eds.), *Clinical handbook of marriage and couples interventions* (pp. 13–1). Chichester, UK: Wiley.

Weiss, R. L., Hops, H., & Patterson, G. R. (1973). A framework for conceptualizing marital conflict, a technology for altering it, some data for evaluating it. In L. A. Hamerlynck, L. C. Handy, & E. I. Mash (Eds.), *Behavior change: Methodology, concepts, and practice* (pp. 309–342). Champaign, IL: Research Press.

Weissman, M. M. (1987). Advances in psychiatric epidemiology: Rates and risks for major depression. *American Journal of Public Health, 77,* 445–451.

Weissman, M. M., & Paykel, E. S. (1974). *The depressed women: A study of social relationships.* Chicago: University of Chicago Press.

Welburn, K. R., Dagg, P., Coristine, M., & Pontefract, A. (2000). Schematic change as a result of an intensive-group therapy day-treatment program. *Psychotherapy, 37,* 189–195.

Welwood, J. (1996). *Love and awakening.* New York: HarperCollins.

Whalen, P. J. (2004). Human amygdala responsivity to masked fearful eye whites. *Science, 306,* 2061.

Whisman, M. A. (2001). The association between depression and marital dissatisfaction. In S. R. H. Beach (Ed.), *Marital and family process in depression: A scientific foundation for clinical practice* (3–24). Washington, DC: American Psychological Association.

Whisman, M. A., Dixon, A. E., & Johnson, B. (1997). Therapists' perspectives of couple problems and treatment issues in couple therapy. *Journal of Family Psychology, 11,* 361–366.

Wolcott, I. H. (1986). Seeking help for marital problems before separation. *Australian Journal of Sex, Marriage and Family, 7,* 154–164.

Wolpe, J. (1977). *Psychotherapy by reciprocal inhibition*. Palo Alto, CA: Stanford University Press.

Wright, J. H., & Beck, A. T. (1993). Family cognitive therapy with inpatients. In J. H. Wright, M. E. Thase, A. T. Beck, & J. W. Ludgate (Eds.), *Cognitive therapy with inpatients* (pp. 176–190). New York: Guilford Press.

Wright, J. H., Thase, M. E., Beck, A. T., & Ludgate, J. W. (Eds.). (1993). *Cognitive therapy with inpatients: Developing a cognitive milieu*. New York: Guilford Press.

Young, J. E. (1990). *Cognitive therapy for personality disorders*. Sarasota, FL: Professional Resource Press.

Young, J. E., Klosko, S., & Weishaar, M. E. (2003). *Schema therapy: A practitioner's guide*. New York: Guilford Press.

Zitter, R., & McCrady, B. (1993). *The Drinking Patterns Questionnaire*. Unpublished questionnaire, Rutgers University, Piscataway, NJ.

Index

Page numbers followed by an *f*, *n*, or *t* indicate figures, notes, or tables.

273